Primary Biliary Cholangitis

Editors

ELIZABETH J. CAREY
CYNTHIA LEVY

CLINICS IN LIVER DISEASE

www.liver.theclinics.com

Consulting Editor
NORMAN GITLIN

August 2018 • Volume 22 • Number 3

ELSEVIER

1600 John F. Kennedy Boulevard • Suite 1800 • Philadelphia, Pennsylvania, 19103-2899

http://www.theclinics.com

CLINICS IN LIVER DISEASE Volume 22, Number 3
August 2018 ISSN 1089-3261, ISBN-13: 978-0-323-61394-1

Editor: Kerry Holland
Developmental Editor: Meredith Madeira

Clinics in Liver Disease (ISSN 1089-3261) is published quarterly by Elsevier Inc., 360 Park Avenue South, New York, NY 10010-1710. Months of issue are February, May, August, and November. Business and Editorial Offices: 1600 John F. Kennedy Blvd., Ste. 1800, Philadelphia, PA 19103-2899. Customer Service Office: 3251 Riverport Lane, Maryland Heights, MO 63043. Periodicals postage paid at New York, NY and additional mailing offices. Subscription prices are $292.00 per year (U.S. individuals), $100.00 per year (U.S. student/resident), $509.00 per year (U.S. institutions), $403.00 per year (international individuals), $200.00 per year (international student/resident), $631.00 per year (international institutions), $338.00 per year (Canadian individuals), $200.00 per year (Canadian student/resident), and $631.00 per year (Canadian institutions). Foreign air speed delivery is included in all *Clinics* subscription prices. All prices are subject to change without notice. **POSTMASTER:** Send address changes to *Clinics in Liver Disease*, Elsevier Health Sciences Division, Subscription Customer Service, 3251 Riverport Lane, Maryland Heights, MO 63043. **Customer Service: Telephone: 1-800-654-2452 (U.S. and Canada); 314-447-8871 (outside U.S. and Canada). Fax: 314-447-8029. E-mail: journalscustomer service-usa@elsevier.com (for print support); journalsonlinesupport-usa@elsevier.com (for online support).**

Reprints. For copies of 100 or more of articles in this publication, please contact the Commercial Reprints Department, Elsevier Inc., 360 Park Avenue South, New York, NY 10010-1710. Tel.: 212-633-3874; Fax: 212-633-3820; E-mail: reprints@elsevier.com.

Clinics in Liver Disease is covered in *MEDLINE/PubMed (Index Medicus)*, Science Citation Index Expanded, Journal Citation Reports/Science Edition, and Current Contents/Clinical Medicine.

Contributors

CONSULTING EDITOR

NORMAN GITLIN, MD, FRCP (LONDON), FRCPE (EDINBURGH), FAASLD, FACP, FACG
Head of Hepatology, Southern California Liver Centers, San Clemente, California, USA

EDITORS

ELIZABETH J. CAREY, MD
Associate Professor of Medicine, Division of Gastroenterology and Hepatology, Mayo Clinic, Phoenix, Arizona, USA

CYNTHIA LEVY, MD
Associate Professor of Medicine, Division of Hepatology, Assistant Director, Schiff Center for Liver Diseases, University of Miami Miller School of Medicine, Miami, Florida, USA

AUTHORS

MARIA T. AGUILAR, MD
Fellow, Division of Gastroenterology and Hepatology, Mayo Clinic, Scottsdale, Arizona, USA

DAVID N. ASSIS, MD
Assistant Professor, Department of Medicine, Section of Digestive Diseases, Yale School of Medicine, New Haven, Connecticut, USA

RUNALIA BAHAR, MD
Department of Internal Medicine, UC Davis School of Medicine, Sacramento, California, USA

ULRICH BEUERS, MD
Professor, Department of Gastroenterology and Hepatology, Tytgat Institute for Liver and Intestinal Research, Academic Medical Center, University of Amsterdam, Amsterdam, The Netherlands

CHRISTOPHER L. BOWLUS, MD
Division of Gastroenterology and Hepatology, UC Davis School of Medicine, Sacramento, California, USA

MARCO CARBONE, MD, PhD
Division of Gastroenterology and Hepatology, Department of Medicine and Surgery, University of Milan Bicocca, Milan, Italy; Academic Department of Medical Genetics, University of Cambridge, Cambridge, United Kingdom

ELIZABETH J. CAREY, MD
Associate Professor of Medicine, Division of Gastroenterology and Hepatology, Mayo Clinic, Phoenix, Arizona, USA

ANDRES F. CARRION, MD
Assistant Professor of Medicine, Director of Hepatology, Division of Gastroenterology and Hepatology, Texas Tech University Health Sciences Center, El Paso, Texas, USA

DAVID M. CHASCSA, MD
Assistant Professor of Medicine, Division of Gastroenterology and Hepatology, Mayo Clinic, Phoenix, Arizona, USA

FRANCESCA COLAPIETRO, MD
Department of Biomedical Sciences, Humanitas University, Milan, Italy

LAURA CRISTOFERI, MD
Division of Gastroenterology and Hepatology, Department of Medicine and Surgery, University of Milan Bicocca, Milan, Italy

MERRILL ERIC GERSHWIN, MD
Division of Rheumatology, Allergy and Clinical Immunology, UC Davis School of Medicine, Davis, California, USA

APARNA GOEL, MD
Division of Gastroenterology and Hepatology, Stanford University Medical Center, Palo Alto, California, USA

ZACHARY D. GOODMAN, MD, PhD
Center for Liver Diseases, Inova Fairfax Hospital, Falls Church, Virginia, USA

GIDEON M. HIRSCHFIELD, FRCP, PhD
Professor, National Institute for Health Research (NIHR) Birmingham Biomedical Research Centre, Institute of Immunology and Immunotherapy, University of Birmingham, Birmingham, United Kingdom

PIETRO INVERNIZZI, MD, PhD
Division of Gastroenterology and Hepatology, Department of Medicine and Surgery, University of Milan Bicocca, Milan, Italy

REMCO KERSTEN, MSc
Department of Gastroenterology and Hepatology, Tytgat Institute for Liver and Intestinal Research, Academic Medical Center, University of Amsterdam, Amsterdam, The Netherlands

WOONG RAY KIM, MD
Division of Gastroenterology and Hepatology, Stanford University Medical Center, Palo Alto, California, USA

PATRICK S.C. LEUNG, PhD
Division of Rheumatology, Allergy and Clinical Immunology, UC Davis School of Medicine, Davis, California, USA

CYNTHIA LEVY, MD
Associate Professor of Medicine, Division of Hepatology, Assistant Director, Schiff Center for Liver Diseases, University of Miami Miller School of Medicine, Miami, Florida, USA

KEITH D. LINDOR, MD
Professor of Medicine, Division of Gastroenterology and Hepatology, Mayo Clinic, Senior Advisor, Office of the Provost, Arizona State University, Phoenix, Arizona, USA

CHUNG H. LIU, BS
Division of Gastroenterology and Hepatology, UC Davis School of Medicine, Sacramento, California, USA

ANA LLEO, MD, PhD
Department of Biomedical Sciences, Humanitas University, Liver Unit, Center for Autoimmune Liver Diseases, Humanitas Clinical and Research Center, Milan, Italy

GEORGE MELLS, MRCP, PhD
Academic Department of Medical Genetics, University of Cambridge, Cambridge, United Kingdom

ALESSANDRA NARDI, PhD
Department of Mathematics, Tor Vergata University of Rome, Rome, Italy

JORDAN D. ROSEN, BS
Department of Dermatology and Cutaneous Surgery, Miami Itch Center, University of Miami Miller School of Medicine, Miami, Florida, USA

MARINA SILVEIRA, MD
Assistant Professor of Medicine, Department of Digestive Diseases, Yale University, New Haven, Connecticut, USA

DAISONG TAN, MD
Division of Liver Pathology Research, Center for Liver Diseases, Inova Fairfax Hospital, Falls Church, Virginia, USA

ATSUSHI TANAKA, MD
Department of Medicine, Teikyo University School of Medicine, Tokyo, Japan

UYEN TO, MD
Hepatology Fellow, Department of Digestive Diseases, Yale University, New Haven, Connecticut, USA

JORRIT VAN NIEKERK, MD
Department of Gastroenterology and Hepatology, Tytgat Institute for Liver and Intestinal Research, Academic Medical Center, University of Amsterdam, Amsterdam, The Netherlands

GWILYM J. WEBB, BMBCh, MA, MRCP
Doctor, National Institute for Health Research (NIHR) Birmingham Biomedical Research Centre, Institute of Immunology and Immunotherapy, University of Birmingham, Birmingham, United Kingdom

KIMBERLY A. WONG, MD
Department of Internal Medicine, UC Davis School of Medicine, Sacramento, California, USA

Contents

> Primary biliary cholangitis (PBC) is considered a model autoimmune disease, characterized by circulating antimitochondrial antibodies and a selective autoimmune destruction of intrahepatic cholangiocytes. PBC is heterogeneous in its presentation, symptomatology, disease progression, and response to therapy. The pathogenesis is still largely unknown, and epidemiologic studies have facilitated the identification of risk factors and the understanding of disease prevalence, geographic variations, heterogeneity, and differences in sex ratio. Recent studies from large international cohorts have better identified prognostic factors, suggesting a change in patient management based on risk-stratification tools to identify subgroups at greatest potential benefit from second-line therapies.

> Both genetic background and environmental factors contribute to primary biliary cholangitis (PBC). Recent innovative technologies, such as genome-wide association studies, identified a remarkable number of susceptible nonhuman leukocyte antigen genes contributing to the development of PBC; however, they are primarily indicators of active immunologic responses commonly involved in autoimmune reactions. Thus, recent studies have focused on epigenetic mechanisms that would link genetic predisposition and environmental triggering factors. In PBC, methylation profiling and altered X chromosome architecture have been intensively explored in conjunction with a striking female predominance. Furthermore, microRNAs have been found to be associated with the etiology of PBC.

> The biliary HCO_3^- umbrella hypothesis states that human cholangiocytes and hepatocytes create a protective apical alkaline barrier against millimolar concentrations of potentially toxic glycine-conjugated bile salts in bile by secreting HCO_3^- into the bile duct lumen. This alkaline barrier may retain bile salts in their polar, deprotonated, and membrane-impermeant state to avoid uncontrolled invasion of apolar toxic bile acids, which initiate apoptosis, autophagy, and senescence. In primary biliary cholangitis, defects of the biliary HCO_3^- umbrella, leading to impaired biliary HCO_3^- secretion, have been identified. Current medical therapies stabilize the putatively defective biliary HCO_3^- umbrella and improve long-term prognosis.

article discusses the background, evaluation, and practical management of these complications of chronic cholestasis.

The evolving research landscape, with advances in the omics technologies, availability of large-scale patient cohorts, and forthcoming availability of novel drugs in primary biliary cholangitis (PBC), is creating a unique opportunity for developing a precision medicine (PM) program. PM has potential to change the paradigm of management. The diagnostic workup of patients with PBC may include information on genetic variants and molecular signature to define a particular subtype of disease and provide an estimate of treatment response and survival. To reach this point, specific interventions, such as sequencing more genomes, creating bigger biobanks, and linking biological information to health data, are needed.

Primary biliary cholangitis (PBC) is a chronic disease that progresses to end-stage liver disease. Ursodeoxycholic acid (UDCA), the standard treatment for PBC for several decades, is associated with improved survival without liver transplant. Approximately 40% of patients do not respond to UDCA. Because of disease variability, there exist several prognostic models that incorporate various factors including biochemical response to UDCA. These models are useful for patient care and counseling as well as risk stratification for research and clinical trials, and the role of these models in the pre-UDCA and UDCA eras is discussed.

Primary biliary cholangitis is a disease characterized by immune-mediated bile duct destruction, followed by inflammation, scarring, and the development of chronic cholestasis and a slow progression to cirrhosis over the course of years. Liver biopsy has traditionally been used in conjunction with clinical evaluation and serologic autoantibody testing to establish the diagnosis, but it is no longer required in typical cases with positive antimitochondrial antibodies. Biopsy remains essential, however, in antimitochondrial antibody–negative patients or suspected overlap syndrome with autoimmune hepatitis, and if an adequate biopsy is performed, precise staging is possible for the assessment of prognosis.

Antimitochondrial antibody (AMA)-negative primary biliary cholangitis (PBC) is a term reserved for the condition with clinical and histopathologic findings consistent with PBC but without positive AMA. There does not seem to be a natural progression from AMA negativity to positivity. Antinuclear and anti–smooth muscle antibodies are frequently found in the absence of histologic autoimmune hepatitis features. The disease course may be more severe than that of AMA-positive PBC. Response to standard therapy for PBC and autoimmune hepatitis varies. Nevertheless, there is insufficient evidence to suggest that AMA-negative PBC is different enough to warrant classification as a separate disease from AMA-positive PBC.

Overlap syndrome of autoimmune hepatitis (AIH) and primary biliary cholangitis (PBC) is typically defined as concomitant or serial presentation with clinical features of both these distinct diseases. The Paris criteria and variations of the International Autoimmune Hepatitis group scoring systems for the diagnosis of AIH have been used to diagnose overlap syndrome. If left untreated, patients with overlap syndrome will have higher rates of portal hypertension, gastrointestinal bleeding, ascites, death, and need for liver transplant. Therefore, early identification is essential in providing appropriate therapy to potentially prevent long-term adverse outcomes in patients with overlap syndrome.

Primary biliary cholangitis (PBC) is an autoimmune cholestatic liver disease diagnosed with elevated alkaline phosphatase in the presence of antimitochondrial antibody. With the introduction and widespread use of ursodeoxycholic acid the proportion of patients with PBC undergoing liver transplant (LT) has decreased. However, up to 40% of patients are ursodeoxycholic acid nonresponders and require second-line treatment or progress to end-stage liver disease requiring LT. Several scoring systems have been developed and validated to assess treatment response and transplant-free survival in patients. Although PBC is a favorable indication for LT, recurrence of PBC may occur and requires biopsy for diagnosis.

CLINICS IN LIVER DISEASE

THE CLINICS ARE AVAILABLE ONLINE!
Access your subscription at:
www.theclinics.com

Preface

Primary Biliary Cholangitis: A New Era

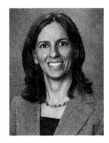
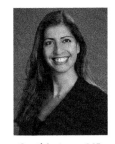

Elizabeth J. Carey, MD   Cynthia Levy, MD
Editors

Primary biliary cholangitis (PBC), first described almost 70 years ago, has entered the spotlight of hepatology attention. With widespread availability of effective treatments for viral hepatitis, attention has turned to the cholestatic liver diseases, which are now active areas of research and discovery. Signs of progress are evident, from the change in name of the disease to the first new medication approved for PBC in 20 years.

This issue of *Clinics in Liver Disease* provides the reader with detailed updates covering a broad range of topics in PBC. Two articles in this issue discuss the epidemiology, genetics, and epigenetics of the disease, highlighting many new discoveries that have occurred in the past decade. Another article focuses on new thoughts on the role of the bicarbonate umbrella in the pathogenesis of PBC and introduces potential new targets for therapy. This is the perfect segue into the following two articles devoted to treatment, including bile acid and non–bile acid therapies as well as an in-depth discussion of drugs in development. Symptom management has always been an important aspect of PBC; one article is devoted to understanding and managing pruritus and the other article is devoted to the chronic complications of cholestasis. The reader will learn to apply principles of precision medicine directly in the management of PBC and understand the proper use of scoring systems and liver histology in this setting. The challenging variant diseases, AMA-negative PBC and PBC-autoimmune hepatitis overlap syndrome, are reviewed in detail. The issue ends with an article on liver transplantation, still the only cure for PBC.

Over the past decade, tremendous advances have been made in the understanding of PBC leading to the advent of new and targeted therapies. Although rare, the absence of a cure and the frequent need for liver transplantation make PBC an important disease for study. The articles in this state-of-the-art issue expertly elucidate recent developments. We thank all the authors not only for their excellent contributions

Clin Liver Dis 22 (2018) xiii–xiv
https://doi.org/10.1016/j.cld.2018.03.012
1089-3261/18/© 2018 Published by Elsevier Inc.

liver.theclinics.com

to this issue but also for their commitment toward further understanding and (some-day) curing this challenging disease.

Elizabeth J. Carey, MD
Division of Gastroenterology and Hepatology
Mayo Clinic
5777 East Mayo Boulevard
Phoenix, AZ 85054, USA

Cynthia Levy, MD
Division of Hepatology
University of Miami
Miller School of Medicine
1500 Northwest 12th Avenue, Suite 1101
Miami, FL 33136, USA

E-mail addresses:
carey.elizabeth@mayo.edu (E.J. Carey)
clevy@med.miami.edu (C. Levy)

Changes in the Epidemiology of Primary Biliary Cholangitis

Ana Lleo, MD, PhD[a,b,*], Francesca Colapietro, MD[a]

KEYWORDS

- Geoepidemiology • Personalized medicine • Female prevalence
- Primary biliary cholangitis

KEY POINTS

- Incidence and prevalence rates of primary biliary cholangitis (PBC) vary widely and seem to be increasing; however, true population-based studies are scarce and therefore large population-based studies combining meticulous case-finding and case-ascertainment strategies are necessary.
- PBC has been classically regarded as a female-predominant disease and, although gender ratios vary, most epidemiologic studies have classically reported a high female-to-male ratio.
- Different lines of evidence support the possibility that PBC could be underdiagnosed in men and that the universally accepted sex ratio is likely an overestimate.
- Like other complex disorders, PBC is heterogeneous in its presentation, symptomatology, disease progression, and response to therapy.
- Using data from epidemiologic studies, it is possible to recognize variant syndromes and to stratify patients according to their risk of critical outcomes.

INTRODUCTION

Primary biliary cholangitis (PBC), previously known as primary biliary cirrhosis,[1] is an auto-immune liver disease characterized by circulating anti-mitochondrial antibodies (AMA) and a selective autoimmune destruction of intrahepatic cholangiocytes, leading to duct destruction and ductopenia, portal fibrosis, and eventually biliary cirrhosis.[2] The patho-genesis of PBC, although largely enigmatic, is characterized by the complex interplay of genetic and environmental factors that leads to immune tolerance breakdown.[3,4]

Epidemiologic studies are essential in the identification of environmental factors that may trigger the disease process in predisposed individuals, similarly to other autoimmune

The authors have nothing to disclose.
[a] Department of Biomedical Sciences, Humanitas University, Via Rita Levi Montalcini 4, Pieve Emanuele, Milan 20090, Italy; [b] Liver Unit, Center for Autoimmune Liver Diseases, Humanitas Clinical and Research Center, Rozzano 20089, Milan, Italy
* Corresponding author. Department of Biomedical Sciences, Humanitas University, Via Rita Levi Montalcini 4, Pieve Emanuele, Milano 20090, Italy.
E-mail address: ana.lleo@humanitas.it

Clin Liver Dis 22 (2018) 429–441
https://doi.org/10.1016/j.cld.2018.03.001
1089-3261/18/© 2018 Elsevier Inc. All rights reserved.

liver.theclinics.com

conditions. However, several issues in PBC epidemiology remain to be addressed and data on the systematic epidemiology of PBC are still uncertain. An increase in PBC prevalence, wide geographic variations, and differences in sex ratio have been reported. Whether PBC epidemiology is truly changing or methodological issues may explain the reported variations, is still a matter of discussion. Indeed, easier access to laboratory screening together with improved diagnostic accuracy, more complete and digitalized medical databases, and lack of a proper epidemiologic design might be responsible for the variability and the limited reproducibility of the available reports.

In this review, we aimed to critically describe the results of available (geo)epidemiologic studies in PBC, to discuss the published data, and to suggest directions for future research.

PREVALENCE AND INCIDENCE RATES

Population-based studies indicated a wide range in the yearly incidence and point prevalence rates in PBC and both seem to be increasing. Further, incidence and prevalence rates in PBC seem to have an uneven distribution throughout the world (**Table 1**). The epidemiology of PBC has been well described in the Western population but population-based studies are scarce in the Asian and African countries.

Table 1
Selected studies of prevalence, incidence, and sex ratio in primary biliary cholangitis

Area	Patients (n)	Prevalence (per Million)	Incidence (Million/Year)	Sex Ratio (M:F)	References
Europe	569	23	54	1:10	Triger et al,[71] 1984
Sweden	111	151	13.3	1:6	Lofgren et al,[72] 1985
Newcastle, UK	347	154	19	1:9	Myszor and James,[19] 1990
Ontario, Canada	225	22	3.3	1:13	Witt-Sullivan et al,[11] 1990
Victoria, Australia	84	19	—	1:11	Watson et al,[10] 1995
Estonia	69	27	2.3	1:22	Remmel et al,[73] 1995
Newcastle, UK	160	240	22	1:10	Metcalf et al,[8] 1997
Norway	21	146	16	1:9	Boberg et al,[74] 1998
Minnesota, USA	46	402	27	1:8	Kim et al,[7] 2000
Newcastle, UK	770	251	31	1:10	Prince et al,[20] 2001
Victoria, Australia	249	51	—	1:9	Sood et al,[18] 2004
Japan	9761	78	—	1:9	Sakauchi et al,[13] 2005
Finland	545	18	1.7	1:7	Rautiainen et al,[75] 2007
Ontario, Canada	137	227	30	1:5	Myers et al,[76] 2009
China	35	492	44	1:8	Liu et al,[77] 2010
Brunei	10	26	10	1:10	Chong et al,[12] 2010
Denmark	722	115	11.2	1:4	Lleo et al,[27] 2016
Lombardia, Italy	2970	160	16.7	1:2	Lleo et al,[27] 2016
Crete, Greece	245	365	20.8	—	Koulentaki et al,[9] 2014
South Korea	2824	47	8.57	1:6	Kim et al,[15] 2016
US	4241	293	—	1:4	Lu et al,[28] 2017
Hong Kong	1016	56	8	1:4	Cheung et al,[14] 2017

Modified from Lleo A, Jepsen P, Morenghi E, et al. Evolving trends in female to male incidence and male mortality of primary biliary cholangitis. Sci Rep 2016;6:25906; with permission.

Importantly, true population-based studies are rare and a population-based approach to case detection has little feasibility for PBC because of its rarity. Therefore, published studies are often the result of combined case-finding and case-ascertainment strategies. Further, regional differences could arise on the basis of medical expertise and awareness. Nearly all studies aimed to establish the number of subjects with a solid diagnosis of PBC in a specific region; it is therefore clear that the number of PBC cases included in the study is largely dependent on several factors, including the location and access to diagnoses in the general population.

Administrative databases can be another good option for epidemiology study of PBC, especially in regions with a universal health insurance system. It obviates the selection bias inherent to studies restricted to just a single or a few health facilities or reference centers. The use of administrative data has been well validated for the Danish model, ensuring registration of any event within the health system of defined geographic boundaries.[5]

Prevalence rates in Europe, North America, Asia, and Australia range from 19.1 to 402 cases per million inhabitants and incidence rates vary between 0.33 and 5.8 cases per million inhabitants per year.[6] Highest prevalence rates are reported in the United States (402 cases per million inhabitants),[7] England (240 cases per million inhabitants),[8] and Greece (365 cases per million inhabitants),[9] whereas the lowest rates are reported in Australia (19 cases per million),[10] Canada (22 cases per million),[11] and Brunei Darussalam, Southeast Asia (26 cases per million inhabitants).[12] Population-based studies from Japan,[13] China,[14] and South Korea[15] have been able to include high numbers of patients and report lower incidence and prevalence rates than Western countries, but a considerable disease burden with more advanced liver disease, including decompensated cirrhosis, hepatocellular carcinoma, and liver transplantation.

The major strength of the most recent studies is the accurately defined numerator and denominator populations by using a validated method for case definition. Moreover, the use of administrative databases limits the selection bias inherent in studies restricted to a few health care providers or tertiary referral centers. However, it cannot be freely compared with other epidemiologic studies,[16–18] even one performed in the same region,[11] due to the use of a completely different method.

Some researchers suggest that incidence of PBC is also growing. Indeed, rates rose from 19 to 31 cases per million population per year in Newcastle-upon-Tyne, UK, between 1989 and 2001.[19,20] Whether these changes are due to a real rise in incidence or are secondary to augmented detection of mild asymptomatic cases remains to be established.

On the basis of data from case-finding studies, a latitudinal geoepidemiological pattern of occurrence of PBC has been proposed,[4] with the disease being most frequent in northern Europe (ie, UK and the Scandinavian countries) and North America. Finally, epidemiologic studies also provide clues for the identification of environmental triggers of PBC, including infectious agents and lifestyle elements that may partly account for differences in geographic distribution. A study published in 1980 revealed a cluster of patients with PBC in Sheffield, UK, where almost all patients with PBC identified had received water from a single source.[21] However, chemical analysis of the water did not identify a potential trigger. Moreover, in New York, a significant association between a cluster of patients with PBC and superfund toxic waste sites contaminated with volatile aromatic hydrocarbons was identified and described.[22]

SEX PREVALENCE IN PRIMARY BILIARY CHOLANGITIS

PBC has been classically regarded as a female-predominant disease and, although gender ratios vary (see **Table 1**), most epidemiologic studies have classically reported female-to-male ratio as high as 10:1. It is therefore considered a prime example of the characteristic sexual dimorphism in autoimmunity. Epidemiologic studies have led to the identification of both genetic factors and environmental elements that are sex specific; these might act as additional players in tolerance breakdown, to explain both the onset and the female predominance of PBC.

We believe that the high female-to-male ratio classically reported in PBC has been, at least in part, influenced by methodological biases. Case-finding studies are based on clinical recognition and the subtle onset and long persistence of PBC at asymptomatic stages leaves wide space to mere speculation for early diagnostic suspicion, which obviously privilege a more straightforward approach to diagnostic tests, such as autoantibodies in women. The opposite bias, favoring men, has been reported in a male-predominant disease (ie, coronary artery disease).[23] Different lines of evidence support the possibility that PBC could be underdiagnosed in men and that the universally accepted sex ratio is likely an overestimate. First, AMA positivity in the general population reports a female preponderance reduced to approximately 2:1.[24,25] Second, Mendes and colleagues[26] reported a 4.3:1.0 ratio among the subjects deceased for PBC during a 20-year period in the United States; however, this may also represent a more rapid progression rate or a worse response to treatment in men. Further, we have recently taken advantage of population-wide records, during the period of 2000 to 2009, in Lombardia, Northern Italy, and Denmark and reported a sex ratio significantly lower than previously cited, a reversal of the usual latitudinal difference in prevalence and a surprisingly higher overall mortality for male patients.[27] We reported that male patients had a significantly worse prognosis than female patients, with a surprisingly higher overall mortality. Cox regression multivariate analysis identified male sex as an independent predictor of all-cause mortality in both Italian (hazard ratio [HR] 2.36) and Danish populations (HR 3.04).[27] Further, recent data from 11 geographically diverse health systems in the United States also reported lower rates of female:male ratio than expected.[28] Finally, Carbone and colleagues[29] showed that men with PBC were significantly less likely to have responded to ursodeoxycholic acid (UDCA) than women; male sex was an independent predictor of nonresponse on multivariate analysis. The same study also reported than men were less likely to be symptomatic, which may be a cause of delay in diagnosis.[29]

FAMILIAL PRIMARY BILIARY CHOLANGITIS

Anecdotal familial PBC cases were reported for the first time more than 40 years ago, including female[30,31] and even male[32] twins. The prevalence of patients with PBC having at least 1 affected relative, was investigated by several groups,[33,34] and the prevalence of PBC among first-degree relatives of known cases described between 1.1% and 6.4%. Nevertheless, these studies were substantially based on case-note review and the criteria for case finding were not clearly illustrated. Furthermore, all studies were performed in tertiary referral centers. Despite these limits, similar results have been reported by 2 case-control studies in which the occurrence of familial PBC was self-reported[16,35] Of note, Jones and colleagues[34] designed a "geographically based population study" and compared prevalence rates within family members with that of the general population of the same geographic area. Interestingly, the authors calculated a risk for a first-degree relative to have PBC as less than 1%, with higher values for female family members. The sibling relative risk, that is, the odds ratio for PBC of a subject with a sibling affected by the disease, was 10.5, among the lowest for autoimmune diseases.

Finally, a 63% concordance rate among monozygotic twins compared with the null concordance among dizygotic pairs has been reported,[32] being the most striking demonstration of the importance of genetic factors for PBC.

RISK FACTORS
Primary Biliary Cholangitis Genetics

Epidemiologic studies indicate that PBC is a heritable condition. This is suggested by twin and familial aggregation studies; a concordance rate of 0.63 in monozygotic twins for PBC is one of the highest reported among autoimmune diseases[32]; moreover, a family history of disease has been reported to vary between 1.33% and 9%.[6] High-throughput whole-genome array technology performed in the past decade has helped define the genetic factors associated with PBC. Data produced from genome-wide association studies (GWAS) and immunochip (iCHIP) in a large cohort of patients suggest that most gene associations are derived from human leukocyte antigens (HLAs),[36] and underline that in past studies there was an underestimation of existing associations.

Apart from HLA associations, genes related to the regulation of components of the immune system also appear to be involved in PBC. So far, 6 large-scale GWAS performed have identified 27 loci non-HLA known to be susceptibility associated with PBC (with $P<5 \times 10^8$)[37] (**Table 2**). The identified risk variants emphasize that immunoregulatory pathways are important in the pathogenesis of PBC. Importantly, such perturbations are shared among a diverse number of autoimmune diseases, suggesting the risk may determine a generalized propensity to autoimmunity not specific to PBC.

The Role of Sex Chromosomes

Even though the female predisposition to develop PBC has been known for a long time, the precise cause of this bias remains unknown, and relatively few hypotheses have been proposed.

Genetic and epigenetic mechanisms have also been demonstrated to have a role in female predominance in PBC, including genetics and epigenetics of sex chromosomes,[38,39] X chromosome monosomy,[40] and skewed X chromosome inactivation.[41] Interestingly, a number of genes involved in immunologic tolerance are located on the X chromosome, which may also partially explain the predominance of autoimmune disease in females in general.[42] Healthy women present 1 X chromosome inactivated by different epigenetic mechanisms, which eventually results in gene silencing. Although X inactivation is random in somatic cells, PBC-affected patients demonstrate preferential loss in cells with X monosomy.[41–43] Finally, it has already been shown that patients with PBC are also characterized by an enhanced X monosomy rate in peripheral blood mononuclear cells, particularly T and B lymphocytes.[44]

Recently, we rigorously defined the X chromosome methylation profile of CD4, CD8, and CD14 cells from patients with PBC and controls. We reported a significant difference in DNA methylation in CD4+ T, CD8+ T, and CD14+ cells in patients with PBC.[39]

The X chromosome is enriched in microRNAs as demonstrated by the fact that 7% of total microRNAs (miRNAs) so far identified are encoded on it. By an epigenetic process, microRNA can regulate the inactivation of the X chromosome in female subjects.[45,46] The result is a suppression of many miRNA-regulated target genes involved in immunosuppressive pathways, which leads to a heightened autoimmune response in women and their predisposition to autoimmune diseases. Numerous studies have demonstrated an overexpression of X-linked miRNA in women affected

Table 2
Non-HLA risk loci identified through genome-wide association studies as associated with primary biliary cholangitis at genome-wide level of significance

Study	Cases (n)	Controls (n)	Loci	Associated Genes	Odds Ratio (95% Confidence Interval)	P
Hirschfield et al,[78] 2009	1031	2713	1p31	IL12RB2	1.51 (1.33–1.70)	2.76×10^{-11}
			3q25	IL12A	1.54 (1.38–1.72)	2.42×10^{-14}
Liu et al,[79] 2010	945	4651	7q32	IRF5-TNPO3	1.57 (1.38–1.77)	8.66×10^{-13}
			17q12	IKZF3, ORMDL3	1.38	1.69×10^{-9}
			19q13	SPIB	1.46	7.97×10^{-11}
Mells et al,[80] 2011	1840	5163	1q31	DENND1B	1.34 (1.25–1.45)	2.06×10^{-14}
			2q32	STAT4, STAT1	1.50 (1.37–1.64)	2.35×10^{-19}
			3q13	CD80	1.35 (1.23–1.47)	2.53×10^{-11}
			3p24	PLCL2	1.20 (1.12–1.27)	2.28×10^{-8}
			4q24	NFKB1	1.26 (1.18–1.34)	4.06×10^{-12}
			5p13	IL7R	1.30 (1.21–1.40)	1.02×10^{-11}
			7p14	ELMO1	1.25 (1.16–1.36)	4.44×10^{-8}
			11q13	RPS6KA4	1.23 (1.15–1.31)	2.06×10^{-10}
			11q23	CXCR5, DDX6	1.37 (1.25–1.50)	2.69×10^{-12}
			12p13	TNFRSF1A	1.22 (1.14–1.30)	1.80×10^{-9}
			14q24	RAD51B	1.29 (1.20–1.39)	1.76×10^{-11}
			14q32	TNFAIP2	1.22 (1.16–1.27)	2.61×10^{-13}
			16p13	CLEC16A, SOCS1	1.29 (1.20–1.38)	2.95×10^{-12}
			16q24	IRF8	1.31 (1.21–1.43)	4.66×10^{-11}
			22q13	TAB1, SYNGR1	1.27 (1.18–1.38)	1.08×10^{-9}
Nakamura et al,[81] 2012	1274	1091	9q32	TNFSF15	1.56 (1.39–1.76)	2.84×10^{-14}
			11q23	POU2AF1	1.39 (1.24–1.56)	2.38×10^{-8}
Juran et al,[82] 2012	2426	5731	13q14	TNFSF11	1.33 (1.20–1.47)	2.18×10^{-8}
Liu et al,[37] 2012	2861	8514	12q24	SH2B3	1.27 (1.19–1.34)	1.18×10^{-14}
			17q21	MAPT	1.25 (1.16–1.35)	2.15×10^{-9}
			19p12	TYK2	1.29 (1.21–1.38)	1.29×10^{-13}

Modified from Gulamhusein AF, Juran BD, Lazaridis KN. Genome-wide association studies in primary biliary cirrhosis. Semin Liver Dis 2015;35(4):394; with permission.

by different autoimmune diseases. However, we still know little about how female-biased X-linked miRNA expression contributes to PBC.

Environmental Factors

The role of environmental factors, such as hormones and nutrition, has been extensively demonstrated in the development of autoimmunity. Given the high sex bias observed in autoimmunity, sex hormones have been the first proposed candidates to have an important role. However, evidence implicates several other factors, which include socioeconomic status, infectious agents, environmental pollutants, vitamin D (dependent on sunlight exposure), nutrition, drugs, and physical and psychological stresses in the pathogenesis of autoimmunity.[47–51] Large-scale epidemiologic studies evaluating environmental factors of PBC demonstrate that lifestyle elements, such as smoking, some cosmetics, and previous pregnancies are associated with an increased risk of PBC.[16]

Moreover, environmental factors should include the microbiome, infectious agents, and chemical compounds.[52] Molecular mimicry has been proposed as a common mechanism that may lead to loss of tolerance, perpetuated by chemical or infectious agents, which could alter tolerance through posttranslational modifications.[53] The vulnerability of one of the major human PBC mitochondrial autoantigens, PDC-E2, to environmental xenobiotic modification may facilitate this mimicry mechanism.[54] Some of the chemicals proposed to be involved in this mechanism are compounds that are widely used, such as perfumes, lipstick, and many common food flavorings. Infections are other environmental factors widely explored as candidates in PBC pathogenesis that can act also through the mechanism of molecular mimicry. Some examples are Mycobacterial hsp65 and *Lactobacillus delbrueckii* that share a common motif with the PDC-E2.[55]

NATURAL HISTORY, COMPLICATIONS, AND TREATMENT BENEFIT

The most important studies regarding the natural history of PBC show that the presentation of the disease has changed over time, and there is a bias in older studies regarding the distinction between symptomatic and asymptomatic patients. In the pre-UDCA era, most patients were diagnosed with advanced liver disease and the main symptom was jaundice, which reflected the progression. As a result, patients with asymptomatic disease had a more benign course than symptomatic patients.[56] However, since the development of diagnostic tools, such as AMA detection, patients with PBC are often asymptomatic at diagnosis, and the prevalent symptoms among patients with PBC are currently fatigue or pruritus, both of which are not associated with disease severity and can be found even in earlier stages. In an Italian study, the proportion of patients asymptomatic at diagnosis increased from 25% between 1973 and 1980 to 46% in the past decade.[57] In the UDCA era, a large community-based study from Newcastle demonstrated that the median survival was similar in asymptomatic and symptomatic groups.[58]

UDCA therapy has a marked impact on clinical outcomes in patients with PBC and extended data indicate that UDCA improves the natural history of PBC, especially when UDCA is administered in early stages. A number of studies[59-61] showed that the survival rate of patients with stage I and stage II disease was similar to the general population. However up to 40% of patients have an insufficient response to UDCA treatment and a significantly increased risk of developing an adverse outcome, such as liver transplantation or death.[62]

Recently, obeticholic acid (OCA) was approved for second-line treatment of patients with PBC who are intolerant of or refractory to UDCA. Estimation of OCA long-term clinical impact and cost-effectiveness has been assessed with a simulation model in an adult population with inadequate response to UDCA[63]; however, long-term follow-up epidemiologic data are needed to confirm the real clinical benefit.

The manifestations of chronic liver disease are attributable to replacement of normal liver by scar tissue. In PBC, it is best captured as a nonsuppurative, granulomatous, lymphocytic cholangitis that leads to cholestasis, ductopenia, and progressive fibrosis. Histologic features relevant to staging chronic biliary diseases include fibrosis, bile duct loss, and copper-associated protein deposits. It is no surprise that the stage of PBC strongly predicts outcome.[56,64] Three European cohorts of patients with PBC have been published reporting causes of death during mean follow-ups of 7.4, 4.8, and 6.0 years respectively.[57,58,65] The 3 studies reported similar length of follow-up and female-to-male ratio, and different causes of death. Most patients in the Italian cohort died of liver failure, whereas only 36.1% of patients in the United Kingdom and 34.4% of patients in the Netherlands died of liver-related causes.

Recently, Harms and colleagues[66] described the incidence of cirrhosis-associated complications and impact on survival in patients with PBC in a large international cohort. The authors showed that up to 15% of UDCA-treated patients with PBC developed major non-neoplastic, cirrhosis-associated hepatic complications within 15 years. Importantly, absence of biochemical response to UDCA was an independent risk factor for these complications.

Further, age and sex have been reported to influence both response to treatment and long-term outcome of patients with PBC.[27,29] Younger patients (age <45 years) are often symptomatic and less likely to respond well to UDCA treatment.[29] Male sex is associated with later diagnosis, more advanced disease at presentation, poorer biochemical response to UDCA, and higher risk of developing hepatocellular carcinoma (HCC).[29,67] The role of male sex in the development of HCC in PBC has been confirmed in 2 independent cohorts of Asian patients with a long follow-up.[68,69] HCC is an infrequent yet critical event in PBC. A large international cohort confirmed male sex to be associated with a higher risk of HCC in PBC; further, advanced liver disease and biochemical nonresponse to UDCA were associated with increased HCC risk in patients with PBC.[67]

PRECISION MEDICINE IN PRIMARY BILIARY CHOLANGITIS

Precision medicine (PM) is a system in which health care is tailored to the individual patient, based on genotypic or phenotypic characteristics correlated to a particular treatment response or disease outcome. The major aim of PM is to address medical interventions to those who will benefit, sparing those who will not. This is especially cost-effective for patients because they will avoid the adverse effects of medication or surgery and the psychological burden of screening, surveillance, or treatment. For obvious reasons, PM is also cost-effective for health care systems, and it is therefore a global priority for health care providers, policy makers, and industries.[70]

Mostly using epidemiologic data it is possible to recognize variant syndromes and to stratify patients with PBC according to their risk of critical outcomes, such as chronic liver failure, variceal hemorrhage and HCC. Importantly, the recently published European Clinical Guidelines[2] include for the first time the recommendation of evaluating all patients with PBC for their risk of developing end-stage complications and, consequently, their potential need for additional treatments.

CONCLUDING REMARKS AND FUTURE DIRECTIONS

Geoepidemiological studies and clustering analysis are essential tools to define the associated risk to single environmental and genetic factors. More importantly, environmentally induced changes have been shown to modify certain diseases giving rise to the key concept of epigenetics. The field of autoimmunity, including PBC, is clearly showing how the findings of basic science influence routine clinical practice in terms of diagnostic procedures, clinical management, and prediction of outcome. However, continuous effort should be performed.

In particular, it will be important to collect additional information on the incidence and prevalence of this rare condition in additional geographic regions, not only in the so-called developed countries. Because the clinical phenotype and the natural history of the disease of PBC differs between patients, it is essential to better define the prognosis of clinical variants of PBC. Further, we are convinced that the study of PBC epidemiology cannot be complete without a careful evaluation of male cases, which should be collected through a multicenter effort to achieve a sufficient number. Indeed, the study of sex differences in PBC will help toward a better definition of the mechanisms leading to the widely different clinical features, in particular allowing a clear definition of cases more likely to progress or to present major complications and to develop novel therapeutic approaches and a personalized management of the single patient.

REFERENCES

1. Beuers U, Gershwin ME, Gish RG, et al. Changing nomenclature for PBC: from 'cirrhosis' to 'cholangitis'. Hepatology 2015;62(5):1620–2.
2. European Association for the Study of the Liver. Electronic address: easloffice@easloffice.eu, European Association for the Study of the Liver. EASL clinical practice guidelines: the diagnosis and management of patients with primary biliary cholangitis. J Hepatol 2017;67(1):145–72.
3. Lleo A, Marzorati S, Anaya JM, et al. Primary biliary cholangitis: a comprehensive overview. Hepatol Int 2017;11(6):485–99.
4. Zhang H, Carbone M, Lleo A, et al. Geoepidemiology, genetic and environmental risk factors for PBC. Dig Dis 2015;33(Suppl 2):94–101.
5. Frank L. Epidemiology. The epidemiologist's dream: Denmark. Science 2003; 301(5630):163.
6. Boonstra K, Beuers U, Ponsioen CY. Epidemiology of primary sclerosing cholangitis and primary biliary cirrhosis: a systematic review. J Hepatol 2012;56(5): 1181–8.
7. Kim WR, Lindor KD, Locke GR 3rd, et al. Epidemiology and natural history of primary biliary cirrhosis in a US community. Gastroenterology 2000;119(6):1631–6.
8. Metcalf JV, Bhopal RS, Gray J, et al. Incidence and prevalence of primary biliary cirrhosis in the city of Newcastle upon Tyne, England. Int J Epidemiol 1997;26(4): 830–6.
9. Koulentaki M, Mantaka A, Sifaki-Pistolla D, et al. Geoepidemiology and space-time analysis of primary biliary cirrhosis in Crete, Greece. Liver Int 2014;34(7): e200–7.
10. Watson RG, Angus PW, Dewar M, et al. Low prevalence of primary biliary cirrhosis in Victoria, Australia. Melbourne Liver Group. Gut 1995;36(6):927–30.
11. Witt-Sullivan H, Heathcote J, Cauch K, et al. The demography of primary biliary cirrhosis in Ontario, Canada. Hepatology 1990;12(1):98–105.
12. Chong VH, Telisinghe PU, Jalihal A. Primary biliary cirrhosis in Brunei Darussalam. Hepatobiliary Pancreat Dis Int 2010;9(6):622–8.
13. Sakauchi F, Mori M, Zeniya M, et al. A cross-sectional study of primary biliary cirrhosis in Japan: utilization of clinical data when patients applied to receive public financial aid. J Epidemiol 2005;15(1):24–8.
14. Cheung KS, Seto WK, Fung J, et al. Epidemiology and natural history of primary biliary cholangitis in the Chinese: a territory-based study in Hong Kong between 2000 and 2015. Clin Transl Gastroenterol 2017;8(8):e116.
15. Kim KA, Ki M, Choi HY, et al. Population-based epidemiology of primary biliary cirrhosis in South Korea. Aliment Pharmacol Ther 2016;43(1):154–62.
16. Gershwin ME, Selmi C, Worman HJ, et al. Risk factors and comorbidities in primary biliary cirrhosis: a controlled interview-based study of 1032 patients. Hepatology 2005;42(5):1194–202.
17. James OF, Bhopal R, Howel D, et al. Primary biliary cirrhosis once rare, now common in the United Kingdom? Hepatology 1999;30(2):390–4.
18. Sood S, Gow PJ, Christie JM, et al. Epidemiology of primary biliary cirrhosis in Victoria, Australia: high prevalence in migrant populations. Gastroenterology 2004;127(2):470–5.

19. Myszor M, James OF. The epidemiology of primary biliary cirrhosis in north-east England: an increasingly common disease? Q J Med 1990;75(276):377–85.

20. Prince MI, Chetwynd A, Diggle P, et al. The geographical distribution of primary biliary cirrhosis in a well-defined cohort. Hepatology 2001;34(6):1083–8.

21. Triger DR. Primary biliary cirrhosis: an epidemiological study. Br Med J 1980; 281(6243):772–5.

22. Ala A, Stanca CM, Bu-Ghanim M, et al. Increased prevalence of primary biliary cirrhosis near Superfund toxic waste sites. Hepatology 2006;43(3):525–31.

23. Adams A, Buckingham CD, Lindenmeyer A, et al. The influence of patient and doctor gender on diagnosing coronary heart disease. Sociol Health Illn 2008; 30(1):1–18.

24. Mattalia A, Quaranta S, Leung PS, et al. Characterization of antimitochondrial antibodies in healthy adults. Hepatology 1998;27(3):656–61.

25. Turchany JM, Uibo R, Kivik T, et al. A study of antimitochondrial antibodies in a random population in Estonia. Am J Gastroenterol 1997;92(1):124–6.

26. Mendes FD, Kim WR, Pedersen R, et al. Mortality attributable to cholestatic liver disease in the United States. Hepatology 2008;47(4):1241–7.

27. Lleo A, Jepsen P, Morenghi E, et al. Evolving trends in female to male incidence and male mortality of primary biliary cholangitis. Sci Rep 2016;6:25906.

28. Lu M, Li J, Haller IV, et al. Factors associated with prevalence and treatment of primary biliary cholangitis in United States health systems. Clin Gastroenterol Hepatol 2017. [Epub ahead of print].

29. Carbone M, Mells GF, Pells G, et al. Sex and age are determinants of the clinical phenotype of primary biliary cirrhosis and response to ursodeoxycholic acid. Gastroenterology 2013;144(3):560–9.e7 [quiz: e13–4].

30. Chohan MR. Primary biliary cirrhosis in twin sisters. Gut 1973;14(3):213–4.

31. Freeman HJ. Primary biliary cirrhosis in genetically identical twins. Gastroenterology 2004;127(5):1645 [author reply: 1645].

32. Selmi C, Mayo MJ, Bach N, et al. Primary biliary cirrhosis in monozygotic and dizygotic twins: genetics, epigenetics, and environment. Gastroenterology 2004;127(2):485–92.

33. Floreani A, Naccarato R, Chiaramonte M. Prevalence of familial disease in primary biliary cirrhosis in Italy. J Hepatol 1997;26(3):737–8.

34. Jones DE, Watt FE, Metcalf JV, et al. Familial primary biliary cirrhosis reassessed: a geographically-based population study. J Hepatol 1999;30(3):402–7.

35. Corpechot C, Chretien Y, Chazouilleres O, et al. Demographic, lifestyle, medical and familial factors associated with primary biliary cirrhosis. J Hepatol 2010; 53(1):162–9.

36. Invernizzi P, Ransom M, Raychaudhuri S, et al. Classical HLA-DRB1 and DPB1 alleles account for HLA associations with primary biliary cirrhosis. Genes Immun 2012;13(6):461–8.

37. Liu JZ, Almarri MA, Gaffney DJ, et al. Dense fine-mapping study identifies new susceptibility loci for primary biliary cirrhosis. Nat Genet 2012;44(10):1137–41.

38. Lleo A, Liao J, Invernizzi P, et al. Immunoglobulin M levels inversely correlate with CD40 ligand promoter methylation in patients with primary biliary cirrhosis. Hepatology 2012;55(1):153–60.

39. Lleo A, Zhang W, Zhao M, et al. DNA methylation profiling of the X chromosome reveals an aberrant demethylation on CXCR3 promoter in primary biliary cirrhosis. Clin Epigenetics 2015;7:61.

40. Invernizzi P, Miozzo M, Battezzati PM, et al. Frequency of monosomy X in women with primary biliary cirrhosis. Lancet 2004;363(9408):533–5.

41. Miozzo M, Selmi C, Gentilin B, et al. Preferential X chromosome loss but random inactivation characterize primary biliary cirrhosis. Hepatology 2007;46(2):456–62.
42. Invernizzi P, Pasini S, Selmi C, et al. Female predominance and X chromosome defects in autoimmune diseases. J Autoimmun 2009;33(1):12–6.
43. Bianchi I, Lleo A, Gershwin ME, et al. The X chromosome and immune associated genes. J Autoimmun 2012;38(2–3):J187–92.
44. Invernizzi P. The X chromosome in female-predominant autoimmune diseases. Ann N Y Acad Sci 2007;1110:57–64.
45. Sharma S, Eghbali M. Influence of sex differences on microRNA gene regulation in disease. Biol sex differences 2014;5(1):3.
46. Hewagama A. Role of X-Chromosome encoded miRNAs in Autoimmunity: Suppressing the suppressor and Female Predisposition. Rheumatol Curr Res 2013;3:118.
47. Tyl RW, Marr MC, Brown SS, et al. Validation of the intact rat weanling uterotrophic assay with notes on the formulation and analysis of the positive control chemical in vehicle. J Appl Toxicol 2010;30(7):694–8.
48. Myers RP, Shaheen AA, Fong A, et al. Validation of coding algorithms for the identification of patients with primary biliary cirrhosis using administrative data. Can J Gastroenterol 2010;24(3):175–82.
49. Grams ME, Plantinga LC, Hedgeman E, et al. Validation of CKD and related conditions in existing data sets: a systematic review. Am J Kidney Dis 2011;57(1):44–54.
50. Ensenberger MG, Thompson J, Hill B, et al. Developmental validation of the PowerPlex 16 HS System: an improved 16-locus fluorescent STR multiplex. Forensic Sci Int Genet 2010;4(4):257–64.
51. Raichur S, Fitzsimmons RL, Myers SA, et al. Identification and validation of the pathways and functions regulated by the orphan nuclear receptor, ROR alpha1, in skeletal muscle. Nucleic Acids Res 2010;38(13):4296–312.
52. Selmi C, De Santis M, Cavaciocchi F, et al. Infectious agents and xenobiotics in the etiology of primary biliary cirrhosis. Dis markers 2010;29(6):287–99.
53. Selmi C, Lu Q, Humble MC. Heritability versus the role of the environment in autoimmunity. J Autoimmun 2012;39(4):249–52.
54. Leung PS, Wang J, Naiyanetr P, et al. Environment and primary biliary cirrhosis: electrophilic drugs and the induction of AMA. J Autoimmun 2013;41:79–86.
55. Bogdanos DP, Baum H, Okamoto M, et al. Primary biliary cirrhosis is characterized by IgG3 antibodies cross-reactive with the major mitochondrial autoepitope and its *Lactobacillus* mimic. Hepatology 2005;42(2):458–65.
56. Roll J, Boyer JL, Barry D, et al. The prognostic importance of clinical and histologic features in asymptomatic and symptomatic primary biliary cirrhosis. N Engl J Med 1983;308(1):1–7.
57. Floreani A, Caroli D, Variola A, et al. A 35-year follow-up of a large cohort of patients with primary biliary cirrhosis seen at a single centre. Liver Int 2011;31(3):361–8.
58. Prince MI, Chetwynd A, Craig WL, et al. Asymptomatic primary biliary cirrhosis: clinical features, prognosis, and symptom progression in a large population based cohort. Gut 2004;53(6):865–70.
59. Corpechot C, Carrat F, Bahr A, et al. The effect of ursodeoxycholic acid therapy on the natural course of primary biliary cirrhosis. Gastroenterology 2005;128(2):297–303.

60. Pares A, Caballeria L, Rodes J. Excellent long-term survival in patients with primary biliary cirrhosis and biochemical response to ursodeoxycholic acid. Gastroenterology 2006;130(3):715–20.

61. Corpechot C, Chazouilleres O, Poupon R. Early primary biliary cirrhosis: biochemical response to treatment and prediction of long-term outcome. J Hepatol 2011;55(6):1361–7.

62. Corpechot C, Abenavoli L, Rabahi N, et al. Biochemical response to ursodeoxycholic acid and long-term prognosis in primary biliary cirrhosis. Hepatology 2008; 48(3):871–7.

63. Samur S, Klebanoff M, Banken R, et al. Long-term clinical impact and cost-effectiveness of obeticholic acid for the treatment of primary biliary cholangitis. Hepatology 2017;65(3):920–8.

64. Poupon RE, Bonnand AM, Chretien Y, et al. Ten-year survival in ursodeoxycholic acid-treated patients with primary biliary cirrhosis. The UDCA-PBC Study Group. Hepatology 1999;29(6):1668–71.

65. Boonstra K, Bokelaar R, Stadhouders PH, et al. Increased cancer risk in a large population-based cohort of patients with primary biliary cirrhosis: follow-up for up to 36 years. Hepatol Int 2014;8(2):266–74.

66. Harms MH, Lammers WJ, Thorburn D, et al. Major hepatic complications in ursodeoxycholic acid-treated patients with primary biliary cholangitis: risk factors and time trends in incidence and outcome. Am J Gastroenterol 2018;113(2):254–64.

67. Trivedi PJ, Lammers WJ, van Buuren HR, et al. Stratification of hepatocellular carcinoma risk in primary biliary cirrhosis: a multicentre international study. Gut 2016;65(2):321–9.

68. Harada K, Hirohara J, Ueno Y, et al. Incidence of and risk factors for hepatocellular carcinoma in primary biliary cirrhosis: national data from Japan. Hepatology 2013;57(5):1942–9.

69. Rong G, Wang H, Bowlus CL, et al. Incidence and risk factors for hepatocellular carcinoma in primary biliary cirrhosis. Clin Rev Allergy Immunol 2015;48(2–3): 132–41.

70. Denecke K, Spreckelsen C. Personalized medicine and the need for decision support systems. Stud Health Technol Inform 2013;186:41–5.

71. Triger DR, Berg PA, Rodes J. Epidemiology of primary biliary cirrhosis. Liver 1984;4(3):195–200.

72. Lofgren J, Jarnerot G, Danielsson D, et al. Incidence and prevalence of primary biliary cirrhosis in a defined population in Sweden. Scand J Gastroenterol 1985; 20(5):647–50.

73. Remmel T, Remmel H, Uibo R, et al. Primary biliary cirrhosis in Estonia. With special reference to incidence, prevalence, clinical features, and outcome. Scand J Gastroenterol 1995;30(4):367–71.

74. Boberg KM, Aadland E, Jahnsen J, et al. Incidence and prevalence of primary biliary cirrhosis, primary sclerosing cholangitis, and autoimmune hepatitis in a Norwegian population. Scand J Gastroenterol 1998;33(1):99–103.

75. Rautiainen H, Salomaa V, Niemela S, et al. Prevalence and incidence of primary biliary cirrhosis are increasing in Finland. Scand J Gastroenterol 2007;42(11): 1347–53.

76. Myers RP, Shaheen AA, Fong A, et al. Epidemiology and natural history of primary biliary cirrhosis in a Canadian health region: a population-based study. Hepatology 2009;50(6):1884–92.

77. Liu H, Liu Y, Wang L, et al. Prevalence of primary biliary cirrhosis in adults referring hospital for annual health check-up in Southern China. BMC Gastroenterol 2010;10:100.
78. Hirschfield GM, Liu X, Xu C, et al. Primary biliary cirrhosis associated with HLA, IL12A, and IL12RB2 variants. N Engl J Med 2009;360(24):2544–55.
79. Liu X, Invernizzi P, Lu Y, et al. Genome-wide meta-analyses identify three loci associated with primary biliary cirrhosis. Nat Genet 2010;42(8):658–60.
80. Mells GF, Floyd JA, Morley KI, et al. Genome-wide association study identifies 12 new susceptibility loci for primary biliary cirrhosis. Nat Genet 2011;43(4):329–32.
81. Nakamura M, Nishida N, Kawashima M, et al. Genome-wide association study identifies TNFSF15 and POU2AF1 as susceptibility loci for primary biliary cirrhosis in the Japanese population. Am J Hum Genet 2012;91(4):721–8.
82. Juran BD, Hirschfield GM, Invernizzi P, et al. Immunochip analyses identify a novel risk locus for primary biliary cirrhosis at 13q14, multiple independent associations at four established risk loci and epistasis between 1p31 and 7q32 risk variants. Hum Mol Genet 2012;21(23):5209–21.

The Genetics and Epigenetics of Primary Biliary Cholangitis

Atsushi Tanaka, MD[a], Patrick S.C. Leung, PhD[b],
Merrill Eric Gershwin, MD[b],*

KEYWORDS

- Autoimmunity • Genome-wide association studies • X chromosome
- X chromosome inactivation • Methylation • microRNA

KEY POINTS

- Although familial studies indicate that genetic predisposition plays a crucial role in the development of primary biliary cholangitis (PBC), epigenetic modifications and environment factors are also involved.
- Genome-wide association studies have not identified non-HLA candidate genes that are specific to the development of PBC and how HLA alleles influence the susceptibility of PBC is unclear.
- Differences in PBC candidate genes between Europe/North America and Japan/China suggest there are unknown genetic risks/protecting factors that are yet to be identified.
- Methylation profiling and altered X chromosome architecture might reveal the reason for the striking female predominance in PBC.
- MicroRNAs are not only important biomarkers for diagnosis or defining treatment responses in PBC, but also demonstrated to be associated with its immunopathology.

INTRODUCTION

Primary biliary cholangitis (PBC) is a chronic cholestatic liver disease; it is an autoimmune reaction targeted to intrahepatic biliary epithelial cells (BECs), eventually resulting in cirrhosis and hepatic failure, without appropriate treatment.[1,2] Histopathologically, it is characterized as chronic nonsuppurative destructive cholangitis with granuloma formation in the liver, and degeneration and necrosis of BECs elicit destructive changes and lead to the disappearance of small or middle-sized intrahepatic bile ducts.[3] PBC is considered as a prototypic autoimmune disease for the following reasons. First,

The authors have nothing to disclose.
a Department of Medicine, Teikyo University School of Medicine, 2-11-1, Kaga, Itabashi-ku, Tokyo 173-8605, Japan; b Division of Rheumatology, Allergy and Clinical Immunology, UC Davis School of Medicine, 451 Health Sciences Drive, Suite 6510, Davis 95616, CA
* Corresponding author. Division of Rheumatology, Allergy and Clinical Immunology, UC Davis School of Medicine, 451 Health Sciences Drive, Suite 6510, Davis 95616, CA.
E-mail address: megershwin@ucdavis.edu

Clin Liver Dis 22 (2018) 443–455
https://doi.org/10.1016/j.cld.2018.03.002
1089-3261/18/© 2018 Elsevier Inc. All rights reserved.

like other autoimmune diseases, PBC mainly affects middle-aged women with a striking female predominance; the male:female ratio is 1:9 (**Table 1**). Second, a high prevalence of other autoimmune diseases, including Sjogren syndrome and chronic thyroiditis, as comorbidities is noted.[4,5] Third, disease-specific autoantibodies, anti-mitochondrial antibodies (AMAs), are detected in the sera of more than 90% of patients with PBC and are scarcely found in patients without PBC.[6,7] Finally, dense infiltrates consisting of T and B lymphocytes are histologically found in the vicinity of affected intrahepatic bile ducts.[8]

Although the etiology of PBC has not yet been completely elucidated, PBC is generally accepted to be a multifactorial disease and is considered to be caused by the interaction of both genetic background and environmental triggers.[9,10] PBC results from the combination of "bad genes and bad luck"; individuals having predisposed genetic factors develop PBC because of environmental triggering effects. Recent innovative technologies, including genome-wide association studies (GWAS), have identified numerous non–human leukocyte antigen (HLA) risk loci contributing to the susceptibility of PBC. However, the results of GWAS are largely disappointing; the relative risk of each gene is rather low, and many of the loci are not associated with protein coding sequences.[11,12] Thus, as in other autoimmune diseases,[13–15] recent studies have been focusing on the epigenetic mechanisms that would link genetic predisposition and environmental triggering factors to elucidate the etiology of PBC. In this review, we summarize recent findings regarding genetic as well as epigenetic mechanisms that would possibly provide promising tools to reveal the molecular etiology of PBC as well as develop new individualized treatment strategies based on the stratification of risk for the progression of the disease.

GENETICS OF PRIMARY BILIARY CHOLANGITIS

Like many other autoimmune diseases,[11,16] PBC has been shown to be associated with genetic predisposing factors that play a crucial role in its development, and possibly progression. Epidemiologic data suggest an increased prevalence of patients

Table 1					
Incidence and prevalence of primary biliary cholangitis (published after 2010)					
Country	No. of Patients	Incidence[a] (95% CI)	Prevalence[a] (95% CI)	Male (%)	Year
Europe and America					
Iceland[66]	168	2.5	38.3	18	2012
Southern Israel[81]	138	2	25.5	5.1	2012
North East England[82]	982	4.51 (4.11–4.91)	NA	10	2014
Netherlands[83]	992	1.1	13.2	14	2014
North Italy[68]	2970	1.67 (1.44–1.91)	11.1 (10.9–11.3)	33	2016
Denmark[68]	722	1.14 (1.06–1.23)	11.5 (11.3–11.8)	21	2016
USA (Wisconsin)[84]	79	4.9	NA	5	2017
Greece[67]	482	NA	58.2	13.5	2017
Asia and Pacific					
Southern China[85]	4	NA	49.2 (12.8–109.3)	25	2010
New Zealand[86]	71	0.8 (0.1–1.6)	9.9 (7.1–12.7)	8	2012
South Korea[40]	2824	0.86	4.75	16	2016

Abbreviations: CI, confidence interval; NA, not applicable.
[a] Per 100,000 population.

with PBC among first-degree relatives and siblings of an index patient, known as familial clustering of PBC.[17–20] In addition, concordance rate of PBC is 63% in monozygotic twins, which is the highest among several autoimmune diseases.[21]

Exploring Susceptibility Genes

Researchers have become interested in identifying inherited factors or genes responsible for the development of PBC. Recently, high-throughput, innovative technologies such as GWAS and immunochip (iCHIP), revealed dozens of risk loci associated with PBC.

In pre-GWAS era, case-control studies were the main tool to identify genetic predisposing factors in PBC. In case-control studies, because encompassing whole genome like in GWAS is impossible and targeted area for searching needs to be limited, HLA alleles have been of particular interest and extensively studied. HLA class II alleles were found to be associated with the development of PBC, especially *DRB1*08* allele family, that is, *DRB1*0801, DRB1*0803, DRB1*14*, and *DPB1*0301* as susceptible and *DRB1*11, DRB1*13* as protective alleles; as expected, these associations vary depending on populations studied.[22–25] Although HLA alleles are definitely crucial in determining the susceptibility of PBC via the alteration of autoantigen presentation, the involvement of HLA alleles in PBC susceptibility is complex; some are susceptible, whereas others are protective, and how HLA alleles influence the susceptibility is largely not clear.

Further, recent GWAS analyses from North America, European countries, Japan, and China have identified HLA alleles that possess the strongest link with susceptibility to PBC and revealed more than 40 non-HLA alleles contributing to PBC susceptibility (see **Table 1**).[26–37] Although risk alleles differ among studies and populations, pathways that involve identified genes are largely shared among populations and are represented as antigen presentation and production of interleukin (IL)-12 (*IRF5, SOCS1, TNFAIP3, NF-κB*, and *IL-12A*), activation of T cells and interferon (IFN)-γ production (*TNFSF15, IL12 R, TYK2, STAT4, SOCS1, NF-κB*, and *TNFAIP3*), and activation of B cells and production of immunoglobulins (*POU2AF1, SPIB, PRKCB, IKZF3*, and *ARID3A*). Therefore, these immune pathways could be important in the pathogenesis of PBC.

However, like other autoimmune diseases, GWAS have not obtained any satisfactory results, and no "smoking gun" has been identified. Importantly, most of the identified non-HLA loci were also found to be susceptible genes in other autoimmune diseases such as rheumatoid arthritis or inflammatory bowel diseases. Therefore, these risk alleles might lead to circumstances in which autoimmune reactions could occur through aberrant production of cytokines and immunoglobulins or uncontrolled signal transduction in T and B lymphocytes. However, these alleles are not sufficient to develop autoimmune reactions exclusively against BECs resulting in chronic cholangitis found in PBC. This is partly because only relatively common (>5%) single-nucleotide polymorphisms were analyzed, and less common, but more important, loci were not investigated in GWAS. Thus, polymorphisms of SLC4A2/anion exchanger 2 (AE2) genes, which are known to be important in protecting BECs against toxic bile acids by providing a bicarbonate layer, were found to be associated with disease progression in a case-control study,[38] but not in GWAS.

Ethnic Difference in Genetics

Epidemiologic studies clearly indicate that the incidence and prevalence of PBC vary across studies (see **Table 1**). For instance, a systematic review in 2012 identified 29 epidemiologic studies of PBC and indicated that the incidence and point prevalence remarkably varied, ranging from 0.39 to 5.8 and from 1.91 to 40.2 per 100 000 population, respectively.[39] Recently, the first large-scale population-based study in Asia was performed in South Korea.[40] This study provided a relatively low prevalence of 4.75 per 100,000 population compared with those reported in European countries and North America, where the prevalence of PBC ranged from 11.1 to 58.2 in 2010. This difference might partly be attributed to methodological issues, such as study design for case-finding or ascertainment.

Candidate genes contributing to the development of PBC are not identical between Europe/North America and Japan/China (**Table 2**). However, the major pathways associated with antigen presentation and IL-12 production, T-cell activation and IFN-γ production, and B cell activation and immunoglobulin production are shared in both; therefore, these pathways definitely play important roles in the development of PBC, irrespective of the difference in genetic backgrounds. Nevertheless, apparent differences among ethnicities in prevalence might suggest unknown genetic risks or protecting factors that have not yet been identified by GWAS. Large-scale, cross-ethnicity GWAS are warranted to address this issue.

EPIGENETIC MODIFICATIONS IN PRIMARY BILIARY CHOLANGITIS
Epigenetic Modifications

Genetic predisposition does not solely determine the susceptibility of PBC. Recent epidemiologic studies revealed a relatively low risk of PBC in first-degree relatives of indicated patients during 8 years of follow-up, suggesting that genetic predisposition alone does not define the risk of PBC.[41] Although studies of monozygotic twins revealed a high concordance rate, discordant pairs were identified.[21] Similar observations were reported in other autoimmune diseases.[42–44] In discordant monozygotic twins, DNA methylation profiles, copy number variation, and gene expression significantly differed between affected and unaffected twins.[45] These results clearly show that epigenetic modifications, as well as environmental triggering factors also play a significant role in PBC.

Epigenetics include any heritable and functional relevant changes in gene activity that are not caused by the changes in nucleotide sequences.[46] In general, 4 mechanisms are regarded as epigenetic mechanisms (**Table 3**): (1) DNA methylation, (2) histone posttranslational modifications, (3) alterations in chromatin/chromosome architecture, and (4) small and noncoding RNA interference.[47] Although studies on epigenetic alterations in PBC are limited and still descriptive, they have provided promising data that indicate the etiologic importance of epigenetics in PBC.[48] Most studies on epigenetic modifications focus on the methylation profiles of the X chromosome to clarify female predominance in PBC and on small and noncoding RNA, microRNAs in particular.

Methylation Profiles of the X Chromosome

Female predominance is another striking feature in PBC.[49] Previous large-scale epidemiologic studies revealed that the male:female ratio was almost 1:10[50–53]; however, this ratio seems to be changing in recent decades, and the number of male patients with PBC is increasing (see **Table 1**). Although the reason for the female predominance is not clear, possible explanations include the alteration in the structure as well as epigenetic modifications of the X chromosome.

As described before, Selmi and colleagues[45] investigated 3 pairs of monozygotic female twins and 8 pairs of sisters discordant for PBC and performed genome-wide analysis of DNA methylation. They found up to 60 differentially methylated regions in affected compared with unaffected twins. Interestingly, 51 of 60 genes were mapped to the X chromosome, which is in agreement with the female predominance of the disease. In addition, 10 copy number variations were found between discordant twins, and

Table 2
Gene list of the main loci detected to be associated with primary biliary cholangitis susceptibility

Chromosome No.	Gene Loci	Europe/North America	Japan/China	RA	IBD	PSC	MS	SLE
1	CD58		Yes	✔			✔	
1	MMEL1, TNFRSF14	Yes		✔	✔	✔	✔	
1	IL12RB2	Yes						
1	DENND1B	Yes			✔			
2	IL1RL2/IL1RL1	Yes			✔			
2	STAT4	Yes	Yes	✔				✔
2	CD28/CTLA4/ICOS		Yes	✔		✔	✔	
2	CCL20(LARC)	Yes						
3	PLCL2	Yes					✔	
3	CD80	Yes	Yes				✔	
3	IL12A, SCHIP1	Yes	Yes				✔	
4	DGK Q	Yes			✔		✔	
4	NF-kB1	Yes	Yes			✔		
4	IL21		Yes			✔		
5	IL7R	Yes	Yes		✔		✔	
5	PAM/C5orf30	Yes		✔				
5	LOC285626/IL12B	Yes			✔		✔	
6	TNFAIP3	Yes		✔	✔		✔	✔
7	ELMO1	Yes			✔		✔	✔
7	IRF5	Yes		✔	✔			✔
9	TNFSF15		Yes		✔			
11	RPS6KA4	Yes			✔		✔	
11	CXCR5	Yes	Yes				✔	✔
11	POU2AF1		Yes					
12	TNFRSF1A	Yes	Yes				✔	
12	SH2B3	Yes		✔		✔		
13	TNFSF11(RANKL)	Yes			✔			
14	RAD51L1	Yes						
14	TNFAIP2	Yes						
15	IL16		Yes					
16	IL21R		Yes					
16	PRKCB		Yes					✔
16	CLEC16A, SOCS1	Yes			✔	✔	✔	
16	CSNK2A2, CCDC113		Yes					
16	IRF8	Yes		✔	✔		✔	
17	IKZF3-ORMDL3	Yes	Yes	✔	✔			
17	MAPT, CRHR1	Yes						
18	TYK2	Yes		✔	✔		✔	
18	ARID3A		Yes					

(continued on next page)

Table 2 (continued)								
Chromosome No.	Gene Loci	Europe/North America	Japan/ China	RA	IBD	PSC	MS	SLE
18	SPIB	Yes						
22	MAP3K7IP1/RPI3, SYNGR1	Yes	Yes	✔				

Abbreviations: IBD, inflammatory bowel diseases; MS, multiple sclerosis; PSC, primary sclerosing cholangitis; RA, rheumatoid arthritis; SLE, systemic lupus erythematosus.
Data for 8 genome-wide association studies (GWAS)/immunochip analyses from European countries and North America from Refs.[26–30,32–34] and 3 GWAS analyses from Japan and China from Refs.[31,35,36]

2 genes were significantly downregulated in PBC. They performed reverse-transcriptase polymerase chain reaction (RT-PCR) and found that these modifications are linked to altered expression levels and revealed that 5 genes (CXCR5, HLA-B, IFI44 L, IFITI, and SMARCA1) were downregulated and 1 (IL6) was unregulated in PBC. The genes mapped to the X chromosome are involved in many cellular pathways. In particular, these genes cause the downregulation of Th2-cytokines such as IFIT1, an interferon type-1 signature represented by IFI44 L. Hypermethylation was also detected in transcription regulators (SMARCA1). However, methylation does not completely correlate with the expression levels of most genes, indicating that other mechanisms, such as allele-specific methylation may be involved in gene transcription.

Data from extensive methylation profiling performed by Lleo and colleagues,[54] indicate another key role of epigenetics in X chromosome modifications in PBC. They isolated CD4+, CD8+, and CD14 + T lymphocytes from PBC and controls. Extracted genomic DNA samples were hybridized to a custom array to determine the methylation status, and bisulfate sequencing was used to confirm the results. The differential expression was validated by RT-PCR. A total of 20, 15, and 9 distinct gene promoters with a significant difference in methylation profile in CD4+, CD8+, and CD14+ T cells were detected in PBC, respectively. Interestingly, the CXCR3 promoter in CD4+ T cells was remarkably demethylated, resulting in significantly elevated expression of CXCR3.[54] CXCR3 is a chemokine receptor for CXCL9, CXCL10, and CXCL11 and plays an important role in regulating leukocyte trafficking.[55] Thus, the hypomethylation of CXCR3 promoter and the consequent increased expression on CD4+ T cells could promote disease progression through enhanced Th1 differentiation and increased recruitment. Indeed, an elevated CXCR3 expression was histologically found in PBC.[56]

In another study by Lleo and colleagues,[57] DNA methylation profiles on the X chromosome were explored, revealing the significance of CD40 ligand (CD40L) with

Table 3 Epigenetic modifications	
Mechanisms	Explanations
DNA methylation	Addition of methyl groups to the DNA to convert certain cytosine residues to 5-methylcytosine
Histone posttranslational modifications	Modifications of the amino acids that make up histone tails of nucleosomes (eg, methylation, acetylation, ubiquitination)
Alterations in chromatin/ chromosome architecture	Remodeling of chromatin/chromosome by protein complexes that can enhance or suppress gene expression
Small and noncoding RNA interference	Silencing of gene expression by using small noncoding RNA transcripts, such as microRNA

elevated immunoglobulin (Ig)M levels in PBC. The interaction of CD40 and CD40L plays a crucial role in immunologic reactions through CD4+ T-cell priming, B-cell terminal maturation, and immunoglobulin class-switch recombination.[58] Serum IgM levels are increased in patients with PBC. Although genetic mutations of CD40L cause an immunodeficiency with elevated serum IgM levels,[59] no gene mutations were detected in CD40L in PBC.[60] Lleo and colleagues[57] showed significantly lower levels of DNA methylation of the CD40L promoter in CD4+ T cells from PBC patients compared with those in controls. Furthermore, this decreased methylation was inversely correlated with serum IgM levels in patients with PBC. These findings clearly indicate that epigenetic modifications, rather than genetic background, play a major role in the elevation of serum IgM in PBC.

Alteration of X Chromosome Architecture

In healthy individuals, X chromosome monosomy, only 1 X chromosome in females, increased in an age-dependent manner. Invernizzi and colleagues[61] assessed the frequency of X monosomy in peripheral blood mononuclear cells (PBMCs) from 100 female patients with PBC and 50 healthy controls. They found that the frequency of X monosomy increased with age in both the groups and was significantly higher in female patients with PBC than in controls. Furthermore, the frequency was higher in T cells and B cells than in monocytes/macrophages, natural killer cells, and polymorphonuclear leukocytes. They also found that this enhanced X monosomy was present in 2 other female-predominant autoimmune diseases, systemic sclerosis and autoimmune thyroiditis,[62] and showed that this X chromosome loss occurs not in a random manner, but in a preferential fashion.[63] Notably, many genes are known to be associated with immunologic tolerance, such as *IL2RG*, *TNFSF5*, and *FOXP3*.[64] Hence, X chromosome loss, that is, haploinsufficiency for specific X-linked genes, is critically involved in the development and female predominance of PBC.

Although specific genes located on the X chromosome and associated with immunopathogenesis of PBC have not yet been determined, Mitchell and colleagues[65] suggested that 2 genes, *CLIC2* and *PIN4*, might be candidates. They analyzed the transcript levels of 125 variable X chromosome inactivation (XCI) status genes in PBMCs of monozygotic female twins discordant for PBC by RT-PCR. Two genes, *CLIC2* and *PIN4*, were consistently downregulated in the affected twin of discordant pairs and exhibited variable escape from the XCI status. Interestingly, there were no significant differences in methylation profiling of *CLIC2* and *PIN4* between samples and no significant correlation with transcript levels. Thus epigenetic modifications affecting PBC might be more complex than methylation differences at X-linked promoters, and variably inactivated X-linked genes might be characterized by partial promoter methylation and bi-allelic transcription.

Recent epidemiologic data suggested that the proportions of male patients with PBC had increased to approximately 15%, indicating male-to-female ratios of 1:6,[39,40,66,67] which is very different from 1:10 in previous studies. Surprisingly, Lleo and colleagues[68] reported that male patients accounted for 21% of PBC cases in Denmark and even up to 33% in Lombardia, Italy. This alteration might be explained by more recognition of male patients with PBC by physicians, but might also indicate that a female predominance in PBC is determined by environmental factors through epigenetic mechanisms described herein, rather than by genetics.[68]

Small and Noncoding RNA Interference

Although only 1% of the mammalian whole genome codes for protein, more than 70% is transcribed to RNA. Noncoding RNAs (ncRNAs) are functional RNA molecules, transcribed from DNA, but not translated into proteins. ncRNAs that can regulate gene expression via epigenetic mechanisms are categorized into 2 main groups: the short ncRNAs (<30 nucleotides) and long ncRNAs (>200 nucleotides). The microRNAs (miR-NAs) included in ncRNAs, are small endogenous RNA molecules that regulate major cellular processes such as apoptosis, differentiation, cell cycle, and immune functions. Thus far, more than 200 miRNAs have been identified to be differentially expressed in PBMCs obtained from patients with PBC (**Table 4**). Although most are characterized as biomarkers for the diagnosis of PBC or for defining treatment responses, very few studies have shown a functional role of miRNAs relevant to immunopathology in this disease.

Padgett and colleagues[69] published the first study regarding miRNAs in PBC in 2009. They used miRNA arrays and explanted livers as specimens and showed that 35 miR-NAs were differentially expressed in PBC, as well as confirmed the downregulation of miR-122a and miR-26a and the increased expression of miR-328 and miR-299-5p by using quantitative PCR. Qin and colleagues[70] also identified 17 miRNAs that were differentially expressed between PBC and controls by using PBMCs. Ninomiya and colleagues[71] performed high-throughput Illumina deep sequencing by using sera from 10 patients with PBC, and then identified 81 miRNAs. Among them, the circulating levels of hsa-miR-505-3p and miR-197-3p were significantly decreased in PBC compared with that in healthy controls, suggesting that these 2 miRNAs might be novel biomarkers of PBC. Moreover, Tan and colleagues[72] used Illumina deep sequencing and proposed an miRNA panel consisting of hsa-miR-122-5p, hsa-miR-141-3p, and hsa-miR-26b-5p for diagnosis; this panel might have higher sensitivity and specificity than conventional diagnostic procedures performed using serum alkaline phosphatase values and AMA. Very recently, Sakamoto and colleagues[73] compared the serum profile of miRNAs between treatment-effective and treatment-resistant patients and found 58 differentially expressed miRNAs that might aid in differentiating treatment responses. Liang and colleagues[74] also performed a comparative study by using both plasma and PBMCs between PBC and healthy controls and identified 16 miRNAs as differentially expressed. They also found that miR-92a expression was closely correlated with the frequency of a subset of IL-17-producing T-helper cells. Based on this, they proposed that the altered expression of miR-92a might be associated with Th17 cell differentiation, although no functional evidence was shown.

Although all of these studies suggested the potential availability of miRNAs as novel biomarkers, only 1 study revealed a functional role of miRNAs in the immunopathogenesis of PBC. BECs in healthy condition are protected against hydrophobic and toxic bile acids by a "bicarbonate umbrella," that is, a biliary bicarbonate layer onto BECs provided

Table 4
MiRNA studies revealing differentially expressed miRNAs in PBC

Author and Year	Number of miRNAs	Specimens	Design
Padgett et al,[69] 2009	35	liver	PBC vs controls
Qin et al,[70] 2013	17	PBMC	PBC vs controls
Ninomiya et al,[71] 2013	81	Sera	PBC vs controls
Tan et al,[72] 2014	126	Sera	PBC vs controls
Sakamoto et al,[73] 2016	58	Sera	Tx effective vs resistant
Liang et al,[74] 2016	16	Sera and PBMC	PBC vs controls

Abbreviations: miRNA, microRNA; PBC, primary biliary cholangitis; PBMC, peripheral blood mononuclear cells; Tx, treatment.

by Cl$^-$/HCO3$^-$ AE2. As described previously, single nuclear polymorphisms of AE2 are associated with disease progression, and AE2/SLC4A2 gene expression was reduced in the liver and PBMCs of patients with PBC.[75] Padgett and colleagues[69] focused on miR-506, which was already shown to be upregulated in the livers as well as BECs from the livers of patients with PBC. Further, they found that miR-506 prevented the translation of AE2 mRNA by binding to the 3'UTR region, leading to decreased AE2 activity in PBC.[76] Definitely, this study provides robust evidence to show that miRNAs play a role in disrupting bicarbonate layer, leading to BEC damage in PBC.

SUMMARY

GWAS have gained considerable insight into the etiology of PBC. Before the GWAS era, our knowledge about genetic predisposition was limited to only HLA loci and a few non-HLA loci, which were arbitrarily selected by researchers. At present, more than 50 susceptible genes that might be associated with the development of PBC have been identified. Nevertheless, GWAS results are overall disappointing; the interactions between genetics and environmental factors are more complex than previously thought.[11,68] In this regard, studies on epigenetic mechanisms performed using high-throughput, innovative technologies are very promising. However, with new treatment options, changing geoepidemiology, and mortality in PBC, novel approaches with increased specificity and sensitivity are needed to further clarify the immunopathogenesis of PBC.[8,77–80] Moreover, more samples from various ethnic backgrounds and more epidemiologic information need to be obtained. A global collaboration is needed to address this issue, and, hopefully, these continuous efforts to elucidate the etiology of PBC might lead to the development of innovative treatment options that can "cure" the disease.

REFERENCES

1. Lindor KD, Gershwin ME, Poupon R, et al. Primary biliary cirrhosis. Hepatology 2009;50(1):291–308.
2. Carey EJ, Ali AH, Lindor KD. Primary biliary cirrhosis. Lancet 2015;386(10003): 1565–75.
3. Lleo A, Marzorati S, Anaya JM, et al. Primary biliary cholangitis: a comprehensive overview. Hepatol Int 2017;11(6):485–99.
4. Selmi C, Gershwin ME. Chronic autoimmune epithelitis in Sjogren's syndrome and primary biliary cholangitis: a comprehensive review. Rheumatol Ther 2017;4(2): 263–79.
5. Zhu Y, Ma X, Tang X, et al. Liver damage in primary biliary cirrhosis and accompanied by primary Sjogren's syndrome: a retrospective pilot study. Cent Eur J Immunol 2016;41(2):182–7.
6. Leung PS, Choi J, Yang G, et al. A contemporary perspective on the molecular characteristics of mitochondrial autoantigens and diagnosis in primary biliary cholangitis. Expert Rev Mol Diagn 2016;16(6):697–705.
7. Marzorati S, Invernizzi P, Lleo A. Making sense of autoantibodies in cholestatic liver diseases. Clin Liver Dis 2016;20(1):33–46.
8. Tsuneyama K, Baba H, Morimoto Y, et al. Primary biliary cholangitis: its pathological characteristics and immunopathological mechanisms. J Med Invest 2017; 64(1.2):7–13.
9. Shuai Z, Wang J, Badamagunta M, et al. The fingerprint of antimitochondrial antibodies and the etiology of primary biliary cholangitis. Hepatology 2017;65(5): 1670–82.

10. Tanaka T, Zhang W, Sun Y, et al. Autoreactive monoclonal antibodies from patients with primary biliary cholangitis recognize environmental xenobiotics. Hepatology 2017;66(3):885–95.

11. Webb GJ, Hirschfield GM. Using GWAS to identify genetic predisposition in hepatic autoimmunity. J Autoimmun 2016;66:25–39.

12. Trivedi PJ, Hirschfield GM. The immunogenetics of autoimmune cholestasis. Clin Liver Dis 2016;20(1):15–31.

13. Limbach M, Saare M, Tserel L, et al. Epigenetic profiling in CD4+ and CD8+ T cells from Graves' disease patients reveals changes in genes associated with T cell receptor signaling. J Autoimmun 2016;67:46–56.

14. Meroni PL, Penatti AE. Epigenetics and systemic lupus erythematosus: unmet needs. Clin Rev Allergy Immunol 2016;50(3):367–76.

15. Pollock RA, Abji F, Gladman DD. Epigenetics of psoriatic disease: a systematic review and critical appraisal. J Autoimmun 2017;78:29–38.

16. Tsou PS, Sawalha AH. Unfolding the pathogenesis of scleroderma through genomics and epigenomics. J Autoimmun 2017;83:73–94.

17. Abu-Mouch S, Selmi C, Benson GD, et al. Geographic clusters of primary biliary cirrhosis. Clin Dev Immunol 2003;10(2–4):127–31.

18. Corpechot C, Chretien Y, Chazouilleres O, et al. Demographic, lifestyle, medical and familial factors associated with primary biliary cirrhosis. J Hepatol 2010; 53(1):162–9.

19. Mantaka A, Koulentaki M, Chlouverakis G, et al. Primary biliary cirrhosis in a genetically homogeneous population: disease associations and familial occurrence rates. BMC Gastroenterol 2012;12:110.

20. Yanagisawa M, Takagi H, Takahashi H, et al. Familial clustering and genetic background of primary biliary cirrhosis in Japan. Dig Dis Sci 2010;55(9):2651–8.

21. Selmi C, Mayo M, Bach N, et al. Primary biliary cirrhosis in monozygotic and dizygotic twins: genetics, epigenetics, and environment. Gastroenterology 2004; 127(2):485–92.

22. Donaldson PT, Baragiotta A, Heneghan MA, et al. HLA class II alleles, genotypes, haplotypes, and amino acids in primary biliary cirrhosis: a large-scale study. Hepatology 2006;44(3):667–74.

23. Invernizzi P, Ransom M, Raychaudhuri S, et al. Classical HLA-DRB1 and DPB1 alleles account for HLA associations with primary biliary cirrhosis. Genes Immun 2012;13(6):461–8.

24. Mella J, Roschmann E, Maier K-P, et al. Association of primary biliary cirrhosis with the allele HLA-DPB1*0301 in a German population. Hepatology 1995;21: 398–402.

25. Onishi S, Sakamaki T, Maeda T, et al. DNA typing of HLA class II genes; DRB1*0803 increases the susceptibility of Japanese to primary biliary cirrhosis. J Hepatol 1994;21:1053–60.

26. Cordell HJ, Han Y, Mells GF, et al. International genome-wide meta-analysis identifies new primary biliary cirrhosis risk loci and targetable pathogenic pathways. Nat Commun 2015;6:8019.

27. Hirschfield GM, Liu X, Han Y, et al. Variants at IRF5-TNPO3, 17q12-21 and MMEL1 are associated with primary biliary cirrhosis. Nat Genet 2010;42(8):655–7.

28. Hirschfield GM, Liu X, Xu C, et al. Primary biliary cirrhosis associated with HLA, IL12A, and IL12RB2 variants. N Engl J Med 2009;360(24):2544–55.

29. Hirschfield GM, Xie G, Lu E, et al. Association of primary biliary cirrhosis with variants in the CLEC16A, SOCS1, SPIB and SIAE immunomodulatory genes. Genes Immun 2012;13(4):328–35.

30. Juran BD, Hirschfield GM, Invernizzi P, et al. Immunochip analyses identify a novel risk locus for primary biliary cirrhosis at 13q14, multiple independent associations at four established risk loci and epistasis between 1p31 and 7q32 risk variants. Hum Mol Genet 2012;21(23):5209–21.

31. Kawashima M, Hitomi Y, Aiba Y, et al. Genome-wide association studies identify PRKCB as a novel genetic susceptibility locus for primary biliary cholangitis in the Japanese population. Hum Mol Genet 2017;26(3):650–9.

32. Liu JZ, Almarri MA, Gaffney DJ, et al. Dense fine-mapping study identifies new susceptibility loci for primary biliary cirrhosis. Nat Genet 2012;44(10):1137–41.

33. Liu X, Invernizzi P, Lu Y, et al. Genome-wide meta-analyses identify three loci associated with primary biliary cirrhosis. Nat Genet 2010;42(8):658–60.

34. Mells GF, Floyd JA, Morley KI, et al. Genome-wide association study identifies 12 new susceptibility loci for primary biliary cirrhosis. Nat Genet 2011;43(4):329–32.

35. Nakamura M, Nishida N, Kawashima M, et al. Genome-wide association study identifies TNFSF15 and POU2AF1 as susceptibility loci for primary biliary cirrhosis in the Japanese population. Am J Hum Genet 2012;91(4):721–8.

36. Qiu F, Tang R, Zuo X, et al. A genome-wide association study identifies six novel risk loci for primary biliary cholangitis. Nat Commun 2017;8:14828.

37. Tang R, Wei Y, Li Y, et al. Gut microbial profile is altered in primary biliary cholangitis and partially restored after UDCA therapy. Gut 2018;67(3):534–41.

38. Poupon R, Ping C, Chretien Y, et al. Genetic factors of susceptibility and of severity in primary biliary cirrhosis. J Hepatol 2008;49(6):1038–45.

39. Boonstra K, Beuers U, Ponsioen CY. Epidemiology of primary sclerosing cholangitis and primary biliary cirrhosis: a systematic review. J Hepatol 2012;56(5):1181–8.

40. Kim KA, Ki M, Choi HY, et al. Population-based epidemiology of primary biliary cirrhosis in South Korea. Aliment Pharmacol Ther 2016;43(1):154–62.

41. Gulamhusein AF, Juran BD, Atkinson EJ, et al. Low incidence of primary biliary cirrhosis (PBC) in the first-degree relatives of PBC probands after 8 years of follow-up. Liver Int 2016;36(9):1378–82.

42. Elboudwarej E, Cole M, Briggs FB, et al. Hypomethylation within gene promoter regions and type 1 diabetes in discordant monozygotic twins. J Autoimmun 2016;68:23–9.

43. Generali E, Ceribelli A, Stazi MA, et al. Lessons learned from twins in autoimmune and chronic inflammatory diseases. J Autoimmun 2017;83:51–61.

44. Xiang Z, Yang Y, Chang C, et al. The epigenetic mechanism for discordance of autoimmunity in monozygotic twins. J Autoimmun 2017;83:43–50.

45. Selmi C, Cavaciocchi F, Lleo A, et al. Genome-wide analysis of DNA methylation, copy number variation, and gene expression in monozygotic twins discordant for primary biliary cirrhosis. Front Immunol 2014;5:128.

46. Aslani S, Mahmoudi M, Karami J, et al. Epigenetic alterations underlying autoimmune diseases. Autoimmunity 2016;49(2):69–83.

47. Wu H, Zhao M, Yoshimura A, et al. Critical link between epigenetics and transcription factors in the induction of autoimmunity: a comprehensive review. Clin Rev Allergy Immunol 2016;50(3):333–44.

48. Marzorati S, Lleo A, Carbone M, et al. The epigenetics of PBC: the link between genetic susceptibility and environment. Clin Res Hepatol Gastroenterol 2016;40(6):650–9.

49. Bae HR, Hodge DL, Yang GX, et al. The interplay of type I and type II interferons in murine autoimmune cholangitis as a basis for sex-biased autoimmunity. Hepatology 2018;67(4):1408–19.

50. Danielsson A, Boqvist L, Uddenfeldt P. Epidemiology of primary biliary cirrhosis in a defined rural population in the northern part of Sweden. Hepatology 1990; 11(3):458–64.

51. Hamlyn AN, Macklon AF, James O. Primary biliary cirrhosis: geographical clustering and symptomatic onset seasonality. Gut 1983;24(10):940–5.

52. Kim WR, Lindor KD, Locke GR 3rd, et al. Epidemiology and natural history of primary biliary cirrhosis in a US community. Gastroenterology 2000;119(6):1631–6.

53. Myszor M, James OF. The epidemiology of primary biliary cirrhosis in north-east England: an increasingly common disease? Q J Med 1990;75(276):377–85.

54. Lleo A, Zhang W, Zhao M, et al. DNA methylation profiling of the X chromosome reveals an aberrant demethylation on CXCR3 promoter in primary biliary cirrhosis. Clin Epigenetics 2015;7(1):61.

55. Lacotte S, Brun S, Muller S, et al. CXCR3, inflammation, and autoimmune diseases. Ann N Y Acad Sci 2009;1173:310–7.

56. Chuang YH, Lian ZX, Cheng CM, et al. Increased levels of chemokine receptor CXCR3 and chemokines IP-10 and MIG in patients with primary biliary cirrhosis and their first degree relatives. J Autoimmun 2005;25(2):126–32.

57. Lleo A, Liao J, Invernizzi P, et al. Immunoglobulin M levels inversely correlate with CD40 ligand promoter methylation in patients with primary biliary cirrhosis. Hepatology 2012;55(1):153–60.

58. Elgueta R, Benson MJ, de Vries VC, et al. Molecular mechanism and function of CD40/CD40L engagement in the immune system. Immunol Rev 2009;229(1): 152–72.

59. Pessach IM, Notarangelo LD. X-linked primary immunodeficiencies as a bridge to better understanding X-chromosome related autoimmunity. J Autoimmun 2009; 33(1):17–24.

60. Higuchi M, Horiuchi T, Kojima T, et al. Analysis of CD40 ligand gene mutations in patients with primary biliary cirrhosis. Scand J Clin Lab Invest 1998;58(5):429–32.

61. Invernizzi P, Miozzo M, Battezzati PM, et al. Frequency of monosomy X in women with primary biliary cirrhosis. Lancet 2004;363(9408):533–5.

62. Invernizzi P, Miozzo M, Selmi C, et al. X chromosome monosomy: a common mechanism for autoimmune diseases. J Immunol 2005;175(1):575–8.

63. Miozzo M, Selmi C, Gentilin B, et al. Preferential X chromosome loss but random inactivation characterize primary biliary cirrhosis. Hepatology 2007;46(2):456–62.

64. Selmi C, Invernizzi P, Miozzo M, et al. Primary biliary cirrhosis: does X mark the spot? Autoimmun Rev 2004;3(7–8):493–9.

65. Mitchell MM, Lleo A, Zammataro L, et al. Epigenetic investigation of variably X chromosome inactivated genes in monozygotic female twins discordant for primary biliary cirrhosis. Epigenetics 2011;6(1):95–102.

66. Baldursdottir TR, Bergmann OM, Jonasson JG, et al. The epidemiology and natural history of primary biliary cirrhosis: a nationwide population-based study. Eur J Gastroenterol Hepatol 2012;24(7):824–30.

67. Gatselis NK, Zachou K, Lygoura V, et al. Geoepidemiology, clinical manifestations and outcome of primary biliary cholangitis in Greece. Eur J Intern Med 2017;42: 81–8.

68. Lleo A, Jepsen P, Morenghi E, et al. Evolving trends in female to male incidence and male mortality of primary biliary cholangitis. Sci Rep 2016;6:25906.

69. Padgett KA, Lan RY, Leung PC, et al. Primary biliary cirrhosis is associated with altered hepatic microRNA expression. J Autoimmun 2009;32(3–4):246–53.

70. Qin B, Huang F, Liang Y, et al. Analysis of altered microRNA expression profiles in peripheral blood mononuclear cells from patients with primary biliary cirrhosis. J Gastroenterol Hepatol 2013;28(3):543–50.

71. Ninomiya M, Kondo Y, Funayama R, et al. Distinct microRNAs expression profile in primary biliary cirrhosis and evaluation of miR 505-3p and miR197-3p as novel biomarkers. PLoS One 2013;8(6):e66086.

72. Tan Y, Pan T, Ye Y, et al. Serum microRNAs as potential biomarkers of primary biliary cirrhosis. PLoS One 2014;9(10):e111424.

73. Sakamoto T, Morishita A, Nomura T, et al. Identification of microRNA profiles associated with refractory primary biliary cirrhosis. Mol Med Rep 2016;14(4):3350–6.

74. Liang DY, Hou YQ, Luo LJ, et al. Altered expression of miR-92a correlates with Th17 cell frequency in patients with primary biliary cirrhosis. Int J Mol Med 2016;38(1):131–8.

75. Medina JF, Martinez A, Vazquez JJ, et al. Decreased anion exchanger 2 immunoreactivity in the liver of patients with primary biliary cirrhosis. Hepatology 1997; 25(1):12–7.

76. Banales JM, Saez E, Uriz M, et al. Up-regulation of microRNA 506 leads to decreased $Cl(-)/HCO(3)$ $(-)$ anion exchanger 2 expression in biliary epithelium of patients with primary biliary cirrhosis. Hepatology 2012;56(2):687–97.

77. Floreani A, Tanaka A, Bowlus C, et al. Geoepidemiology and changing mortality in primary biliary cholangitis. J Gastroenterol 2017;52(6):655–62.

78. Tanaka A, Leung PS, Young HA, et al. Toward solving the etiological mystery of primary biliary cholangitis. Hepatol Commun 2017;1(4):275–87.

79. Mousa HS, Carbone M, Malinverno F, et al. Novel therapeutics for primary biliary cholangitis: toward a disease-stage-based approach. Autoimmun Rev 2016; 15(9):870–6.

80. Trivedi PJ, Hirschfield GM, Gershwin ME. Obeticholic acid for the treatment of primary biliary cirrhosis. Expert Rev Clin Pharmacol 2016;9(1):13–26.

81. Delgado JS, Vodonos A, Delgado B, et al. Primary biliary cirrhosis in Southern Israel: a 20 year follow up study. Eur J Intern Med 2012;23(8):e193–8.

82. McNally RJ, James PW, Ducker S, et al. No rise in incidence but geographical heterogeneity in the occurrence of primary biliary cirrhosis in north East England. Am J Epidemiol 2014;179(4):492–8.

83. Boonstra K, Kunst AE, Stadhouders PH, et al. Rising incidence and prevalence of primary biliary cirrhosis: a large population-based study. Liver Int 2014;34(6): e31–8.

84. Kanth R, Shrestha RB, Rai I, et al. Incidence of primary biliary cholangitis in a rural midwestern population. Clin Med Res 2017;15(1–2):13–8.

85. Liu H, Liu Y, Wang L, et al. Prevalence of primary biliary cirrhosis in adults referring hospital for annual health check-up in Southern China. BMC Gastroenterol 2010;10:100.

86. Ngu JH, Gearry RB, Wright AJ, et al. Low incidence and prevalence of primary biliary cirrhosis in Canterbury, New Zealand: a population-based study. Hepatol Int 2012;6(4):796–800.

Role of Bile Acids and the Biliary HCO$_3^-$ Umbrella in the Pathogenesis of Primary Biliary Cholangitis

Jorrit van Niekerk, MD[1], Remco Kersten, MSc[1], Ulrich Beuers, MD*

KEYWORDS

- PBC • Bile salts • Bicarbonate • Bicarbonate umbrella • Pathogenesis

KEY POINTS

- In primary biliary cholangitis, defects of the biliary HCO$_3^-$ umbrella leading to impaired biliary HCO$_3^-$ secretion have been identified.
- Current therapies stabilize the putatively defective biliary HCO$_3^-$ umbrella in patients with primary biliary cholangitis improving their long-term prognosis by different molecular mechanisms of action.
- Biliary HCO$_3^-$ secretion is thought to be pivotal in humans protecting cholangiocytes against uncontrolled entry of glycine-conjugated bile acids, sustaining bile flow and facilitating disposal of xenobiotics and endobiotics.

INTRODUCTION

The pathogenesis of primary biliary cholangitis (PBC), but also other chronic fibrosing cholangiopathies, remains incompletely understood.[1] In search of a possible pathophysiologic explanation, evidence from experimental, clinical, and genetic studies led us to introduce the biliary HCO$_3^-$ umbrella hypothesis,[2] stating that cholangiocytes (and hepatocytes) create a protective apical alkaline barrier stabilized by the glycocalyx[3] by secreting bicarbonate (HCO$_3^-$) into the bile duct lumen. This alkaline

Disclosure: J. van Niekerk and R. Kersten have nothing to disclose and have no conflicts of interest. Dr U. Beuers is supported by grants for investigator-initiated studies from Dr. Falk GmbH and Intercept, received consulting fees from Intercept and Novartis, and lecture fees from Falk Foundation, Gilead, Intercept, Novartis, Shire, and Zambon.
Department of Gastroenterology and Hepatology, Tytgat Institute for Liver and Intestinal Research, Academic Medical Center, University of Amsterdam, Meibergdreef 9, Amsterdam 1105 AZ, The Netherlands
[1] Contributed equally.
* Corresponding author. Department of Gastroenterology and Hepatology, Tytgat Institute for Liver and Intestinal Research, Academic Medical Center, University of Amsterdam, C2-327, Meibergdreef 9, Amsterdam 1100 DE, The Netherlands.
E-mail address: u.h.beuers@amc.uva.nl

barrier would retain bile salts in their polar, membrane-impermeant state. A defective apical HCO_3^- secretory apparatus would weaken the alkaline barrier, leading to partial protonation particularly of glycine-conjugated (pK_a 4) rather than taurine-conjugated (pK_a 1–2) bile salts in humans, rendering the resulting glycine-conjugated bile acids apolar and capable of crossing the cholangiocyte membrane independent of bile salt transporter activity,[4] thereby inducing apoptosis and senescence in cholangiocytes.[4,5] In support of the biliary HCO_3^- umbrella hypothesis, we showed in vitro that bile salt toxicity is pH dependent and that knockdown of the anion exchanger 2 (AE2) sensitizes human cholangiocytes to bile salt-induced apoptosis.[4] In PBC, expression of cholangiocellular AE2, the apical Cl^-/HCO_3^- exchanger, and type III inositoltrisphosphate receptor (InsP$_3$R3), both crucial for adequate biliary HCO_3^- secretion, are defective.[6–9] Consequently, biliary HCO_3^- secretion in PBC is impaired.[8]

Herein, we critically review the most recent evidence regarding the biliary HCO_3^- umbrella hypothesis by assessing biliary HCO_3^- transport mechanisms of cholangiocytes and different factors that affect the biliary HCO_3^- umbrella. We discuss apical and basolateral cholangiocyte membrane transporters and channels that might be involved in the formation of the HCO_3^--rich layer at the apical membrane of biliary duct epithelia in cooperation with local neurohormonal and nuclear factors. Their possible role in the pathogenesis of PBC and other fibrosing cholangiopathies is also discussed. Therapeutic interventions stabilizing the biliary HCO_3^- umbrella are described.

BILE FORMATION AND MODIFICATION

Bile formation is a complex biological process that is primarily performed by hepatocytes, whereas cholangiocytes facilitate and modify biliary bile by secretory and absorptive mechanisms.[10] Bile salts are the major solutes in bile and are synthesized from cholesterol via 17 enzymatic steps in different intracellular compartments including the cytosol, endoplasmic reticulum, mitochondria, and peroxisomes. The major pathway of bile salt synthesis is initiated by hydroxylation of cholesterol by cholesterol 7α-hydroxylase (CYP7A1), a member of the cytochrome P450 family. Human hepatocytes conjugate bile salts before secretion into bile mainly with glycine and to a lesser amount with taurine.[4] Notably, the glycine/taurine ratio of conjugated bile salts is shifted toward membrane-impermeable taurine conjugates in bile of untreated patients with PBC readapting to the glycine/taurine ratio of healthy individuals after effective treatment with ursodeoxycholic acid (UDCA).[11]

Other compounds excreted in bile are phospholipids, cholesterol, and potentially harmful lipophilic endogenous and exogenous substances, such as bilirubin or xenobiotics. The adenosine triphosphate (ATP)-dependent secretion of bile salts and these organic compounds is followed by osmotic passage of water and electrolytes. Canalicular bile is modified downstream, by adjusting the levels of HCO_3^-, Cl^-, water, and pH by periportal hepatocytes and cholangiocytes. Bile formation is regulated by a complex interplay of numerous intracellular signaling pathways and membrane receptors, transporters, and channels in hepatocytes and cholangiocytes.[10]

Biliary HCO_3^- secretion is pivotal in humans and is thought to serve a number of functions: (1) to sustain bile flow, (2) to facilitate disposal of xenobiotics and endobiotics, (3) to generate an alkaline tide for digestion of nutrients in the intestine, and (4) to form a 'biliary HCO_3^- umbrella'.[2–4] Biliary HCO_3^- secretion is tightly regulated by cellular signaling pathways and membrane receptors, transporters, and channels.[10] Recruitment of transporters is mediated by microvesicles, multivesicular bodies, and exosomes.[12] Additionally, nuclear receptors and microRNAs (miRNAs) regulate expression of numerous genes to enhance or decrease expression of proteins contributing to this HCO_3^- efflux.[9,13] In this regard, molecular physiology of biliary HCO_3^- secretion and contributing factors of the biliary HCO_3^- umbrella in human and rodent cholangiocytes are discussed hereafter.

PRIMARY CILIA

Cholangiocytes are highly specialized epithelial cells, aligned throughout the biliary tree, connected with tight junctions, and maintain a barrier with a distinct cellular polarity. Microvilli derive from the apical plasma membrane to increase surface and facilitate tissue homeostasis. The primary cilium (**Fig. 1**) modulates intracellular signaling.[14] The size and shape of primary cilia is maintained by fibrocystin, a receptor-like protein. Cilia exhibit mechanosensory, osmosensory, and chemosensory functions and extend above the presumed level of the biliary HCO_3^- umbrella, where they can sense changes in bile flow, composition, and osmolality to adjust biliary HCO_3^- secretion.[14] The bending of primary cilia by luminal flow induces an increase in intracellular Ca^{2+} levels by a mechanosensory complex, polycystin 1, and a

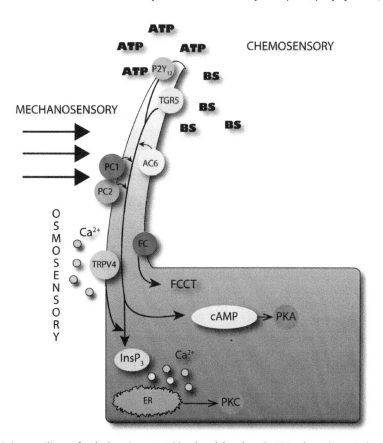

Fig. 1. Primary cilium of a cholangiocyte. AC6, adenylyl cyclase 6; ATP, adenosine trisphosphate; BS, bile salts; Ca^{2+}, calcium; cAMP, cyclic adenosine monophosphate; ER, endoplasmatic reticulum; FC, fibrocystin; FCCT, fibrocystin c-terminal tail; $InsP_3$, inositol trisphosphate; $P2Y_{12}$, purinergic G protein-coupled receptor; PC1, polycystin-1; PC2, polycystin-2; PKA, protein kinase A; PKC, protein kinase C; TGR5, Takeda G-protein–coupled receptor 5; TRPV4, transient receptor potential cation channel subfamily V member 4.

Ca^{2+} channel. Intracellular cyclic adenosine monophosphate (cAMP) levels are adjusted by cilia bending via adenylyl cyclase 6, an enzyme that is expressed in cilia axonemes and converses ATP to cAMP and pyrophosphate.[12] Osmosensation is facilitated by TRPV4, an ion channel located on primary cilia. Hypotonicity induces ciliary TRPV4- and thus Ca^{2+}-dependent ATP release and HCO_3^- secretion in cholangiocytes.[15] Adjusting intracellular Ca^{2+} levels by targeting ciliary TRPV4 is currently under investigation, but limited by side effects.[16]

The purinergic receptor, P2Y12, is the only P2Y isoform, out of a family of 12, that is located on primary cilia of cholangiocytes.[14] This receptor is a chemosensor and an important player in the regulation of HCO_3^- secretion. It senses ATP at the luminal site after a choleretic stimulus. ATP is released into bile by cholangiocytes through different mechanisms, including vesicular exocytosis and cystic fibrosis transmembrane conductance regulator (CFTR)-mediated transport.[14] Deciliated cholangiocytes lack the power to downregulate cAMP signaling via P2Y12.[17]

Takeda G-protein–coupled receptor 5 (TGR5) is another chemosensor located at the primary cilia. It responds to unconjugated and conjugated bile salts, with taurolithocholate being the most potent agonist to regulate target genes implicated in hepatocyte and cholangiocyte bile salt transport and metabolism.[18] Notably, the activation of TGR5 in ciliated cholangiocytes decreases cAMP after binding to $G\alpha i$-protein instead of increasing cAMP levels after binding to the $G\alpha s$-protein in nonciliated cells.[19,20] Thus, ciliary, but not otherwise localized TGR5 might dampen the cholangiocyte secretory response upon extracellular choleretic stimuli. Murine TGR5 also induced antiinflammatory and antiapoptotic effects, in ciliated cholangiocytes facilitated by the extracellular signal-regulated kinase 1/2 pathway and in nonciliated cholangiocytes via inhibition of mitogen-activated protein kinase activation.[21] Thus, localization of the TGR5 receptor determines its function.

In summary, primary cilia (see **Fig. 1**) are crucial for biliary homeostasis and, when deficient, are a major cause of disease. Cholangiociliopathies, such as autosomal dominant polycystic kidney disease and autosomal recessive polycystic kidney disease are caused by gene mutations in the genes encoding polycystin 1, a Ca^{2+} channel, and fibrocystin, respectively. Defects in primary cilia seem to result in decreased Ca^{2+} and increased cAMP levels, causing cholangiocyte hyperproliferation, abnormal cell–matrix interactions, and altered fluid secretion/absorption, capable of resulting in cystogenesis, and disturbed biliary HCO_3^- secretion.[22]

THE APICAL CHOLANGIOCYTE MEMBRANE
Sodium-Independent Anion Exchanger 2

Biliary HCO_3^- secretion by human cholangiocytes into the bile duct lumen is carried out by AE2 (*SLC4A2*), which is mostly expressed at the apical membrane in vivo.[7,23] The AE2 transporter family is part of the SLC4 superfamily or HCO_3^- transporter family, expressed in epithelial secretory cells of, for example, the stomach, bile ducts, colon, kidney, or testis, where the direction of chloride and HCO_3^- exchange is determined by their transmembrane chemical gradient. AE2-mediated biliary HCO_3^- secretion promotes bile flow, maintains an alkaline environment, and retains bile salts in their polar, deprotonated, and membrane-impermeant state.[2,4] AE2 serves also as a regulator of intracellular pH and osmolality in cholangiocytes.

Cholangiocellular AE2 expression, both on a messenger RNA (mRNA) and a protein level, and biliary HCO_3^- secretion are impaired in PBC,[6–9] an effect mainly mediated by miR-506.[9,24] Intriguingly, miR-506 overexpression in vitro mimicked PBC-like features in human cholangiocytes and induced activation and proliferation of PBC immunocytes in coculture with cholangiocytes.[24] Impaired HCO_3^- secretion of cholangiocytes may allow uncontrolled invasion of glycine-conjugated bile acid monomers at high micromolar concentrations (as in bile)[4] reinforcing impairment of AE2 expression by induction of reactive oxygen species (ROS) and enhanced chemokine- and cytokine-mediated bile duct inflammation.[25]

UDCA, standard treatment in PBC, restored AE2 mRNA and protein expression in association with improvement of cholestasis.[6,7] *SLC4A2* allelic variants were associated with the development and/or progression of PBC in French and Japanese PBC patient cohorts, respectively,[26,27] but not in large genome-wide association studies. Additionally, knockdown of AE2 in human cholangiocytes by short hairpin RNA led to an intracellular alkalization,[4] which stimulates expression and activity of soluble adenylyl cyclase (sAC), an evolutionarily conserved HCO_3^- sensor and Ca^{++}- and HCO_3^--inducible mediator of bile salt-induced apoptosis in human cholangiocytes.[28] Accordingly, bile salt-induced apoptosis was inhibited by a specific sAC inhibitor or by sAC knockdown in vitro.[28]

AE2 knockout ($AE2^{-/-}$) mice were shown to develop antimitochondrial antibodies, mild portal inflammation and fibrosis, but—in contrast with humans—no cirrhosis.[29] Biliary HCO_3^- secretion was not impaired in $AE2^{-/-}$ mice in comparison with wild-type littermates, and isolated cholangiocytes from $AE2^{-/-}$ mice showed no intracellular alkalization.[30] The difference in pH regulation between murine and human cholangiocytes is most likely explained by the expression of an additional sodium HCO_3^- cotransporter (NBC) in mouse cholangiocytes, which is absent in human cholangiocytes.[30]

Loading of intracellular HCO_3^- occurs through basolateral Na^+-dependent $Cl^-/$ HCO_3^- cotransport in humans[31] and by Na^+/HCO_3^- cotransport (NBC; discussed elsewhere in this article) in rodents.[30,32] Carbonic anhydrase (CA)-mediated HCO_3^- formation by hydration of CO_2 and subsequent H^+ extrusion through Na^+/H^+ exchange also occurs both in human and mouse cholangiocytes.

Taken together, these data suggest that AE2 deficiency may play a crucial role in the pathogenesis of PBC.

Apical Sodium-Dependent Bile Salt Transporter

Bile salts are the major organic constituents of bile. They are synthesized in the hepatocytes, secreted by the bile salt export pump (BSEP, ABCB11) to the canalicular space and transported along the biliary tree and small intestine to the ileum to regulate digestion of fat and absorption of fat-soluble vitamins. Intestinal bile salts also play an important role in the modulation of glucose and lipid metabolism or defense against small intestinal bacterial overgrowth, among other functions. In the ileum, bile salts are taken up by the ileal ASBT, are bound to the intestinal bile acid binding protein and released into mesenteric venous blood mainly by the ileal basolateral transporter OSTα/β, to reach via the portal circulation the liver for uptake by the sodium taurocholate cotransporting polypeptide and organic anion transporting polypeptides and, ultimately, resecretion into the bile—known as the enterohepatic circulation of bile salts.[10,33]

ASBT is not only expressed in ileocytes, but also in cholangiocytes and renal tubular cells. Cholangiocyte ASBT regulation and function is incompletely understood in humans. ASBT is electrogenic, requires 2 sodium ions for conjugated bile salt uptake,[34,35] resides inside the cytoplasm, and is inserted into the apical membrane in a secretin-/cAMP-dependent manner in rat cholangiocytes.[36] ASBT insertion occurs by vesicular transport and its degradation seems to be, just like that of sodium taurocholate cotransporting polypeptide in hepatocytes, mediated by the ubiquitin-proteasome system.[37]

Cholangiocellular ASBT has been proposed to serve as a shunt for bile salts to absorb and subsequently secrete them in the periductular plexus for reuptake and secretion by hepatocytes to maintain bile salt–dependent flow. However, it has also been speculated that ASBT, as a bile salt sensor, might modulate intracellular signaling pathways in cholangiocytes and choleresis in a taurocholate-dependent manner.[38] Previously, we speculated that, physiologically, it would rather have a detrimental effect when large amounts of human biliary bile salts present as bile salt monomers at millimolar concentrations in human bile are taken up via ASBT-facilitated transport by human cholangiocytes.[2] In our model of the "biliary HCO_3^- umbrella", we questioned the role of ASBT as a relevant apical bile salt transporter in human cholangiocytes, considering the potentially detrimental effect for cholangiocytes being exposed to high millimolar levels of potentially toxic human bile salts compared with low millimolar concentrations in the intestine and colon, and to low micromolar concentrations in the systemic circulation. We, therefore, concluded that ASBT may have a bile salt sensor function in human cholangiocytes rather than the function of an efficient bile salt transporter.[2] Studies are under way to further elucidate the role of ASBT in human cholangiocytes.

Aquaporine 1

Water transport in cholangiocytes is regulated by aquaporines, which are arranged in tetramers, to mediate a bidirectional passive movement of water in response to osmotic gradients at the apical and basolateral membrane of the cell.[14] Cholangiocytes are home to aquaporine 4 (AQP4) at the basolateral membrane and AQP1 at the apical membrane.[39] The localization of AQP1 at the apical membrane of the cholangiocytes is mediated by intracellular vesicle transport together with CFTR and AE2 in response to choleretic stimuli. This vesicular colocalization of transporters enhances the accepted paradigm of biliary secretion of HCO_3^- secretion driven by a Cl^- gradient, which is mediated by CFTR and TMEM16A, accompanied by passive movement of water in response to this osmotic gradient.[40]

Cl⁻ Channels

Cystic fibrosis transmembrane conductance regulator and anoctamin-1

Chloride and bicarbonate are predominant anions found in bile. The equilibrium between chloride and bicarbonate is mediated by the interplay of the chloride channels TMEM16A and CFTR and the Cl^-/HCO_3^- exchanger AE2.[14,41] The activation of CFTR after a choleretic stimulus, via the cAMP/PKA pathway, leads to its phosphorylation. Subsequently, CFTR generates a chloride gradient to enhance alkaline efflux of biliary HCO_3^- by AE2 and facilitate water secretion by AQP1 to adjust biliary pH.[2,42] The CFTR gene, located on chromosome 7, is mutated in cystic fibrosis, leading to dysregulation of epithelial fluid transport in the lung, pancreas, liver, and biliary tree. CFTR dysfunction may lead to diminished biliary HCO_3^- secretion and ultimately to CF-associated liver disease with secondary sclerosing cholangitis and biliary cirrhosis. Notably, $CFTR^{-/-}$ mice develop milder liver abnormalities compared with humans, most likely owing to their less toxic hydrophilic bile salt pool suggesting that cholangiocellular exposure to hydrophobic bile salts represents a key pathogenic factor in cystic fibrosis–associated liver disease.

CFTR also has a function as a "hub" protein to regulate biliary ATP excretion and vesicle trafficking to the apical membrane. ATP itself, after apical secretion, can stimulate the apical P2Y receptors of neighboring cells in a paracrine fashion. Subsequently, inositol 1,4,5-trisphosphate (IP_3) activates its receptor InsP3R3, to release Ca^{2+} from IP_3-sensitive endoplasmic Ca^{2+} stores near the apical membrane.[43]

Subapical $[Ca^{2+}]_i$ increase activates the Ca^{2+}/Cl^- channel TMEM16A and, thereby, chloride secretion.[44]

TMEM16A is located on the human chromosome 11q13, consists of 5 isoforms (A, B, C, D, and E) and is expressed in all secretory epithelia including cholangiocytes. TMEM16A regulates anion permeability via protein kinase C alpha (PKCα)- and Ca^{2+}-dependent mechanisms, leading to the dominant chloride gradient that drives AE2-mediated Cl^-/HCO_3^- exchange.[45]

UDCA, the standard treatment for patients with PBC, which is also applied in various other cholestatic liver diseases owing to its potent anticholestatic effects, stimulates PKCα- and Ca^{2+}-dependent Cl^- and HCO_3^- secretion of cholangiocytes via activation of TMEM16A,[42,46] a mechanism of action similar to that unraveled for hepatocytes 2 decades ago.[47–50]

Insulin Receptor

Insulin receptors are localized in the apical membrane of cholangiocytes and are activated by insulin and insulin-like growth factor present in bile.[51] Insulin affects secretin-induced HCO_3^- secretion in rat cholangiocytes after bile duct ligation (BDL), by increasing $[Ca^{2+}]_i$ and activating PKCα. Thus, the insulin secreted by hepatocytes can modulate downstream cholangiocyte secretion in a paracrine manner.[51] Whether alterations in bile formation in diabetics may be related to altered insulin effects on ductal secretion remains a matter of speculation (**Fig. 2**).

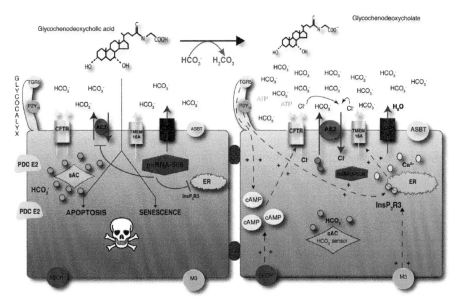

Fig. 2. The biliary HCO_3^- umbrella in health (*right*) and in PBC (*left*). AE2, anion exchanger 2; AQP1, aquaporine 1; ASBT, apical sodium dependent bile salt transporter; ATP, adenosine trisphosphate; Ca^{2+}, calcium; cAMP, cyclic adenosine monophosphate; CFTR, cystic fibrosis transmembrane conductance regulator; Cl^-, chloride; ER, endoplasmatic reticulum; H_2CO_3, carbonic acid; HCO_3^-, bicarbonate; $InsP_3R3$, type III inositol 1,4,5-trisphosphate receptor; M3, muscarinic receptor 3; miRNA-506, microRNA 506; $P2Y_{12}$, purinergic G protein-coupled receptor type 12; PDC-E2, E2 subunit of the pyruvate dehydrogenase complex; sAC, soluble adenylyl cyclase; SECR, secretin receptor; TGR5, the G-protein–coupled receptor 5; TMEM16A, anoctamin1.

Sodium Hydrogen Exchanger and Sodium-Dependent Cl^-/HCO_3^- Exchanger

Sodium hydrogen exchangers are phosphoproteins controlled by protein kinases in response to choleretic stimuli. They regulate acid–base homeostasis and fluid absorption. Na^+/H^+ exchange is responsible for NaCl absorption at the apical membrane of cholangiocytes and is only activated at a pH of less than 7.0. Moreover, together with the basolateral sodium-dependent Cl^-/HCO_3^- exchanger and CA, HCO_3^- efflux by AE2 is counterbalanced to maintain the demanded HCO_3^- concentration at the apical membrane of the cholangiocyte.[4] NHE cholangiocellular activities are impaired in PBC compared with healthy controls, contributing to a defective biliary HCO_3^- umbrella.[52]

Sodium Bicarbonate Cotransporters

Transport of HCO_3^- in rodents is facilitated by NBC isoforms, part of the SLC4 superfamily like AE2.[53] In $AE2^{-/-}$ mice, apical NBC1 proved to be responsible for basal pH maintenance and HCO_3^- secretion, negatively regulated by cAMP and ATP, suggesting that NBC1 in $AE2^{-/-}$ mice may compensate for AE2 loss.[30] In humans, NBC isoforms have so far not been identified at the apical cholangiocyte membrane.

Type III Inositoltrisphosphate Receptor and Other Modulators of Cytosolic Free Calcium

Cytosolic free calcium $[Ca^{2+}]_i$ in cholangiocytes, like many other cells, is modulated by recruitment of calcium from intracellular calcium stores and extracellular calcium influx on one hand and membrane Ca^{2+} extrusion pumps on the other hand. Type III $InsP_3$ receptor ($InsP_3R3$), an endoplasmic reticulum, calcium-selective cation channel regulated by $InsP_3$ and Ca^{2+}, resides in the apical region of human cholangiocytes, where it spatially regulates subapical Ca^{2+} signaling to support HCO_3^- and chloride secretion.[43] $InsP_3R3$ can be activated after stimulation of either G protein-coupled receptors or receptor tyrosine kinases.

Notably, the expression of $InsP_3R3$ is diminished in PBC and other cholangiopathies[54] as well as animal models where, like in humans, impaired Ca^{2+} signaling is associated with decreased secretion of chloride and HCO_3^- into the bile.[54] miR-506 mediates the downregulation of $InsP_3R3$ expression in cholangiocytes. miR-506 binds $InsP_3R3$ mRNA $3'$ untranslated region and promotes the reduction of $InsP_3R3$ mRNA and protein expression.[55] Furthermore, $InsP_3R3$ can be downregulated by transcription factor NRF2, which is activated by ROS.[56] ROS independently can downregulate AE2 expression, as mentioned.[25] Taken together, these results suggest a close interplay between $InsP_3R3$ and AE2 and their expression control by miR-506 and ROS, leading to impaired apical HCO_3^- secretion in PBC.

Potassium Channels

Two potassium channels are responsible for cholangiocyte hyperpolarization, namely SK-2, a small apical/basolateral conductance Ca^{2+}-sensitive K^+ channel and IK1, a basolateral inward rectifier potassium current channel. Supposedly, IK1 and Ca^{2+}-sensitive K^+ channel channels work in parallel with TMEM16A and CFTR to regulate cholangiocyte secretion in response to extracellular nucleotides and increasing $[Ca^{2+}]_i$.[44,57]

Epithelial Sodium Channels

Inward Na^+ transport facilitates movement of water across the cell membrane and provides an electrical driving force for outward Cl^- currents.[58] $ENaC\alpha$ is localized in the apical cholangiocyte membrane and is activated by protease activity and bile flow resulting in at least a transient increase of Na^+ influx and absorption of H_2O at the apical membrane by AQP. ATP has an inhibitory effect on ENaC activity and a stimulating effect on TMEM16A activity. The exact role of ENaC in PBC and other cholangiopathies remains uncertain.

Takeda G-Protein–Coupled Receptor 5

The membrane-bound bile acid receptor TGR5 is found in cholangiocytes at the apical membrane and at the primary cilia (discussed elsewhere in this article).[19,59] Activation of TGR5 by hydrophobic bile salts in nonciliated cholangiocytes occurs after binding the Gαs-protein leading to cAMP-mediated Cl^-/HCO_3^- exchange and choleresis.[19,20] In gallbladder epithelial cells, TGR5 mediates the endosomal recruitment of ASBT and CFTR toward the apical membrane, increasing transport capacity.[60] TGR5 also mediates antiinflammatory pathways by reducing nuclear factor-κB activity and cytokine expression, and antiapoptotic pathways by phosphorylation of the cellular death receptor CD95.[18] Still, activation of TGR5 also induced proliferative effects questioning its future role as a therapeutic target in cholestatic liver diseases.[21]

ENZYMES, NUCLEAR RECEPTORS, AND TRANSCRIPTION FACTORS
Alkaline Phosphatase

Serum alkaline phosphatase (AP) is a diagnostic marker of cholestasis (together with elevated γ-glutamyl transferase and/or conjugated bilirubin), a surrogate marker of prognosis in PBC and also primary sclerosing cholangitis and an increasingly accepted measure of therapeutic response in PBC.[61] In cholestasis, serum AP is thought to be increased by retrograde reflux from biliary epithelia and enhanced synthesis, as well as aberrant basolateral release from hepatocytes. Hepatic AP is an ectophosphatase with the ability to enzymatically dephosphorylate ATP and to determine P2 receptor function at the apical membrane of the cholangiocyte. In vivo studies showed that in BDL rats AP administration decreases bile flow and biliary HCO_3^- secretion.[62] Hepatic APs efficacy in dephosphorylating ATP depends on extracellular pH. Higher pH means higher enzymatic activity of AP to dephosphorylate ATP. Thereby, a negative feedback loop controls local pH at the apical cholangiocyte membrane by modulating the ATP-mediated activation of TMEM16A and subsequent biliary HCO_3^- export.

Galactoside 2-Alpha-ʟ-fucosyltransferase 2

The cholangiocyte glycocalyx is a 20- to 40-nm apical membrane-bound barrier of glycoproteins[2,4] that possibly forms a trap for apically released HCO_3^-.[3] Synthesis and stability of this glycoprotein barrier depends on various enzymes, among them FUT2, which catalyzes the transfer of fucose to glycoproteins and glycolipids. In genome-wide association studies, FUT2 polymorphisms were linked to primary sclerosing cholangitis and independently to elevated serum levels of AP and γ-glutamyl transferase.[63,64] Fut2$^{-/-}$ mice developed portosystemic shunting resulting in microcirculatory disturbances, mild periductal fibrosis, and vulnerability toward human bile salts.[65] Human biliary epithelial cells were prone to pH-dependent toxicity by chenodeoxycholate and glycochenodeoxycholate after removal of sialic acid residues from the glycocalyx.[2,4] These results support the idea that the glycocalyx may form a biliary surface microclimate pH regulatory system at the apical cholangiocyte membrane[2] and might thereby contribute to stabilization of the biliary HCO_3^- umbrella in biliary epithelia.

Sphingosine-1-Phosphate Receptor 2

The G-protein–coupled receptor S1PR2 is stimulated by S1P and mostly hydrophilic bile salts in mice and upregulated in cholestasis.[66] S1PR2 knockout reduced inflammation, cholangiocyte proliferation, and cholestatic liver injury in mice after BDL.[67] Studies on the role of human cholangiocellular S1PR2 in chronic cholangiopathies seem attractive.

MicroRNAs

miRNAs are single stranded, noncoding, 22 to 23 nucleotides long RNA sequences residing in the cytoplasm. In hepatocytes, miR-33 is a potent modulator of various transporters (ABCA1, ABCG5, ABCG8, ABCB11, and ATP8B1). The silencing of miR-33 led to increased bile flow and cholesterol secretion in mice.[68] MiR-21 is increased in mouse cholangiocytes after BDL and in transforming growth factor-β receptor$^{-/-}$ mice leading to an increased synthesis of tumor necrosis factor-α and interferon-γ.[69]

In advanced PBC, miR-139-5p is downregulated, associated with increased levels of tumor necrosis factor-α,[70] thereby possibly affecting the stability of the biliary HCO_3^- umbrella (discussed elsewhere in this article).

Most relevant for PBC, miR-506 is upregulated in PBC cholangiocytes (discussed elsewhere in this article; see **Fig. 2**).[9] miR-506 expression in human cholangiocytes is enhanced by proinflammatory cytokines, including interleukin-8, interleukin-12, and tumor necrosis factor-α, all of which are overexpressed in PBC.[24] MiR-506 in human cholangiocytes downregulates AE2 and $InsP_3R3$ expression,[9,55] inhibits cAMP- and $InsP_3R3$-mediated fluid secretion in isolated bile duct units,[55] and stimulates sAC-dependent HCO_3^--sensitive bile acid–induced apoptosis[28] and aberrant expression of PDC-E2–like peptides on the plasma membrane.[24] $InsP_3R3$ loss in cholangiocytes results in a disrupted HCO_3^- secretion after secretin and acetylcholine (ACh) stimulation. Conversely, inhibition of miR-506 by anti–miR-506 enhances AE2 activity and improves Cl^-/HCO_3^- exchange.[9] It is noteworthy that the gene for miR-506 is located on the X-chromosome, where there is a clear female preponderance in PBC. This led to the recent hypothesis that an initial disease trigger in PBC might induce an X-linked epigenetic change, leading to a female-biased activation of the miR-506–$InsP_3R3$–AE2–sAC axis.[71] Thus, miR-506 mimics PBC-like features in human cholangiocytes in vitro and may play a crucial role in the control of intracellular levels and biliary secretion of HCO_3^- to stabilize the biliary HCO_3^- umbrella. Therapeutic targeting of miR-506 in PBC and possibly other chronic fibrosing cholangiopathies seems, therefore, attractive.

Peroxisome Proliferator-Activated Receptor Alpha/Delta

Peroxisome proliferator-activated receptors (PPARs) consist of 3 isoforms (α, β/δ, γ) that form heterodimer complexes with retinoid X receptor and then bind to peroxisome proliferator response elements to regulate expression levels of many genes involved in cell differentiation and metabolism. PPAR-α is expressed in the liver, kidney, adipose tissue, and other tissues containing high levels of fatty acids. PPARs are involved in bile salt synthesis by inhibiting CYP7A1 expression and inducing CYP3A4 expression, and enhance biliary phosphatidylcholine secretion,[72] thereby facilitating biliary mixed micelle formation and potentially relieving the biliary HCO_3^- umbrella by reducing bile salt monomer levels in bile.[73] The promising effects of bezafibrate and fenofibrate in the treatment of patients with PBC inadequately responding to UDCA may be related in part to these molecular mechanisms. PPAR agonists like bezafibrate represent an attractive therapeutic option in PBC, but also other fibrosing cholangiopathies.[73]

Farnesoid X Receptor and Fibroblast Growth Factor 19

The bile salt-activated nuclear receptor farnesoid X factor receptor (FXR) plays a pivotal role in bile salt homeostasis, glucose and lipid metabolism.[73,74] FXR is expressed in various cell types including hepatocytes, cholangiocytes, enterocytes, or renal tubular cells and was initially discovered in the ileal enterocyte, where it binds with retinoid X receptor as heterodimer to influence target gene transcription via short heterodimer partner in the same cell or via human fibroblast growth factor 19 (FGF19) secreted into blood and binding to FGF receptor 4/β-klotho on the target cell membrane to activate c-Jun N-terminal Kinase and mitogen-activated protein kinase/extracellular signal-regulated kinase 1/2 pathways, resulting in repression of CYP7A1 and CYP27 in hepatocytes. FGF19 also stimulates hepatocyte growth factor and wound healing in biliary epithelia. In the human liver, high levels of FGF19 mRNA were first detected in severe extrahepatic cholestasis, decreasing after biliary drainage.[75] Subsequently, FGF19 was also identified in the liver tissue of patients with PBC and FGF19 levels were positively correlated with disease severity,[76] suggesting that hepatic FGF19 expression is rather a universal response to cholestasis.

In cholangiocytes, FXR also exerts protective effects against bile salt induced cell injury. In experimental hypoxia mimicking cold ischemia during liver transplantation, FXR was markedly downregulated, leading to the upregulation of ASBT expression, downregulation of OSTα/β expression, accumulation of intracellular bile salts, and induction of bile salt-induced apoptosis.[77] Thus, targeting FXR in PBC and other fibrosing cholangiopathies is an attractive strategy for protection of both hepatocytes and cholangiocytes.[73,74]

Soluble Adenylyl Cyclase

Unlike AC transmembrane isoforms, sAC is located in the cytosol, mitochondria, and nucleus of various cell types, including cholangiocytes.[28] sAC is not activated by hormones, G-proteins, or forskolin, but by HCO_3^- and calcium and is fine-tuned by ATP, which implicates that sAC is a pH sensor.[78] In cholangiocytes of patients with PBC, AE2 expression and activity was decreased, HCO_3^- secretion was diminished, and intracellular pH was increased.[9] We demonstrated that AE2 knockdown in human cholangiocytes is associated with pH-dependent bile salt-induced apoptosis, but in addition also etoposide-induced apoptosis.[4] This led us to speculate that apoptosis in human AE2-deficient cholangiocytes is a result not only of accumulation of intracellular bile salts, but also HCO_3^-.[28] Indeed, sAC mediates cAMP release and Ca^{2+} release from intracellular stores to regulate bile salt–induced apoptosis by intrinsic apoptotic pathways including cytochrome C and caspase 3 release and DNA fragmentation, which can all be reversed by sAC inhibition.[28] Thus, sAC represents an attractive therapeutic target in PBC to prevent pH- and bile salt–mediated apoptosis.[28]

Vitamin D Receptor

Vitamin D is hydroxylated to 25-hydroxy vitamin D in hepatocytes and subsequently excreted into bile, absorbed in the intestine and again hydroxylated in the kidney to 1,25-dihydroxy vitamin D, the biologically active form of vitamin D, which is recirculating in the enterohepatic circulation. Vitamin D receptor (VDR) is abundant in hepatocytes, Kupffer cells, stellate cells, and cholangiocytes. VDR bound to 1,25-dihydroxy vitamin D heterodimerizes with retinoid X receptor and binds to VDR-responsive elements in the promoter region of vitamin D–responsive genes. VDR can also be activated by the most hydrophobic and toxic human bile salt, lithocholate. VDR induces antiinflammatory, antibacterial, antiproliferative, prodifferentiative, and immunomodulatory effects and strengthens the innate immune response by various mechanisms.[79] Notably, VDR is strongly expressed in human biliary epithelium and stimulates formation of cathelicidin, a major antimicrobial peptide contributing to a microbial-free environment in bile.[80] In vitro, the therapeutic bile salt UDCA and 1,25-dihydroxy vitamin D had additive effects on VDR-dependent catheli-cidin expression in cholangiocytes, whereas the major human hydrophobic bile salt, chenodeoxycholic acid, stimulated cathelicidin expression via FXR-dependent mech-anisms.[80] UDCA therapy in PBC led to enhanced expression of VDR and catheli-cidin.[80] In hepatocytes, VDR activation inhibits bile acid synthesis by inhibiting CYP7A1 via the c-RAF/MEK1/2/extracellular signal-regulated kinase 1/2 pathway.[81] Taken together, these and other findings make VDR a highly attractive therapeutic target for PBC and other chronic fibrosing cholangiopathies.

Carbonic Anhydrases

CAs catalyze the reversible hydration of CO_2 to HCO_3^- and H^+ and are the major source of secreted HCO_3^- in cholangiocytes and critical for pH regulation. Twelve CA isoforms with a tissue-specific distribution have been described in humans. Among these, CA-II is most abundant in biliary epithelia, but not other liver cells. Notably, immunization with human CA-II led to cholangitis in a susceptible mouse strain compared with sham-immunized littermates; adoptive splenocyte transfer from CA-II immunized mice led to cholangitis in recipient susceptible mice.[82] Thus, cholangiocellular CA isoforms deserve more attention as potential therapeutic targets in PBC and other fibrosing cholangiopathies.

Purinergic Receptors

Purinergic receptors (P2Y, P2X) are ubiquitously expressed. P2Y receptors have been localized not only on cilia (discussed elsewhere in this article), but in addition both on apical and basolateral membranes of rat cholangiocytes and are G-coupled proteins that are stimulated by biliary (apical) or blood (basolateral) ATP and derivatives (aden-osine diphosphate, uridine 5'-triphosphate, and uridine 5'-diphosphate). Activation of P2Y receptors leads to either calcium release from IP3-sensitive cellular stores (P2Y1, 2, 4, 6, 11) or inhibition of ACs and decreased intracellular cAMP levels (P2Y12, 13, 14). A P2Y-induced increase in Cl^- efflux via TMEM16A stimulates biliary HCO_3^- secretion.[83] Thus, biliary P2Y receptors might represent a therapeutic target in chronic fibrosing cholangiopathies stabilizing the biliary HCO_3^- umbrella.

BASOLATERAL MEMBRANE
Secretin Receptor

The hormone secretin is released postprandially from S cells, mainly of the duodenum, into the mesenteric and portal venous blood. Secretin is an important driving force for cholangiocellular secretion of chloride, HCO_3^- and water.[84] In rodents, the SR, a G-protein–coupled receptor activating AC, is expressed on the basolateral membrane of large, but not small cholangiocytes. Various complementary pathways have been identified for secretin induced HCO_3^- secretion in rodents after binding to SR: (i) acti-vating AC8, thereby increasing cAMP, inducing PKA phosphorylation and stimulating CFTR-mediated Cl^- transport, which activates AE2, resulting in secretin induced HCO_3^- secretion[85]; (ii) activating CFTR (see i), which stimulates ATP secretion; luminal ATP then activates apical P2Y receptors in a paracrine fashion, leading to subapical InsP3R3 activation, $[Ca^{2+}]_i$ increase and activation of the Ca^{2+}-sensitive Cl^- channel TMEM16A and subsequent activation of AE2, resulting in secretin induced HCO_3^- secretion[43]; (iii) inducing cAMP- and microtubule-dependent movement of intracel-lular vesicles containing CFTR, AE2, and AQP1, which colocalize into the apical membrane, resulting in secretin induced HCO_3^- secretion[40]; and (iv) stimulation of

ASBT translocation into the apical membrane in normal and BDL rodent cholangio-cytes[36] and possibly thereby stimulation of cholehepatic shunting and/or signaling of bile salts, possibly contributing to HCO_3^- formation.[10,33]

Notably, patients with PBC showed an absent HCO_3^- secretion response to secretin as determined by PET, a process reversed by UDCA, suggesting a potential role of impaired secretin-induced HCO_3^- secretion in the pathogenesis of PBC.[8]

Muscarinic Acetylcholine Receptor Type 3

ACh is the primary neurotransmitter of the parasympathic nerve system, which is most active during digestion, coordinating the ACh response with the actions of secretin. ACh acts on basolateral M3R, present on small and large cholangiocytes.[86] The M3R is G-protein coupled and mobilizes phosphoinositides to generate IP_3, stimulate $InsP_3Rs$ and induce $[Ca^{2+}]_i$ increases. Ca^{2+}-sensitive calcineurin subsequently activates AC8, thereby increasing cAMP. This pathway does not affect basal AE2 activity, but enhances secretin-induced AE2 activity and secretin induced HCO_3^- secretion.[54,86] M3R knockout in mice leads to impaired bile formation, most likely owing to impaired HCO_3^- secretion, and enhanced susceptibility to cholestatic liver injury.[87] A defective ACh–bicarbonate response is also suggested to play a role in nonanastomotic strictures after liver transplantation and, thereby, liver denervation.[2] Bile has a higher bile salt/phospholipid ratio just after liver transplantation, which increases the risk of NAS.[88] Vagotomy has previously been demonstrated in BDL rats to decrease M3R expression, SR gene expression, secretin-induced cAMP increases, and ACh potentiation of the secretin-induced HCO_3^- secretion.[89] Because adrenergic denervation decreases secretin induced bicarbonate secretion,[90] combined adrenergic and cholinergic denervation possibly make cholangiocytes vulnerable to the toxic bile composition after liver transplantation.[2,88]

Notably, M3R antibodies are found in up to 93% of patients with PBC.[91] Their functional relevance in PBC is unknown, but M3R antibodies have been shown to be associated with salivary dysfunction in Sjögren's syndrome, which has a high cooccurrence with PBC. Thus, one might speculate that M3R antibodies could impair ACh-potentiated secretin-induced bicarbonate secretion in PBC.

Other Basolateral Receptors, Cytokines, and Chemokines

Numerous additional receptors, but also cytokines and chemokines, have been identified as putative modifiers of biliary secretion particularly in rodents. It is beyond the scope of this review to explain in detail all the findings summarized in **Table 1**.

THERAPEUTIC INTERVENTIONS POTENTIALLY STABILIZING A DEFECTIVE BILIARY HCO_3^- UMBRELLA
Ursodeoxycholic Acid

UDCA (13–15 mg/kg/d) is the standard treatment for patients with PBC and intrahepatic cholestasis of pregnancy.[92] UDCA is a posttranscriptional secretagogue with choleretic, but also potent anticholestatic effects in hepatocytes and cholangiocytes by activating complex signaling chains after entry into the cell involving modulation of $[Ca^{2+}]_i$, $PKC\alpha$, PKA, PI_3K, and MEK leading to vesicular insertion of transporters into the apical membrane and, thereby, enhanced secretory capacity.[42,46–50,73,93,94] Patients with PBC were shown to have an impaired secretin-induced HCO_3^- secretion, which was restored by UDCA treatment,[8] in part by enhancing the impaired AE2 expression in PBC.[6,7]

Table 1
Basolateral receptors, carriers and cytokines/chemokines potentially affecting the biliary HCO_3^- umbrella

Agonist	Receptor	Model	Effect on Basal Secretion of HCO_3^-/Cl^-	Effect on Secretion of Secretin Induced HCO_3^-/Cl^-	Relevance for PBC or Other Cholangiopahies
Phenylephrine	α1	BDL rat	No effect	Potentiation	Role in NAS after LTx?
UK14,304	α2	BDL rat	No effect	Inhibition	?
Dobutamine (chronic infusion)	β1	BDL rat (adrenergically denervated)	No effect	Potentiation	Role in NAS after LTx?
Clenbuterol	β2	BDL rat (adrenergically denervated)	No effect	Potentiation	Role in NAS after LTx?
Quinelorane	Dopamine 2 receptor	BDL rat	No effect	Inhibition	?
8-hydroxyd-DPAT	Serotonin 1A	BDL rat	No effect	Inhibition	?
Anpirtoline	Serotonin 1B	BDL rat	No effect	Inhibition	?
Melatonin	MT1	BDL rat	Attenuated	Inhibition	?
GABA	GABA_A GABA_B GABA_C	BDL rat	No (net) effect	Net effect: inhibition Large cholangiocytes: inhibition Small cholangiocytes: potentiation	?
Endothelin 1	ET-A ET-B	BDL rat Normal rat	No effect Augmented	Inhibition Not determined	?

Endothelin 3	ET-B	Normal rat	Augmented	Not determined	?
Gastrin	CCK-B	BDL rat	No effect	Inhibition	?
Somatostatin	SSTR2	BDL rat	Attenuated	Inhibition	?
Vasoactive Intestinal Peptide	VPAC1	Normal and BDL rat isolated perfused liver	Augmented	Not determined	?
Bombesin	Bombesin receptor	Normal rat IBDU	Augmented	Not determined	?
VEGF-A	VEGFR-2 VEGFR-3	Hepatic artery ligated BDL rat	Augmented	Potentiated	Role in NAS after LTx?
TNF-α	TNFR1 TNFR2	Actinomycin D treated BDL rat	No effect	Inhibition	Elevated in PBC serum
IFN-γ	IFNγ-R	Isolated human cholangiocyte Cirrhotic mouse	Attenuated Not determined	Inhibition	Elevated in PBC serum
IL-5	IL-5R	Isolated rat BEC	No effect	Inhibition[a]	Elevated in PBC serum
IL-6[b]	IL-6R	IBDU rat	No effect	Inhibition[c]	Elevated in PBC serum
IL-1[b]	IL-1R	IBDU rat	No effect	Inhibition[c]	Elevated in PBC serum

Abbreviations: IBDU, isolated bile duct units; IFN, interferon; IL, interleukin; LTx, liver transplantation; NAS, nonanastomotic stricturing; PBC, primary biliary cholangitis; TNF, tumor necrosis factor; VEGF, vascular endothelial growth factor; VEGFR, vascular endothelial growth factor receptor.

[a] Inhibition of NECA stimulated Cl currents.

[b] Effect only in combination with one of the following: TNF-α, IFN-γ, IL-5, IL-6, IL-1.

[c] Inhibition of forskolin stimulated AE2 activity.

UDCA also induces CFTR-dependent cholangiocellular ATP release in mouse cholangiocytes resulting from vesicular insertion of CFTR into the apical membrane[42] and CFTR-independent hepatocellular ATP release into bile in the isolated perfused rat liver[95] potentially leading to stimulated ATP/P2Y-mediated HCO_3^- secretion as outlined above.[43] Unconjugated UDCA induces biliary secretion of S-nitrosoglutathione in perfused rat liver. S-Nitrosoglutathione induces ATP release through PKB and PI_3K in cultured cholangiocytes.[96]

In summary, stabilizing the biliary HCO_3^- umbrella seems to be a key mechanism and site of action of UDCA in PBC.[73]

Norursodeoxycholic Acid

Norursodeoxycholic acid, the C_{23} homologue of UDCA, is effective in treating cholestasis in Mdr2$^{-/-}$ mice[97] and shows moderate anticholestatic effects in patients with primary sclerosing cholangitis.[98] Norursodeoxycholic acid greatly induces HCO_3^- secretion in humans[99] and rodents,[100] putatively by cholehepatic shunting of norursodeoxycholic acid,[100] leading to enhanced biliary HCO_3^- formation and stabilization of the biliary HCO_3^- umbrella.

Corticosteroids

Combination therapy of budesonide with UDCA was more effective in improving liver biochemistry and histologic features than UDCA monotherapy in patients with stages I through III PBC incompletely responding to UDCA.[101,102] In rat cholangiocytes, dexamethasone or budesonide increase AE2 expression, AE2 activity, and HCO_3^- secretion.[103] In human cholangiocytes, the cotreatment of dexamethasone with UDCA, by acting on the glucocorticoid receptor, increases transcription of an alternate AE2 promoter and AE2 activity.[104] Thus, corticosteroids may stabilize the biliary HCO_3^- umbrella independent of their antiinflammatory effects.[73,74]

Obeticholic Acid

Obeticholic acid is a semisynthetic bile acid analogue that potently activates FXR. Obeticholic acid is meanwhile accepted for second-line treatment of patients with PBC incompletely responding to UDCA alone.[105] Obeticholic acid has anticholestatic, antiinflammatory, and antifibrotic effects in experimental and clinical studies.[73,74] Among the beneficial effects of FXR agonists in experimental cholestasis, stimulation of biliary HCO_3^- secretion has been described as a key mechanism of action. It remains unclear whether this also is valid for patients with PBC.

Fibrates

Fibrates have been shown to be effective anticholestatic drugs in combination with UDCA for patients who do respond inadequately to UDCA alone.[73,74] Fibrates are ligands of PPAR. Among other effects, PPAR-α downregulates CYP7A1 and, thereby, bile acid synthesis, and upregulates CYP3A4, which detoxifies bile salts.[106] PPAR-α also stimulates hepatocellular expression of multidrug resistance protein 3, and, thereby, biliary phosphatidylcholine secretion preventing damage to the biliary epithelium.[107] Thus, fibrates might indirectly stabilize the biliary HCO_3^- umbrella by phosphatidylcholine-mediated chaperoning of biliary bile salt monomers.

ACKNOWLEDGMENTS

The authors gratefully acknowledge the continuous support within the working group, particularly of Ronald Oude Elferink, Stan van de Graaf, Jung-Chin Chang,

Dagmar Tolenaars and Coen Paulusma. This work was supported by a grant for an investigator-initiated study from Dr. Falk GmbH and a South-African PSC Patient Foundation.

REFERENCES

1. Hirschfield GM, Gershwin ME. The immunobiology and pathophysiology of primary biliary cirrhosis. Annu Rev Pathol 2013;8:303–30.
2. Beuers U, Hohenester S, de Buy Wenniger LJ, et al. The biliary HCO3⁻ umbrella: a unifying hypothesis on pathogenetic and therapeutic aspects of fibrosing cholangiopathies. Hepatology 2010;52(4):1489–96.
3. Maillette de Buy Wenniger LJ, Hohenester S, Maroni L, et al. The cholangiocyte glycocalyx stabilizes the 'biliary HCO3 umbrella': an integrated line of defense against toxic bile acids. Dig Dis 2015;33(3):397–407.
4. Hohenester S, Wenniger LM, Paulusma CC, et al. A biliary HCO3⁻ umbrella constitutes a protective mechanism against bile acid-induced injury in human cholangiocytes. Hepatology 2012;55(1):173–83.
5. Sasaki M, Miyakoshi M, Sato Y, et al. Increased expression of mitochondrial proteins associated with autophagy in biliary epithelial lesions in primary biliary cirrhosis. Liver Int 2013;33(2):312–20.
6. Prieto J, Qian C, Garcia N, et al. Abnormal expression of anion exchanger genes in primary biliary cirrhosis. Gastroenterology 1993;105(2):572–8.
7. Medina JF, Martinez A, Vazquez JJ, et al. Decreased anion exchanger 2 immunoreactivity in the liver of patients with primary biliary cirrhosis. Hepatology 1997;25(1):12–7.
8. Prieto J, Garcia N, Marti-Climent JM, et al. Assessment of biliary bicarbonate secretion in humans by positron emission tomography. Gastroenterology 1999;117(1):167–72.
9. Banales JM, Saez E, Uriz M, et al. Up-regulation of microRNA 506 leads to decreased Cl-/HCO3⁻ anion exchanger 2 expression in biliary epithelium of patients with primary biliary cirrhosis. Hepatology 2012;56(2):687–97.
10. Boyer JL. Bile formation and secretion. Compr Physiol 2013;3(3):1035–78.
11. Dilger K, Hohenester S, Winkler-Budenhofer U, et al. Effect of ursodeoxycholic acid on bile acid profiles and intestinal detoxification machinery in primary biliary cirrhosis and health. J Hepatol 2012;57(1):133–40.
12. Masyuk AI, Masyuk TV, Splinter PL, et al. Cholangiocyte cilia detect changes in luminal fluid flow and transmit them into intracellular Ca2+ and cAMP signaling. Gastroenterology 2006;131(3):911–20.
13. O'Hara SP, Mott JL, Splinter PL, et al. MicroRNAs: key modulators of posttranscriptional gene expression. Gastroenterology 2009;136(1):17–25.
14. Tabibian JH, Masyuk AI, Masyuk TV, et al. Physiology of cholangiocytes. Compr Physiol 2013;3(1):541–65.
15. Gradilone SA, Masyuk AI, Splinter PL, et al. Cholangiocyte cilia express TRPV4 and detect changes in luminal tonicity inducing bicarbonate secretion. Proc Natl Acad Sci U S A 2007;104(48):19138–43.
16. Gradilone SA, Masyuk TV, Huang BQ, et al. Activation of Trpv4 reduces the hyperproliferative phenotype of cystic cholangiocytes from an animal model of ARPKD. Gastroenterology 2010;139(1):304–14.e2.
17. Masyuk AI, Gradilone SA, Banales JM, et al. Cholangiocyte primary cilia are chemosensory organelles that detect biliary nucleotides via P2Y12 purinergic receptors. Am J Physiol Gastrointest Liver Physiol 2008;295(4):G725–34.

18. Sato H, Macchiarulo A, Thomas C, et al. Novel potent and selective bile acid derivatives as TGR5 agonists: biological screening, structure-activity relationships, and molecular modeling studies. J Med Chem 2008;51(6):1831–41.

19. Keitel V, Ullmer C, Haussinger D. The membrane-bound bile acid receptor TGR5 (Gpbar-1) is localized in the primary cilium of cholangiocytes. Biol Chem 2010;391(7):785–9.

20. Masyuk AI, Huang BQ, Radtke BN, et al. Ciliary subcellular localization of TGR5 determines the cholangiocyte functional response to bile acid signaling. Am J Physiol Gastrointest Liver Physiol 2013;304(11):G1013–24.

21. Reich M, Deutschmann K, Sommerfeld A, et al. TGR5 is essential for bile acid-dependent cholangiocyte proliferation in vivo and in vitro. Gut 2016;65(3): 487–501.

22. Santos-Laso A, Izquierdo-Sanchez L, Lee-Law PY, et al. New advances in polycystic liver diseases. Semin Liver Dis 2017;37(1):45–55.

23. Martinez-Anso E, Castillo JE, Diez J, et al. Immunohistochemical detection of chloride/bicarbonate anion exchangers in human liver. Hepatology 1994;19: 1400–6.

24. Erice O, Munoz-Garrido P, Vaquero J, et al. MicroRNA-506 promotes primary biliary cholangitis-like features in cholangiocytes and immune activation. Hepatology 2018;67(4):1420–40.

25. Hisamoto S, Shimoda S, Harada K, et al. Hydrophobic bile acids suppress expression of AE2 in biliary epithelial cells and induce bile duct inflammation in primary biliary cholangitis. J Autoimmun 2016;75:150–60.

26. Poupon R, Ping C, Chretien Y, et al. Genetic factors of susceptibility and of severity in primary biliary cirrhosis. J Hepatol 2008;49(6):1038–45.

27. Aiba Y, Nakamura M, Joshita S, et al. Genetic polymorphisms in CTLA4 and SLC4A2 are differentially associated with the pathogenesis of primary biliary cirrhosis in Japanese patients. J Gastroenterol 2011;46(10):1203–12.

28. Chang JC, Go S, de Waart DR, et al. Soluble adenylyl cyclase regulates bile salt-induced apoptosis in human cholangiocytes. Hepatology 2016;64(2): 522–34.

29. Salas JT, Banales JM, Sarvide S, et al. Ae2a,b-deficient mice develop antimitochondrial antibodies and other features resembling primary biliary cirrhosis. Gastroenterology 2008;134(5):1482–93.

30. Uriarte I, Banales JM, Saez E, et al. Bicarbonate secretion of mouse cholangiocytes involves Na^+-HCO_3^- cotransport in addition to Na^+-independent Cl^-/HCO_3^- exchange. Hepatology 2010;51(3):891–902.

31. Strazzabosco M, Joplin R, Zsembery A, et al. Na/-dependent and -independent Cl^-/HCO_3^- exchange mediate cellular HCO_3^- transport in cultured human intrahepatic bile duct cells. Hepatology 1997;25(4):976–85.

32. Strazzabosco M, Mennone A, Boyer JL. Intracellular pH regulation in isolated rat bile duct epithelial cells. J Clin Invest 1991;87:1503–12.

33. Hofmann AF. Bile acids: trying to understand their chemistry and biology with the hope of helping patients. Hepatology 2009;49(5):1403–18.

34. Balakrishnan A, Polli JE. Apical sodium dependent bile acid transporter (ASBT, SLC10A2): a potential prodrug target. Mol Pharm 2006;3(3):223–30.

35. Lionarons DA, Boyer JL, Cai SY. Evolution of substrate specificity for the bile salt transporter ASBT (SLC10A2). J Lipid Res 2012;53(8):1535–42.

36. Alpini G, Glaser S, Baiocchi L, et al. Secretin activation of the apical Na+-dependent bile acid transporter is associated with cholehepatic shunting in rats. Hepatology 2005;41(5):1037–45.

37. Xia X, Roundtree M, Merikhi A, et al. Degradation of the apical sodium-dependent bile acid transporter by the ubiquitin-proteasome pathway in cholangiocytes. J Biol Chem 2004;279(43):44931–7.

38. Alpini G, Glaser S, Rodgers R. Functional expression of the apical Na^+-dependent bile acid transporter in large but not small rat cholangiocytes. Gastroenterology 1997;113:1734–40.

39. Marinelli RA, Pham L, Tietz PS. Expression of aquaporin-4 water channels in rat cholangiocytes. Hepatology 2000;31(6):1313–7.

40. Tietz PS, Marinelli RA, Chen XM, et al. Agonist-induced coordinated trafficking of functionally related transport proteins for water and ions in cholangiocytes. J Biol Chem 2003;278(22):20413–9.

41. Fitz JG, Basavappa S, McGill J, et al. Regulation of membrane chloride currents in rat bile duct epithelial cells. J Clin Invest 1993;91(1):319–28.

42. Fiorotto R, Spirli C, Fabris L, et al. Ursodeoxycholic acid stimulates cholangiocyte fluid secretion in mice via CFTR-dependent ATP secretion. Gastroenterology 2007;133(5):1603–13.

43. Minagawa N, Nagata J, Shibao K, et al. Cyclic AMP regulates bicarbonate secretion in cholangiocytes through release of ATP into bile. Gastroenterology 2007;133(5):1592–602.

44. Dutta AK, Woo K, Doctor RB, et al. Extracellular nucleotides stimulate Cl- currents in biliary epithelia through receptor-mediated IP3 and Ca2+ release. Am J Physiol Gastrointest Liver Physiol 2008;295(5):G1004–15.

45. Dutta AK, Khimji AK, Liu S, et al. PKCalpha regulates TMEM16A-mediated Cl(-) secretion in human biliary cells. Am J Physiol Gastrointest Liver Physiol 2016; 310(1):G34–42.

46. Li Q, Dutta A, Kresge C, et al. Bile acids stimulate cholangiocyte fluid secretion by activation of membraneTMEM16A Cl(-) channels. Hepatology 2018. [Epub ahead of print].

47. Beuers U, Nathanson MH, Isales CM, et al. Tauroursodeoxycholic acid stimulates hepatocellular exocytosis and mobilizes extracellular Ca++ mechanisms defective in cholestasis. J Clin Invest 1993;92(6):2984–93.

48. Beuers U, Throckmorton DC, Anderson MS, et al. Tauroursodeoxycholic acid activates protein kinase C in isolated rat hepatocytes. Gastroenterology 1996; 110(5):1553–63.

49. Beuers U, Bilzer M, Chittattu A, et al. Tauroursodeoxycholic acid inserts the apical conjugate export pump, Mrp2, into canalicular membranes and stimulates organic anion secretion by protein kinase C-dependent mechanisms in cholestatic rat liver. Hepatology 2001;33(5):1206–16.

50. Wimmer R, Hohenester S, Pusl T, et al. Tauroursodeoxycholic acid exerts anticholestatic effects by a cooperative cPKC alpha-/PKA-dependent mechanism in rat liver. Gut 2008;57(10):1448–54.

51. Lesage GD, Marucci L, Alvaro D, et al. Insulin inhibits secretin-induced ductal secretion by activation of PKC alpha and inhibition of PKA activity. Hepatology 2002;36(3):641–51.

52. Melero S, Spirli C, Zsembery A, et al. Defective regulation of cholangiocyte Cl-/ HCO_3^- and Na+/H+ exchanger activities in primary biliary cirrhosis. Hepatology 2002;35(6):1513–21.

53. Pushkin A, Kurtz I. SLC4 base (HCO_3^-, $CO_3\ 2^-$) transporters: classification, function, structure, genetic diseases, and knockout models. Am J Physiol Renal Physiol 2006;290(3):F580–99.

54. Shibao K, Hirata K, Robert ME, et al. Loss of inositol 1,4,5-trisphosphate receptors from bile duct epithelia is a common event in cholestasis. Gastroenterology 2003;125(4):1175–87.

55. Ananthanarayanan M, Banales JM, Guerra MT, et al. Post-translational regulation of the type III inositol 1,4,5-trisphosphate receptor by miRNA-506. J Biol Chem 2015;290(1):184–96.

56. Weerachayaphorn J, Amaya MJ, Spirli C, et al. Nuclear factor, erythroid 2-like 2 regulates expression of type 3 inositol 1,4,5-trisphosphate receptor and calcium signaling in cholangiocytes. Gastroenterology 2015;149(1):211–22.e10.

57. Dutta AK, Khimji AK, Kresge C, et al. Identification and functional characterization of TMEM16A, a Ca2+-activated Cl- channel activated by extracellular nucleotides, in biliary epithelium. J Biol Chem 2011;286(1):766–76.

58. Li Q, Kresge C, Bugde A, et al. Regulation of mechanosensitive biliary epithelial transport by the epithelial Na(+) channel. Hepatology 2016;63(2):538–49.

59. Kawamata Y, Fujii R, Hosoya M, et al. A G protein-coupled receptor responsive to bile acids. J Biol Chem 2003;278(11):9435–40.

60. Keitel V, Cupisti K, Ullmer C, et al. The membrane-bound bile acid receptor TGR5 is localized in the epithelium of human gallbladders. Hepatology 2009;50(3):861–70.

61. Poupon R. Liver alkaline phosphatase: a missing link between choleresis and biliary inflammation. Hepatology 2015;61(6):2080–90.

62. Alvaro D, Benedetti A, Marucci L, et al. The function of alkaline phosphatase in the liver: regulation of intrahepatic biliary epithelium secretory activities in the rat. Hepatology 2000;32(2):174–84.

63. Chambers JC, Zhang W, Sehmi J, et al. Genome-wide association study identifies loci influencing concentrations of liver enzymes in plasma. Nat Genet 2011;43(11):1131–8.

64. Folseraas T, Melum E, Rausch P. Extended analysis of a genome-wide association study in primary sclerosing cholangitis detects multiple novel risk loci. J Hepatol 2012;57(2):366–75.

65. Maroni L, Hohenester SD, van de Graaf SF, et al. Knockout of the primary sclerosing cholangitis-risk gene Fut2 causes liver disease in mice. Hepatology 2017;66:542–54.

66. Nagahashi M, Takabe K, Liu R, et al. Conjugated bile acid-activated S1P receptor 2 is a key regulator of sphingosine kinase 2 and hepatic gene expression. Hepatology 2015;61(4):1216–26.

67. Wang Y, Aoki H, Yang J, et al. The role of sphingosine 1-phosphate receptor 2 in bile acid-induced cholangiocyte proliferation and cholestasis-induced liver injury in mice. Hepatology 2017;65(6):2005–18.

68. Allen RM, Marquart JC, Albert J. miR-33 controls the expression of biliary transporters, and mediates statin- and diet-induced hepatotoxicity. EMBO Mol Med 2012;4:882–95.

69. Ando Y, Yang GX, Kenny TP, et al. Overexpression of microRNA-21 is associated with elevated pro-inflammatory cytokines in dominant-negative TGF-beta receptor type II mouse. J Autoimmun 2013;41:111–9.

70. Katsumi T, Ninomiya M, Nishina T, et al. MiR-139-5p is associated with inflammatory regulation through c-FOS suppression, and contributes to the progression of primary biliary cholangitis. Lab Invest 2016;96(11):1165–77.

71. Chang JC, Go S, Verhoeven AJ, et al. Role of the bicarbonate-responsive soluble adenylyl cyclase in cholangiocyte apoptosis in primary biliary cholangitis; a new hypothesis. Biochim Biophys Acta 2018;1864(4 Pt B):1232–9.

72. Ghonem NS, Ananthanarayanan M, Soroka CJ, et al. Peroxisome proliferator-activated receptor alpha activates human multidrug resistance transporter 3/ATP-binding cassette protein subfamily B4 transcription and increases rat biliary phosphatidylcholine secretion. Hepatology 2014;59(3):1030–42.

73. Beuers U, Trauner M, Jansen P, et al. New paradigms in the treatment of hepatic cholestasis: from UDCA to FXR, PXR and beyond. J Hepatol 2015;62(1 Suppl):S25–37.

74. Trauner M, Fuchs CD, Halilbasic E, et al. New therapeutic concepts in bile acid transport and signaling for management of cholestasis. Hepatology 2017;65(4):1393–404.

75. Schaap FG, van der Gaag NA, Gouma DJ, et al. High expression of the bile salt-homeostatic hormone fibroblast growth factor 19 in the liver of patients with extrahepatic cholestasis. Hepatology 2009;49(4):1228–35.

76. Wunsch E, Milkiewicz M, Wasik U, et al. Expression of hepatic fibroblast growth factor 19 is enhanced in primary biliary cirrhosis and correlates with severity of the disease. Sci Rep 2015;5:13462.

77. Cheng L, Tian F, Tian F, et al. Repression of Farnesoid X receptor contributes to biliary injuries of liver grafts through disturbing cholangiocyte bile acid transport. Am J Transplant 2013;13(12):3094–102.

78. Zippin JH, Chen Y, Straub SG, et al. $CO2/HCO_3^-$- and calcium-regulated soluble adenylyl cyclase as a physiological ATP sensor. J Biol Chem 2013;288(46):33283–91.

79. Adorini L, Penna G. Control of autoimmune diseases by the vitamin D endocrine system. Nat Clin Pract Rheumatol 2008;4(8):404–12.

80. D'Aldebert E, Biyeyeme Bi Mve MJ, Mergey M, et al. Bile salts control the anti-microbial peptide cathelicidin through nuclear receptors in the human biliary epithelium. Gastroenterology 2009;136(4):1435–43.

81. Han SI, Li Q, Ellis E, et al. A novel bile acid-activated vitamin D receptor signaling in human hepatocytes. Mol Endocrinol 2010;24(6):1151–64.

82. Ueno Y, Ishii M, Takahashi S, et al. Different susceptibility of mice to immune-mediated cholangitis induced by immunization with carbonic anhydrase II. Lab Invest 1998;78(5):629–37.

83. Dranoff JA, Masyuk AI, Kruglov EA, et al. Polarized expression and function of P2Y ATP receptors in rat bile duct epithelia. Am J Physiol Gastrointest Liver Physiol 2001;281(4):G1059–67.

84. Sato K, Meng F, Giang T, et al. Mechanisms of cholangiocyte responses to injury. Biochim Biophys Acta 2018;1864(4 Pt B):1262–9.

85. McGill JM, Basavappa S, Gettys TW, et al. Secretin activates Cl- channels in bile duct epithelial cells through a cAMP-dependent mechanism. Am J Physiol 1994;266(4 Pt 1):G731–6.

86. Alvaro D, Alpini G, Jezequel AM, et al. Role and mechanisms of action of acetyl-choline in the regulation of rat cholangiocyte secretory functions. J Clin Invest 1997;100(6):1349–62.

87. Durchschein F, Krones E, Pollheimer MJ, et al. Genetic loss of the muscarinic M3 receptor markedly alters bile formation and cholestatic liver injury in mice. Hepatol Res 2018;48(3):E68–77.

88. Buis CI, Geuken E, Visser DS, et al. Altered bile composition after liver transplantation is associated with the development of nonanastomotic biliary strictures. J Hepatol 2009;50(1):69–79.

89. LeSagE G, Alvaro D, Benedetti A, et al. Cholinergic system modulates growth, apoptosis, and secretion of cholangiocytes from bile duct-ligated rats. Gastroenterology 1999;117(1):191–9.

90. Glaser S, Alvaro D, Francis H, et al. Adrenergic receptor agonists prevent bile duct injury induced by adrenergic denervation by increased cAMP levels and activation of Akt. Am J Physiol Gastrointest Liver Physiol 2006;290(4): G813–26.

91. Berg CP, Blume K, Lauber K, et al. Autoantibodies to muscarinic acetylcholine receptors found in patients with primary biliary cirrhosis. BMC Gastroenterol 2010;10:120.

92. European Association for the Study of the Liver. EASL clinical practice guidelines: management of cholestatic liver diseases. J Hepatol 2009;51(2): 237–67.

93. Beuers U. Drug insight: mechanisms and sites of action of ursodeoxycholic acid in cholestasis. Nat Clin Pract Gastroenterol Hepatol 2006;3(6):318–28.

94. Haussinger D, Kurz AK, Wettstein M, et al. Involvement of integrins and Src in tauroursodeoxycholate-induced and swelling-induced choleresis. Gastroenterology 2003;124(5):1476–87.

95. Nathanson MH, Burgstahler AD, Masyuk A, et al. Stimulation of ATP secretion in the liver by therapeutic bile acids. Biochem J 2001;358(Pt 1):1–5.

96. Rodriguez-Ortigosa CM, Banales JM, Olivas I, et al. Biliary secretion of S-nitrosoglutathione is involved in the hypercholeresis induced by ursodeoxycholic acid in the normal rat. Hepatology 2010;52(2):667–77.

97. Fickert P, Wagner M, Marschall HU, et al. 24-norUrsodeoxycholic acid is superior to ursodeoxycholic acid in the treatment of sclerosing cholangitis in Mdr2 (Abcb4) knockout mice. Gastroenterology 2006;130(2):465–81.

98. Fickert P, Hirschfield GM, Denk G, et al. norUrsodeoxycholic acid improves cholestasis in primary sclerosing cholangitis. J Hepatol 2017;67(3):549–58.

99. Hofmann AF, Zakko SF, Lira M, et al. Novel biotransformation and physiological properties of norursodeoxycholic acid in humans. Hepatology 2005;42(6): 1391–8.

100. Yoon YB, Hagey LR, Hofmann AF, et al. Effect of side-chain shortening on the physiologic properties of bile acids: hepatic transport and effect on biliary secretion of 23-nor-ursodeoxycholate in rodents. Gastroenterology 1986;90(4): 837–52.

101. Leuschner M, Maier KP, Schlichting J, et al. Oral budesonide and ursodeoxycholic acid for treatment of primary biliary cirrhosis: results of a prospective double-blind trial. Gastroenterology 1999;117(4):918–25.

102. Rautiainen H, Karkkainen P, Karvonen AL, et al. Budesonide combined with UDCA to improve liver histology in primary biliary cirrhosis: a three-year randomized trial. Hepatology 2005;41(4):747–52.

103. Alvaro D, Gigliozzi A, Marucci L, et al. Corticosteroids modulate the secretory processes of the rat intrahepatic biliary epithelium. Gastroenterology 2002; 122(4):1058–69.

104. Arenas F, Hervias I, Uriz M, et al. Combination of ursodeoxycholic acid and glucocorticoids upregulates the AE2 alternate promoter in human liver cells. J Clin Invest 2008;118(2):695–709.

105. Nevens F, Andreone P, Mazzella G, et al. A placebo-controlled trial of obeticholic acid in primary biliary cholangitis. N Engl J Med 2016;375(7):631–43.

106. Honda A, Ikegami T, Nakamuta M, et al. Anticholestatic effects of bezafibrate in patients with primary biliary cirrhosis treated with ursodeoxycholic acid. Hepatology 2013;57(5):1931–41.
107. Ghonem NS, Boyer JL. Fibrates as adjuvant therapy for chronic cholestatic liver disease: its time has come. Hepatology 2013;57(5):1691–3.

Current Treatment Options for Primary Biliary Cholangitis

Kimberly A. Wong, MD[a], Runalia Bahar, MD[a], Chung H. Liu, BS[b], Christopher L. Bowlus, MD[b],*

KEYWORDS

- Autoimmune liver disease • Therapy • Bile acids • Farnesoid X receptor

KEY POINTS

- Forty percent of patients with primary biliary cholangitis do not have an adequate response to first-line treatment with ursodeoxycholic acid and remain at risk for progression.
- The farnesoid X receptor agonist obeticholic acid added to ursodeoxycholic acid can improve serum alkaline phosphatase, a strong surrogate marker of clinical outcomes.
- The peroxisome proliferator activated receptor agonists fenofibrate and bezafibrate have potential benefit for patients with an incomplete response to ursodeoxycholic acid but further study is needed to demonstrate safety.
- New farnesoid X receptor agonists, fibroblast growth factor 19 analogues, and peroxisome proliferator activated receptor agonists are in development and may offer additional second-line agents.

INTRODUCTION

Primary biliary cholangitis (PBC), previously known as primary biliary *cirrhosis*, is a progressive, rare autoimmune inflammatory disease of the interlobular bile ducts, leading to cholestasis and secondary damage of hepatocytes that may ultimately progress to cirrhosis and liver failure.[1] A prototypical autoimmune disease, PBC affects predominantly middle-aged women in whom loss of tolerance to specific

Disclosure Statement: Dr C.L. Bowlus discloses grant funding from Intercept Pharmaceuticals, Bristol-Myers Squibb, Cymabay, Gilead Biosciences, GlaxoSmithKline, Shire Pharmaceuticals, Takeda Pharmaceuticals, NGM Biosciences, and TARGET Pharmasolutions; and service on advisory boards for Intercept Pharmaceuticals, Bristol Myers Squibb, GlaxoSmithKline, and Conatus; and speakers' bureau for Intercept Pharmaceuticals. Drs K.A. Wong, R. Bahar and C.H. Liu have nothing to disclose.
[a] Department of Internal Medicine, UC Davis School of Medicine, 4150 V Street, PSSB 3000, Sacramento, CA 95817, USA; [b] Division of Gastroenterology and Hepatology, UC Davis School of Medicine, 4150 V Street, PSSB 3500, Sacramento, CA 95817, USA
* Corresponding author. Division of Gastroenterology and Hepatology, UC Davis School of Medicine, 4150 V Street, PSSB 3500, Sacramento, CA 95817.
E-mail address: clbowlus@ucdavis.edu

Clin Liver Dis 22 (2018) 481–500
https://doi.org/10.1016/j.cld.2018.03.003
1089-3261/18/© 2018 Elsevier Inc. All rights reserved.

epitopes on mitochondrial antigens leads to the development of antimitochondrial antibodies (AMA) and immunologic destruction of the biliary epithelial cells of small size bile ducts. However, immune-based therapies have failed to show effectiveness in PBC to date and current treatments are based on bile acid physiology, both first-line treatment with ursodeoxycholic acid (UDCA) and second-line treatment with obeticholic acid (OCA).

PBC is typically suspected when liver tests are abnormal and the diagnosis can be made when at least 2 of 3 criteria are met, including[2,3] persistent elevation of alkaline phosphatase for more than 6 months with normal imaging of the biliary tract; serologic reactivity to AMA or PBC-specific antinuclear antibodies, such as anti-Sp100, anti-Gp 210; and/or histologic features of nonsuppurative obstructive cholangitis, also known as florid duct lesions, involving the interlobular bile ducts. Approximately 5% to 10% of patients with PBC will not have AMA, so-called AMA-negative PBC, and require liver biopsy for diagnosis, but compared with individuals with AMA reactivity, the clinical features and disease progression are similar.[4,5] Another 8% to 10% of patients with PBC may have features of autoimmune hepatitis (AIH) as well, the so-called PBC/AIH overlap syndrome.[6,7] The diagnosis of PBC/AIH overlap is controversial, but the Paris criteria are the most widely accepted and require a diagnosis of PBC plus an at least 2 of the following to be met: alanine aminotransferase (ALT) or more than 5 times the upper limit of normal (ULN); immunoglobulin G of more than 2 times the ULN or anti–smooth muscle antibodies of more than 1:80; and histologic evidence of periportal or periseptal lymphocytic piecemeal necrosis.[6] Presentation with fibrosis seems to be more common among patients with PBC/AIH overlap and the rates of progression to liver failure, complications of portal hypertension, and death have been reported to be higher in PBC/AIH overlap compared with PBC without AIH.[8]

In the absence of treatment, PBC is a slowly progressive disease with the majority of patients advancing 1 histologic stage every 2 years[9] and median survival of symptomatic and asymptomatic patients of 7.5 years and 16 years, respectively.[10] Notably, most asymptomatic patients develop symptoms over the course of 4.5 to 17.8 years[10–15] and survival among patients with PBC without symptoms is still worse compared with a similar control population.[16] The Mayo risk score predicts short-term survival of patients with PBC in the absence of therapeutic intervention and depends on patient age, serum bilirubin, serum albumin, prothrombin time, presence of edema, and use of diuretic therapy.[17,18] In addition to the risk of cirrhosis and its inherent complications, approximately 50% of patients with PBC suffer from symptoms of fatigue and pruritus. Thus, the optimal management of PBC should address not only the progression of liver disease, but also the symptoms (fatigue and pruritus) as well as associated conditions, such as keratoconjunctivitis sicca, xerostomia, osteoporosis, and hypothyroidism. However, for the purposes of this review, we focus on those treatment options that target the liver disease.

HISTORICAL PERSPECTIVE OF PRIMARY BILIARY CHOLANGITIS TREATMENT

Several barriers to drug development have slowed treatments for PBC. First, PBC is a rare condition, meaning that recruitment of sufficient numbers of patients to power clinical trials has been challenging. This factor has also made PBC a less attractive indication for industry, although there have been recent changes in their financial calculus, leading to a rapid growth in PBC clinical trials. Second, the slow progressive nature of PBC requires large, long-term trials to demonstrate effects on hard clinical outcomes such as liver transplantation and survival. This situation is exacerbated by the increasing identification of patients with PBC at early stages of disease who are unlikely to reach a clinical outcome within the time frame of a clinical trial. Third, as treatments are developed, the pool of patients available for clinical trials diminishes and only the most refractory cases become available for development of novel and perhaps more efficacious treatments. With these limitations in mind, the efficacy of PBC treatments has largely be based on surrogate clinical endpoints, the single exception being UDCA.

Ursodeoxycholic Acid

UDCA was the first drug approved by the US Food and Drug Administration (FDA) for use in PBC and remains the first-line therapy for all patients with PBC. UDCA protects cholangiocytes against the cytotoxicity of hydrophobic bile acids, stimulates the hepatobiliary secretion of bile acids, increases the hydrophilicity index of the circulating bile pool, and may have immunomodulatory and antiinflammatory effects.[19] Despite several Cochrane reviews[20] in conflict with the overwhelming evidence, UDCA at a dose of 13 to 15 mg/kg/d improves biochemical indices, delays histologic progression, and most probably improves survival without transplantation. An early prospective study of 15 patients found UDCA to improve liver tests and pruritus.[21] Since that report, there have been 16 randomized, controlled trials of UDCA involving more than 1400 patients with PBC.[20] Notably, these studies varied by UDCA dose, treatment duration, disease stage, and outcomes measured. The results of studies of adequate duration ($\geq$2 years) and with adequate doses of UDCA (13–15 mg/kg/d) have consistently shown biochemical and histologic benefits of UDCA (**Table 1**). The notable UDCA studies include a randomized, placebo-controlled trial of 146 patients treated for 2 years in which UDCA was effective in reducing treatment failure defined as a doubling in bilirubin or development of severe complications as well as improving bilirubin, Mayo risk score, and mean histologic score.[22] In addition, during a 2-year open-label phase after the placebo-controlled trial, the previously placebo-treated patients had significantly worse transplant-free survival compared with the UDCA-treated patients with PBC.[23] These results were further corroborated by randomized, placebo-controlled trials of 222 patients and 192 patients treated for 2 years, both of which demonstrated that patients treated with UDCA had positive effects on serum bilirubin and other liver biochemistries; however, the studies were not adequately powered to determine a difference in liver transplantation or death.[24,25] Similarly, Combes and colleagues[26] found UDCA even at 11 mg/kg/d for 2 years delayed histologic progression of disease, but only among those with an entry bilirubin of less than 2 mg/dL. The longest randomized, placebo-controlled trial included 180 patients treated for 4 years in which UDCA treatment was associated with a delayed time to treatment failure defined as death; liver transplantation; histologic progression by 2 stages or to cirrhosis; development of varices, ascites, or encephalopathy; doubling of bilirubin; marked worsening of fatigue or pruritus; inability to tolerate the drug; or voluntary withdrawal for any reason.[27]

Combined data from these clinical trials have demonstrated that patients treated with UDCA had delayed histologic progression of disease when UDCA was initiated at early stages of disease[28] and improved transplant-free survival in those treated with UDCA at late stages of disease.[28] Further, Corpechot and colleagues[29] used a Markov model of clinical trial data to demonstrate that UDCA therapy was associated with a 5-fold lower rate of histologic progression from early stage disease to extensive fibrosis or cirrhosis.

Overall, the safety of UDCA has been established in these trials as well as several other trials investigating other indications.[20,30] No significant differences in serious

Table 1
Studies of UDCA in primary biliary cholangitis

Author	Study Design	Inclusion Criteria	Duration	No. of Patients	UDCA Dose	Main Result
Improved clinical parameters						
Poupon et al,[21] 1987	Prospective trial	Patients with PBC	2 y	15	13–15 mg/kg/d	Improvement in GGT, AP, ALT, bilirubin, decreased pruritus
Poupon et al,[22] 1991	Double-blind, randomized, placebo-controlled trial	Biopsy-proven PBC	2 y	146	13–15 mg/kg/d	Improvement in bilirubin, AP, ALT, AST, GGT, cholesterol, IgM, antimitochondrial-antibody titer; improvement in Mayo risk score; improvement in mean histologic score
Lindor et al,[27] 1994	Double-blind, placebo-controlled trial	Patients with PBC	2 y	180	13–15 mg/kg/d	Delayed time to treatment failure[a]
Improved histology						
Poupon et al,[28] 2003	Combined data from 4 trials	Patients with PBC with liver biopsy specimens	Variable	367	Variable	Decreased periportal necroinflammation, improved ductal proliferation, delayed histologic progression when initiated at earlier stages
Corpechot et al,[29] 2000	Randomized, double-blind, placebo-controlled trial	Patients with PBC	4 y	103	13–5 mg/kg/d	5-Fold lower progression rate from early stage disease
Angulo et al,[31] 1999	Study of patients enrolled in prior placebo-controlled trials	Patients with PBC with liver biopsy specimens	5–9 y	67	13–15 mg/kg/d	Decreased rate of progression to cirrhosis
Combes et al,[26] 1995	Randomized, placebo-controlled trial	PBC ≥6 mo duration, liver biopsy	2 y	151	10–12 mg/kg/d	Decreased bilirubin, improved histology, decreased complications and liver transplantation or death

Study	Study design	Patient population	Duration	No. of Patients	Dose	Outcomes
Heathcote et al,[24] 1994	Randomized, placebo-controlled trial	Patients with PBC confirmed by liver biopsy and antimitochondrial antibody positive	2 y	222	14 mg/kg/d	Decreased bilirubin, AP, AST, ALT, cholesterol, IgM, improved histologic features, however no difference in liver transplantation or death
Pares et al,[25] 2000	Randomized, double-blind, placebo-controlled trial	Patients with PBC, biopsy proven	2 y	192	14–16 mg/kg/d	Improved histology, however no change in time to death or liver transplantation
Improved transplant-free survival						
Poupon et al,[23] 1994	Randomized placebo-controlled trial	Biopsy-proven PBC	4 y[b]	145	13–15 mg/kg/d	Decreased disease progression and death, reduced need for transplantation
Poupon et al,[111] 1997	Combined data from 3 trials	Biopsy-proven PCB, elevated AP, positive antimitochondrial antibodies	2–4 y	548	Variable	Improved survival free of liver transplantation in moderate to severe disease

Abbreviations: ALT, alanine aminotransferase; AP, alkaline phosphatase; AST, aspartate aminotransferase; GGT, gamma-glutamyl transferase; IgM, immunoglobulin M; PBC, primary biliary cholangitis; UDCA, ursodeoxycholic acid.

[a] Treatment failure: death, liver transplantation, histologic progression by 2 stages or to cirrhosis, development of varices, ascites, or encephalopathy, doubling of bilirubin, marked worsening of fatigue or pruritus, inability to tolerate the drug, voluntary withdrawal for any reason.

[b] Initially a 2-y study; however, owing to the benefit of UDCA, all patients received UDCA in an open trial and were monitored for 2 more years.

adverse events have been identified in any clinical trials. Diarrhea was the most common adverse event in trials of UDCA for gallstones, occurring in 2% to 9% of patients, but has not been seen in trials of PBC. Abdominal pain, nausea, and vomiting have been reported but in less than 5% of patients with PBC. Initiating UDCA at lower doses and titrating may decrease the risk of these symptoms.

In summary, data from clinical trials in which UDCA is given at adequate doses for at least 2 years have found biochemical and histologic benefits, but improvements in clinical outcomes, particularly transplant-free survival, require trials of at least 4 years' duration. This finding is not surprising, given that while the disease progresses even to cirrhosis, the time to liver decompensation and liver-related death may be years. In addition, the timing of liver transplantation is confounded by factors that vary with era and geography. Further, those patients with early disease may be more likely to respond to treatment, but are unlikely to have a clinical event even if untreated over several years of observation.

SECOND-LINE THERAPIES

After the introduction of UDCA, long-term observation of patients with PBC treated with UDCA demonstrated a lower rate of progression to cirrhosis[31] and there was a decrease in the number and percentage of liver transplants performed for PBC despite a trend toward increasing incidence.[32–34] However, there remained a group of patients with PBC who continued to progress despite UDCA treatment. Although the Mayo risk score was found to still have usefulness in predicting survival for those receiving UDCA,[35] several long-term observational cohorts of UDCA-treated patients with PBC were used to develop new models to predict long-term transplant-free survival. These criteria, including the Rotterdam criteria, Barcelona criteria, Paris I and Paris II criteria, or Toronto criteria, introduced the concept of a biochemical response to UDCA and demonstrated that patients who met these response criteria had a better clinical outcome and in many cases a transplant-free survival that was not significantly different from a matched control population.[2,36] More recently, continuous models such as the UK-PBC and GLOBE scores, have demonstrated excellent specificity and sensitivity for predicting transplant-free survival up to 10 to 15 years.[37,38] In addition, these scores quantify the relative risk of clinical outcomes rather than the qualitative biochemical response criteria. These models all assess prognosis based on either changes in or absolute levels of blood tests after 1-year of UDCA treatment. Although there are several minor differences in the calculations and variables included in the models, all of the models have found that the primary drivers of transplant-free survival are serum bilirubin and serum alkaline phosphatase.

Although nearly all patients with PBC will have some biochemical response with improvement in the serum alkaline phosphatase, 30% to 40% will have an inadequate biochemical response to UDCA and remain at risk of disease progression. This risk correlates with increasing serum alkaline phosphatase of more than 2 times the ULN and bilirubin even when it is below the ULN.[39] Patients with PBC who have an inadequate response to UDCA or those few who are intolerant to UDCA should be candidates for second-line therapies (**Fig. 1**).

Obeticholic Acid

OCA is conditionally approved by the FDA for patients with an inadequate response to UDCA or for patients unable to tolerate UDCA. OCA is a derivative of chenodeoxycholic acid, the natural occurring ligand of the farnesoid X receptor (FXR), which mediates the synthesis and enterohepatic circulation of bile acids. OCA is 100 times more

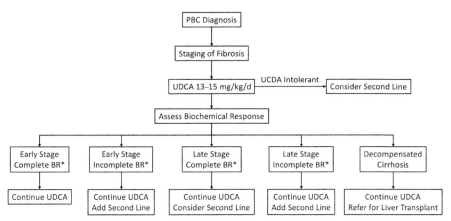

Fig. 1. Treatment algorithm for primary biliary cholangitis (PBC). After the diagnosis of PBC, staging of fibrosis can be achieved by liver biopsy or noninvasive methods such as vibration controlled transient elastography. First-line treatment with ursodeoxycholic acid (UDCA) should be given to all patients with PBC. *After 12 months, biochemical response (BR) should be assessed by the GLOBE score or other criteria. Second-line therapy should be considered according to the biochemical response and the stage of fibrosis. Obeticholic acid should be considered unless there is severe pruritus or other contraindication to its use. A fibrate may be an acceptable alternative second line agent, but it not currently approved by the US Food and Drug Administration for this indication.

potent as an FXR ligand compared with chenodeoxycholic acid. In the liver, FXR activation decreases the conversion of cholesterol to bile acids and increases the transport of bile acids out of hepatocytes. Activation of FXR in the ileum decreases bile acid reabsorption and increases expression of fibroblast growth factor 19, which acts in the liver to further decrease bile acid synthesis. OCA may also have antifibrotic properties and may improve portal hypertension.[40–42]

The initial phase II studies of OCA evaluated its use as monotherapy in patients with PBC and as add-on therapy to UDCA in patients with PBC with an inadequate response to UDCA (**Table 2**). In an international double-blind, placebo-controlled trial, placebo was compared with OCA at 10 and 50 mg/d for 3 months in 53 patients with PBC with persistently increased alkaline phosphatase levels who had not been taking UDCA for at least 6 months.[43] The groups that received OCA at 10 or 50 mg/d had a significant decrease from baseline in alkaline phosphatase (−53.9%; 95% confidence interval [CI], −62.6 to −29.3 and −37.2%, 95% CI, −54.8 to 24.6, respectively) compared with placebo (−0.8%; 95% CI, −6.4 to 8.7). Pruritus was the most common adverse event leading to discontinuation of 15% and 38% of patients receiving 10 and 50 mg OCA, respectively.

In the second phase II trial of OCA in PBC, 165 patients with PBC with a serum alkaline phosphatase 1.5 to 10.0 times the ULN despite UDCA treatment were randomized to 10, 25, or 50 mg OCA or placebo while continuing UDCA.[44] All OCA-treated groups had significantly greater reductions from baseline in serum alkaline phosphatase compared with placebo with the mean relative decrease of 24% (95% CI, −30% to −18%), 25% (95% CI, −30% to −20%), and 21% (95% CI, −30% to −12%) for the 10, 25, and 50 mg OCA groups, respectively, compared with 3% (95% CI, −7% to 2%) in the placebo group. Groups that received OCA also had significant improvements in γ-glutamyl transferase and ALT, but only 7% of OCA-treated patients completely normalized their alkaline phosphatase. Pruritus was again the only adverse

Table 2
Studies of OCA in primary biliary cholangitis

Author	Study Design	Inclusion Criteria	Duration	Number of Patients	OCA Dose	Use of UDCA	Main Result
Kowdley et al,[43] 2017	Randomized, double-blind, placebo-controlled phase II study	Patients with PBC with AP 1.5–10× ULN, off UDCA >3 mo	3 mo	60	10, 50 mg/d	No	Decrease in AP, ALT, bilirubin, IgM, dose-dependent increase in pruritus
Hirschfield et al,[44] 2015	Randomized, double-blind, placebo-controlled trial	AP 1.5–10× ULN	3 mo	165	10, 25, 50 mg/d	Yes	Decrease in AP, GGT, ALT
Hirschfield et al,[44] 2015	Open label	Long-term safety extension	Study stopped after all patients had ≥23 mo in LTSE	78	10–50 mg/d	Yes	Further decrease in AP in 10, 25 mg group; worsened pruritus after titration to 25 mg
Nevens et al,[45] 2016	Randomized, double-blind, placebo-controlled trial	AP 1.5–10.0× ULN	12 mo	216	5, 10 mg/d	Yes	AP of <1.67 ULN with a reduction of ≥15% from baseline, normal total bilirubin

Abbreviations: ALT, alanine aminotransferase; AP, alkaline phosphatase; GGT, gamma-glutyl transferase; IgM, immunoglobulin M; LTSE, long term safety extension; OCA, obeticholic acid; PBC, primary biliary cholangitis; UDCA, ursodeoxycholic acid; ULN, upper limit of normal.

event more frequent in the OCA group compared with the placebo group and was seen in terms of both frequency and severity of pruritus. In addition, there was a dose–response effect with the greatest frequency and severity seen in the 50 mg OCA group. Seventy-eight patients continued in a 12-month open-label extension with 61 patients completing the study, at which time the mean final daily dose was 20 mg.

The pivotal phase III study evaluated the effects of 12 month treatment of OCA in patients with PBC with an inadequate response to UDCA, defined by a serum alkaline phosphatase of 1.67 times the ULN or a bilirubin greater than 1 times the ULN but less than 2 times the ULN, or intolerant of UDCA.[45] Patients were randomized in a double-blind fashion (1:1:1) to receive placebo daily, OCA 10 mg/d, or OCA 5 mg/d with a titration to 10 mg after 6 months based on response and tolerability. The primary endpoint measured after 12 months of treatment was the combination of a serum alkaline phosphatase of less than 1.67 times ULN with a reduction of at least 15% from baseline and a normal total bilirubin. More than 90% of the 216 patients with PBC received UDCA as background therapy. The primary endpoint was met by 47% and 46% of patients in the 10 mg and 5 to 10 mg OCA groups, respectively, compared with 10% in the placebo group ($P<.001$). In addition, significant decreases in alkaline phosphatase and total bilirubin occurred in the OCA-treated groups compared with the placebo group. There was no change in noninvasive measures of fibrosis. Pruritus was more common in the OCA group and was reported in 68% and 56% of patients in the 10 mg and 5 to 10 mg OCA-treatment arms, respectively, compared with 38% in the placebo arm. In addition, the severity of pruritus in the 10 mg treated patients was reported to be more severe compared with placebo up to 6 months of treatment, but then were not significantly different at 12 months. Discontinuation owing to pruritus occurred in 10% of the 10 mg OCA-treated patients compared with 1% in the 5 to 10 mg OCA group and none in the placebo group. After the initial 12 months of the trial, patients were given the option to continue in an open-label long-term extension starting at 5 mg OCA and increasing to 10 mg OCA as tolerated. The majority of patients (91%) entered the extension phase and results to date support ongoing efficacy of OCA through 2 years.

The results of these studies led to the conditional approval of OCA for patients with PBC with an inadequate response to UDCA or who are intolerant to UDCA with an initial starting dose of 5 mg and increasing to 10 mg after 3 months based on tolerability. The definition of inadequate response is left open to clinical judgment.

Notably, the FDA-approved prescribing guidance advised that patients with Child-Pugh B and C cirrhosis should initiate dosing of OCA at 5 mg once weekly, which can be increased to the maximum approved dose of OCA 10 mg twice weekly. This dosing was based on modeling of the pharmacokinetic of OCA and not on any experimental evidence in patients with PBC with advanced cirrhosis. Importantly, a recent FDA safety announcement was made related to 19 patients with PBC with Child-Pugh B or C cirrhosis who had received an incorrect dose of OCA and subsequently developed severe liver injury and/or death.

In summary, data on OCA clearly demonstrate its ability to improve liver biochemistries, including total bilirubin which are associated with improved clinical outcomes, but long-term, randomized trials are needed to confirm that this translates into clinically meaningful endpoints such as transplant-free and overall survival. Given the limited options for patients with PBC with an incomplete response to UDCA, OCA should be considered, particularly in those without significant pruritus.

Fibrates

Fibrates have anticholestatic effects mediated through the peroxisome proliferator-activated receptor alpha-UDP-glucuronosyltransferases signaling axis. Thus, fibrates have been extensively studied as therapeutic agents because of their potential ability to decrease bile acid synthesis and bile acid-related hepatic inflammation.[46,47] Numerous small pilot studies and case reports have shown that fibrates, including fenofibrate in the United States and bezafibrate in Europe and Japan, improve liver biochemistries, liver stiffness measurements, and pruritus in patients with PBC (**Table 3**).[48–72] Metaanalyses have demonstrated that fibrates improve liver biochemistries without an increase in adverse effects.[73,74] These data have been further supported by a recently completed phase III randomized, placebo-controlled trial (BEZURSO). Patients with an inadequate response to UDCA by Paris-2 criteria were treated with bezafibrate 400 mg/d or placebo for 2 years. The primary endpoint was normal total bilirubin, alkaline phosphatase, AST, ALT, albumin, and prothrombin time at 2 years. The primary endpoint was reached more frequently in the bezafibrate group than in the placebo group (30% vs 0%, respectively).[72] Notably, there were significant beneficial relative changes from baseline to 2 years in serum alkaline phosphatase, ALT, total bilirubin, and albumin. Although these studies have shown a clinical benefit of fibrate therapy in PBC, a recent Cochrane review did not find evidence for an effect of bezafibrate (either alone or in combination with UDCA) on mortality, liver-related morbidity, or adverse events.[75] It is also important to note that prior studies have noted serious side effects with fibrate therapy, including hepatotoxicity and elevated creatinine and creatinine kinase.[44,76] Laboratory parameters must be closely monitored and dosing adjustment must be made while patients are on fibrate therapy. Further studies are needed to determine if these biochemical improvements translate to significant decreases in liver-related death or need for liver transplantation.[77]

IMMUNOSUPPRESSANT AGENTS

Despite the vast literature supporting the concept of PBC as an autoimmune disease, immunosuppressive agents have failed to find a role in the treatment of PBC, except in cases of PBC/AIH overlap in which AIH component is treated the same as AIH without PBC. The reason for this lack of efficacy is unclear, but may be due to the predominance of bile acid-mediated injury once bile duct injury occurs or ongoing immune activation by the environmental or autoantigen that is, resistant to immunosuppressants studied to date.

Corticosteroids, including budesonide and prednisone, have been trialed in patients who do not sufficiently improve on UDCA monotherapy.[78] Two prospective randomized controlled studies have shown budesonide to be associated with improvements in liver chemistries and liver histology,[79,80] although a third open-label study found a nonstatistically significant worsening of the Mayo score in patients receiving budesonide.[81] Adverse effects, including adrenal insufficiency and decreased bone mineral density,[81] are of concern and, thus, budesonide is not recommended for the treatment of PBC. Despite promising results of open-label studies of methotrexate on liver chemistries and liver histology,[82–84] a large randomized, double-blind, placebo-controlled trial of 265 patients over a median of 7.6 years comparing methotrexate and UDCA with placebo and UDCA was terminated early owing to futility.[85] Other immunosuppressants including mycophenolate mofetil,[86,87] azathioprine,[88–90] and the B-cell–depleting monoclonal antibody rituximab[91,92] have failed to demonstrate efficacy in patients with PBC.

Table 3
Studies of fibrates in a minimum of 20 patients with primary biliary cholangitis

Author	Study Design	Inclusion Criteria	Duration	No. of Patients	Fenofibrate/ Bezafibrate Dose	Main Result
Han et al,[50] 2012	Prospective case series	Patients with PBC treated with UDCA for ≥1 y	3–6 mo	22	Fenofibrate 200 mg/d	Decrease/normalization AP; Decrease AST, ALT, GGT, cholesterol, TG
Levy et al,[52] 2011	Pilot study	Patients with PBC with AP >2× ULN	12 mo	20	Fenofibrate 160 mg/d	Decrease AP, AST, IgM, IL-1, IL-2, increase ApoAII, ApoCII
Lens et al,[48] 2014	Prospective case series	Patients with PBC treated with UDCA and abnormal AP	12 mo	30	Bezafibrate 400 mg/d	Decrease/normalization AP; Decrease ALT, GGT, cholesterol, TG, pruritus, liver stiffness unchanged
Iwasaki et al,[56] 2008	Two prospective randomized-controlled trials	Noncirrhotic patients with PBC	52 wk	Study 1: 45 Study 2: 21	Bezafibrate 400 mg/d	Study 1: bezafibrate monotherapy as effective as UDCA; Study 2: bezafibrate + UDCA improved biochemical markers in patients with incomplete response to UDCA
Kita et al,[57] 2006	Prospective case series	Patients with PBC	6 mo	22	Bezafibrate 400 mg/d	Decrease AP, GGT, IgM
Kanda et al,[63] 2006	Randomized trial	Patients with PBC with elevated AP while on UDCA	6 mo	11 UDCA + bezafibrate, 11 UDCA	Bezafibrate 400 mg/d	Decrease AP, GGT
Kurihara et al,[68] 2000	Randomized trial	Biopsy-proven PBC	12 mo	12 bezafibrate, 12 UDCA	Bezafibrate 400 mg/d	Decrease AP, GGT, IgM, bezafibrate more effective than UDCA

(continued on next page)

Table 3
(continued)

Author	Study Design	Inclusion Criteria	Duration	No. of Patients	Fenofibrate/ Bezafibrate Dose	Main Result
Nakai et al,[69] 2000	Randomized trial	Patients with PBC with prior UDCA treatment	12 mo	10 UDCA + bezafibrate, 13 UDCA	Bezafibrate 400 mg/d	Decrease AP, GGT, IgM
Corpechot et al,[72] 2017	Randomized, placebo-controlled trial	Patients with PBC with inadequate response to UDCA by Paris-2 criteria	24 mo	100	Bezafibrate 400 mg/d	Normalization of bilirubin, AP, AST, ALT, albumin, PT
Reig et al,[71] 2017	Prospective study	Patients with PBC treated with UDCA with AP >1.5× ULN	38 mo	48	Bezafibrate 400 mg/d	54% of patients with normalized AP, improvement in jaundice, pruritus, liver stiffness; all but 1 case reported improvement in pruritus

Abbreviations: ALT, alanine aminotransferase; AP, alkaline phosphatase; GGT, gamma-glutamyl transferase; IgM, immunoglobulin M; IL, interleukin; PBC, primary biliary cholangitis; PT, prothrombin time; TG, triglycerides; UDCA, ursodeoxycholic acid; ULN, upper limit of normal.

TREATMENT OF ASSOCIATED CONDITIONS
Hyperlipidemia

Hypercholesterolemia is found in 75% to 95% of patients with PBC, although the clinical significance of this finding is uncertain.[93] Statin therapy is recommended for patients with PBC with hyperlipidemia and known risk factors for atherosclerotic disease. Several studies have demonstrated the safety and efficacy of statin therapy in PBC.[94–98] Statins have also been studied as potential therapeutic targets in PBC. The expression of MHC-II antigens on biliary epithelial cells leads to the activation of CD4 T-lymphocytes and destruction of intrahepatic bile ducts.[99,100] Statins, which are 3-hydroxy-3-methyl-glutaryl-coenzyme A reductase inhibitors, reduce MHC-II expression on biliary epithelial cells.[101] Small case series noted decreased alkaline phosphatase, and biochemical and histopathologic improvements in patients with PBC treated with statins.[96,102,103] However, subsequent studies failed to demonstrate a clinical benefit of statin therapy in PBC. A retrospective cohort study found no changes in alkaline phosphatase or Mayo risk score after treatment with atorvastatin, despite a significant decrease in total cholesterol and low-density lipoprotein cholesterol.[94] Another prospective cohort study did not find any improvement in alkaline phosphatase in patients with PBC that were treated with atorvastatin.[104]

Bone Disease

The population of patients with PBC have many risk factors for bone disease in addition to cholestasis, which can further increase this risk. Overall, osteoporosis is seen in 20% to 44% of patients with PBC, and the incidence increases with the progression of liver disease.[105] The development of osteoporosis in PBC has been thought to be associated with decreased bone formation and increased bone resorption in the setting of cholestasis and cirrhosis.[106] Malnutrition and vitamin deficiencies, particularly vitamins D and K, also contribute to the development of osteoporosis in PBC.[107] The diagnosis of osteoporosis is made with a dual energy x-ray absorptiometry scan of the lumbar spine and femur. Initiation of therapy should be evaluated on a case-by-case basis. Factors that may affect the decision to start treatment include the duration and severity of liver disease, severity of cholestasis, qualification for liver transplantation, or the occurrence of a fragility fracture. When the decision to start therapy is based on dual energy x-ray absorptiometry imaging, therapy should be initiated at an earlier stage when bone mineral density is between 1.0 and 2.5 standard deviations below the norm. Therapy should start with supplementation to achieve 1000 to 1500 mg of elemental calcium per day and vitamin D intake of 400 to 800 IU/d. Although data are currently limited, studies to date have shown that bisphosphonate therapy in PBC results in improved bone density, with minimal side effects.[108–110]

SUMMARY

All patients with PBC should be treated with UDCA at 13 to 15 mg/kg/d and monitored for a biochemical response using any of the available criteria. If there is an incomplete response to UDCA, then second-line therapies should be considered, namely OCA. If OCA is not tolerated or otherwise contraindicated, growing evidence supports the use of a fibrate, but their safety has not been firmly established and caution should be used. For the small number of patients intolerant of UDCA, these second-line agents may also be considered. Other factors such as advanced fibrosis should also be used to determine appropriate candidates for second line treatment even if biochemical response if met. However, in patients with PBC with decompensated cirrhosis, medical treatment is unlikely to significantly impact the course of their disease and the unknown risk of second-line therapies in these patients should give caution. Instead, liver transplantation should be considered for these patients.

REFERENCES

1. Selmi C, Bowlus CL, Gershwin ME, et al. Primary biliary cirrhosis. Lancet 2011; 377(9777):1600–9.
2. European Association for the Study of the Liver. easl clinical practice guidelines: the diagnosis and management of patients with primary biliary cholangitis. J Hepatol 2017;67(1):145–72.
3. Lindor KD, Gershwin ME, Poupon R, et al. Primary biliary cirrhosis. Hepatology 2009;50(1):291–308.
4. Siddique A, Kowdley KV. Approach to a patient with elevated serum alkaline phosphatase. Clin Liver Dis 2012;16(2):199–229.
5. Carey EJ, Ali AH, Lindor KD. Primary biliary cirrhosis. Lancet 2015;386(10003): 1565–75.
6. Chazouilleres O, Wendum D, Serfaty L, et al. Primary biliary cirrhosis-autoimmune hepatitis overlap syndrome: clinical features and response to therapy. Hepatology 1998;28(2):296–301.
7. Heurgue A, Vitry F, Diebold MD, et al. Overlap syndrome of primary biliary cirrhosis and autoimmune hepatitis: a retrospective study of 115 cases of autoimmune liver disease. Gastroenterol Clin Biol 2007;31(1):17–25.
8. Silveira MG, Talwalkar JA, Angulo P, et al. Overlap of autoimmune hepatitis and primary biliary cirrhosis: long-term outcomes. Am J Gastroenterol 2007;102(6): 1244–50.
9. Locke GR 3rd, Therneau TM, Ludwig J, et al. Time course of histological progression in primary biliary cirrhosis. Hepatology 1996;23(1):52–6.
10. Mahl TC, Shockcor W, Boyer JL. Primary biliary cirrhosis: survival of a large cohort of symptomatic and asymptomatic patients followed for 24 years. J Hepatol 1994;20(6):707–13.
11. Long RG, Scheuer PJ, Sherlock S. Presentation and course of asymptomatic primary biliary cirrhosis. Gastroenterology 1977;72(6):1204–7.
12. Mitchison HC, Lucey MR, Kelly PJ, et al. Symptom development and prognosis in primary biliary cirrhosis: a study in two centers. Gastroenterology 1990;99(3): 778–84.
13. Nyberg A, Loof L. Primary biliary cirrhosis: clinical features and outcome, with special reference to asymptomatic disease. Scand J Gastroenterol 1989;24(1):57–64.
14. Springer J, Cauch-Dudek K, O'Rourke K, et al. Asymptomatic primary biliary cirrhosis: a study of its natural history and prognosis. Am J Gastroenterol 1999;94(1):47–53.
15. Prince M, Chetwynd A, Newman W, et al. Survival and symptom progression in a geographically based cohort of patients with primary biliary cirrhosis: follow-up for up to 28 years. Gastroenterology 2002;123(4):1044–51.
16. Balasubramaniam K, Grambsch PM, Wiesner RH, et al. Diminished survival in asymptomatic primary biliary cirrhosis. A prospective study. Gastroenterology 1990;98(6):1567–71.
17. Kim WR, Dickson ER. Predictive models of natural history in primary biliary cirrhosis. Clin Liver Dis 1998;2(2):313–31, ix.
18. Dickson ER, Grambsch PM, Fleming TR, et al. Prognosis in primary biliary cirrhosis: model for decision making. Hepatology 1989;10(1):1–7.

19. Poupon R. Ursodeoxycholic acid and bile-acid mimetics as therapeutic agents for cholestatic liver diseases: an overview of their mechanisms of action. Clin Res Hepatol Gastroenterol 2012;36(Suppl 1):S3–12.

20. Rudic JS, Poropat G, Krstic MN, et al. Ursodeoxycholic acid for primary biliary cirrhosis. Cochrane Database Syst Rev 2012;(12):CD000551.

21. Poupon R, Chretien Y, Poupon RE, et al. Is ursodeoxycholic acid an effective treatment for primary biliary cirrhosis? Lancet 1987;1(8537):834–6.

22. Poupon RE, Balkau B, Eschwege E, et al. A multicenter, controlled trial of ursodiol for the treatment of primary biliary cirrhosis. UDCA-PBC Study Group. N Engl J Med 1991;324(22):1548–54.

23. Poupon RE, Poupon R, Balkau B. Ursodiol for the long-term treatment of primary biliary cirrhosis. The UDCA-PBC Study Group. N Engl J Med 1994;330(19): 1342–7.

24. Heathcote EJ, Cauch-Dudek K, Walker V, et al. The Canadian multicenter double-blind randomized controlled trial of ursodeoxycholic acid in primary biliary cirrhosis. Hepatology 1994;19(5):1149–56.

25. Pares A, Caballeria L, Rodes J, et al. Long-term effects of ursodeoxycholic acid in primary biliary cirrhosis: results of a double-blind controlled multicentric trial. UDCA-Cooperative Group from the Spanish Association for the Study of the Liver. J Hepatol 2000;32(4):561–6.

26. Combes B, Carithers RL Jr, Maddrey WC, et al. A randomized, double-blind, placebo-controlled trial of ursodeoxycholic acid in primary biliary cirrhosis. Hepatology 1995;22(3):759–66.

27. Lindor KD, Dickson ER, Baldus WP, et al. Ursodeoxycholic acid in the treatment of primary biliary cirrhosis. Gastroenterology 1994;106(5):1284–90.

28. Poupon RE, Lindor KD, Pares A, et al. Combined analysis of the effect of treatment with ursodeoxycholic acid on histologic progression in primary biliary cirrhosis. J Hepatol 2003;39(1):12–6.

29. Corpechot C, Carrat F, Bonnand AM, et al. The effect of ursodeoxycholic acid therapy on liver fibrosis progression in primary biliary cirrhosis. Hepatology 2000;32(6):1196–9.

30. Hempfling W, Dilger K, Beuers U. Systematic review: ursodeoxycholic acid–adverse effects and drug interactions. Aliment Pharmacol Ther 2003;18(10): 963–72.

31. Angulo P, Batts KP, Therneau TM, et al. Long-term ursodeoxycholic acid delays histological progression in primary biliary cirrhosis. Hepatology 1999;29(3): 644–7.

32. Kuiper EM, Hansen BE, Metselaar HJ, et al. Trends in liver transplantation for primary biliary cirrhosis in The Netherlands 1988-2008. BMC Gastroenterol 2010; 10:144.

33. Lee J, Belanger A, Doucette JT, et al. Transplantation trends in primary biliary cirrhosis. Clin Gastroenterol Hepatol 2007;5(11):1313–5.

34. Lu M, Li J, Haller IV, et al. Factors associated with prevalence and treatment of primary biliary cholangitis in United States Health systems. Clin Gastroenterol Hepatol 2017. [Epub ahead of print].

35. Angulo P, Lindor KD, Therneau TM, et al. Utilization of the Mayo risk score in patients with primary biliary cirrhosis receiving ursodeoxycholic acid. Liver 1999; 19(2):115–21.

36. Pares A, Caballeria L, Rodes J. Excellent long-term survival in patients with primary biliary cirrhosis and biochemical response to ursodeoxycholic Acid. Gastroenterology 2006;130(3):715–20.

37. Lammers WJ, Hirschfield GM, Corpechot C, et al. Development and validation of a scoring system to predict outcomes of patients with primary biliary cirrhosis receiving ursodeoxycholic acid therapy. Gastroenterology 2015;149(7): 1804–12.e4.

38. Cheung KS, Seto WK, Fung J, et al. Prognostic factors for transplant-free survival and validation of prognostic models in Chinese patients with primary biliary cholangitis receiving ursodeoxycholic acid. Clin Transl Gastroenterol 2017;8(6): e100.

39. Lammers WJ, van Buuren HR, Hirschfield GM, et al. Levels of alkaline phosphatase and bilirubin are surrogate end points of outcomes of patients with primary biliary cirrhosis: an international follow-up study. Gastroenterology 2014;147(6): 1338–49.e5 [quiz: e1315].

40. Fiorucci S, Antonelli E, Rizzo G, et al. The nuclear receptor SHP mediates inhibition of hepatic stellate cells by FXR and protects against liver fibrosis. Gastroenterology 2004;127(5):1497–512.

41. Fiorucci S, Rizzo G, Antonelli E, et al. Cross-talk between farnesoid-X-receptor (FXR) and peroxisome proliferator-activated receptor gamma contributes to the antifibrotic activity of FXR ligands in rodent models of liver cirrhosis. J Pharmacol Exp Ther 2005;315(1):58–68.

42. Verbeke L, Farre R, Trebicka J, et al. Obeticholic acid, a farnesoid X receptor agonist, improves portal hypertension by two distinct pathways in cirrhotic rats. Hepatology 2014;59(6):2286–98.

43. Kowdley KV, Luketic V, Chapman R, et al. A randomized trial of obeticholic acid monotherapy in patients with primary biliary cholangitis. Hepatology 2017;66(1):S89.

44. Hirschfield GM, Mason A, Luketic V, et al. Efficacy of obeticholic acid in patients with primary biliary cirrhosis and inadequate response to ursodeoxycholic acid. Gastroenterology 2015;148(4):751–61.e8.

45. Nevens F, Andreone P, Mazzella G, et al. A placebo-controlled trial of obeticholic acid in primary biliary cholangitis. N Engl J Med 2016;375(7):631–43.

46. Suraweera D, Rahal H, Jimenez M, et al. Treatment of primary biliary cholangitis ursodeoxycholic acid non-responders: a systematic review. Liver Int 2017; 37(12):1877–86.

47. Hegade VS, Khanna A, Walker LJ, et al. Long-term fenofibrate treatment in primary biliary cholangitis improves biochemistry but not the UK-PBC risk score. Dig Dis Sci 2016;61(10):3037–44.

48. Lens S, Leoz M, Nazal L, et al. Bezafibrate normalizes alkaline phosphatase in primary biliary cirrhosis patients with incomplete response to ursodeoxycholic acid. Liver Int 2014;34(2):197–203.

49. Honda A, Ikegami T, Nakamuta M, et al. Anticholestatic effects of bezafibrate in patients with primary biliary cirrhosis treated with ursodeoxycholic acid. Hepatology 2013;57(5):1931–41.

50. Han XF, Wang QX, Liu Y, et al. Efficacy of fenofibrate in Chinese patients with primary biliary cirrhosis partially responding to ursodeoxycholic acid therapy. J Dig Dis 2012;13(4):219–24.

51. Takeuchi Y, Ikeda F, Fujioka S, et al. Additive improvement induced by bezafibrate in patients with primary biliary cirrhosis showing refractory response to ursodeoxycholic acid. J Gastroenterol Hepatol 2011;26(9):1395–401.

52. Levy C, Peter JA, Nelson DR, et al. Pilot study: fenofibrate for patients with primary biliary cirrhosis and an incomplete response to ursodeoxycholic acid. Aliment Pharmacol Ther 2011;33(2):235–42.

53. Hazzan R, Tur-Kaspa R. Bezafibrate treatment of primary biliary cirrhosis following incomplete response to ursodeoxycholic acid. J Clin Gastroenterol 2010;44(5):371–3.
54. Liberopoulos EN, Florentin M, Elisaf MS, et al. Fenofibrate in primary biliary cirrhosis: a pilot study. Open Cardiovasc Med J 2010;4:120–6.
55. Walker LJ, Newton J, Jones DE, et al. Comment on biochemical response to ursodeoxycholic acid and long-term prognosis in primary biliary cirrhosis. Hepatology 2009;49(1):337–8 [author reply: 338].
56. Iwasaki S, Ohira H, Nishiguchi S, et al. The efficacy of ursodeoxycholic acid and bezafibrate combination therapy for primary biliary cirrhosis: a prospective, multicenter study. Hepatol Res 2008;38(6):557–64.
57. Kita R, Takamatsu S, Kimura T, et al. Bezafibrate may attenuate biliary damage associated with chronic liver diseases accompanied by high serum biliary enzyme levels. J Gastroenterol 2006;41(7):686–92.
58. Ohmoto K, Yoshioka N, Yamamoto S. Long-term effect of bezafibrate on parameters of hepatic fibrosis in primary biliary cirrhosis. J Gastroenterol 2006;41(5):502–3.
59. Nakamuta M, Enjoji M, Kotoh K, et al. Long-term fibrate treatment for PBC. J Gastroenterol 2005;40(5):546–7.
60. Akbar SM, Furukawa S, Nakanishi S, et al. Therapeutic efficacy of decreased nitrite production by bezafibrate in patients with primary biliary cirrhosis. J Gastroenterol 2005;40(2):157–63.
61. Itakura J, Izumi N, Nishimura Y, et al. Prospective randomized crossover trial of combination therapy with bezafibrate and UDCA for primary biliary cirrhosis. Hepatol Res 2004;29(4):216–22.
62. Dohmen K, Mizuta T, Nakamuta M, et al. Fenofibrate for patients with asymptomatic primary biliary cirrhosis. World J Gastroenterol 2004;10(6):894–8.
63. Kanda T, Yokosuka O, Imazeki F, et al. Bezafibrate treatment: a new medical approach for PBC patients? J Gastroenterol 2003;38(6):573–8.
64. Ohira H, Sato Y, Ueno T, et al. Fenofibrate treatment in patients with primary biliary cirrhosis. Am J Gastroenterol 2002;97(8):2147–9.
65. Yano K, Kato H, Morita S, et al. Is bezafibrate histologically effective for primary biliary cirrhosis? Am J Gastroenterol 2002;97(4):1075–7.
66. Kurihara T, Maeda A, Shigemoto M, et al. Investigation into the efficacy of bezafibrate against primary biliary cirrhosis, with histological references from cases receiving long term monotherapy. Am J Gastroenterol 2002;97(1):212–4.
67. Ohmoto K, Mitsui Y, Yamamoto S. Effect of bezafibrate in primary biliary cirrhosis: a pilot study. Liver 2001;21(3):223–4.
68. Kurihara T, Niimi A, Maeda A, et al. Bezafibrate in the treatment of primary biliary cirrhosis: comparison with ursodeoxycholic acid. Am J Gastroenterol 2000;95(10):2990–2.
69. Nakai S, Masaki T, Kurokohchi K, et al. Combination therapy of bezafibrate and ursodeoxycholic acid in primary biliary cirrhosis: a preliminary study. Am J Gastroenterol 2000;95(1):326–7.
70. Miyaguchi S, Ebinuma H, Imaeda H, et al. A novel treatment for refractory primary biliary cirrhosis? Hepatogastroenterology 2000;47(36):1518–21.
71. Reig A, Sese P, Pares A. Effects of bezafibrate on outcome and pruritus in primary biliary cholangitis with suboptimal ursodeoxycholic acid response. Am J Gastroenterol 2018;113(1):49–55.
72. Corpechot C, Chazouilleres O, Rousseau D, et al. A 2-year multicenter, double-blind, randomized, placebo-controlled study of bezafibrate for the treatment of

primary biliary cholangitis in patients with inadequate biochemical response to ursodeoxycholic acid therapy (Bezurso). J Hepatol 2017;66(1):S89.

73. Zhang Y, Chen K, Dai W, et al. Combination therapy of bezafibrate and urso-deoxycholic acid for primary biliary cirrhosis: a meta-analysis. Hepatol Res 2015;45(1):48–58.

74. Zhang Y, Li S, He L, et al. Combination therapy of fenofibrate and ursodeoxy-cholic acid in patients with primary biliary cirrhosis who respond incompletely to UDCA monotherapy: a meta-analysis. Drug Des Devel Ther 2015;9:2757–66.

75. Rudic JS, Poropat G, Krstic MN, et al. Bezafibrate for primary biliary cirrhosis. Cochrane Database Syst Rev 2012;(1):CD009145.

76. Davidson MH, Armani A, McKenney JM, et al. Safety considerations with fibrate therapy. Am J Cardiol 2007;99(6A):3C–18C.

77. Bowlus CL, Kenney JT, Rice G, et al. Primary biliary cholangitis: medical and specialty pharmacy management update. J Manag Care Spec Pharm 2016; 22(10-a-s Suppl):S3–15.

78. Mitchison HC, Bassendine MF, Malcolm AJ, et al. A pilot, double-blind, controlled 1-year trial of prednisolone treatment in primary biliary cirrhosis: he-patic improvement but greater bone loss. Hepatology 1989;10(4):420–9.

79. Leuschner M, Maier KP, Schlichting J, et al. Oral budesonide and ursodeoxy-cholic acid for treatment of primary biliary cirrhosis: results of a prospective double-blind trial. Gastroenterology 1999;117(4):918–25.

80. Rautiainen H, Karkkainen P, Karvonen AL, et al. Budesonide combined with UDCA to improve liver histology in primary biliary cirrhosis: a three-year ran-domized trial. Hepatology 2005;41(4):747–52.

81. Angulo P, Jorgensen RA, Keach JC, et al. Oral budesonide in the treatment of patients with primary biliary cirrhosis with a suboptimal response to ursodeoxy-cholic acid. Hepatology 2000;31(2):318–23.

82. Kaplan MM, Bonder A, Ruthazer R, et al. Methotrexate in patients with primary biliary cirrhosis who respond incompletely to treatment with ursodeoxycholic acid. Dig Dis Sci 2010;55(11):3207–17.

83. Bonis PA, Kaplan M. Methotrexate improves biochemical tests in patients with primary biliary cirrhosis who respond incompletely to ursodiol. Gastroenterology 1999;117(2):395–9.

84. Babatin MA, Sanai FM, Swain MG. Methotrexate therapy for the symptomatic treatment of primary biliary cirrhosis patients, who are biochemical incomplete responders to ursodeoxycholic acid therapy. Aliment Pharmacol Ther 2006; 24(5):813–20.

85. Combes B, Emerson SS, Flye NL, et al. Methotrexate (MTX) plus ursodeoxy-cholic acid (UDCA) in the treatment of primary biliary cirrhosis. Hepatology 2005;42(5):1184–93.

86. Talwalkar JA, Angulo P, Keach JC, et al. Mycophenolate mofetil for the treatment of primary biliary cirrhosis in patients with an incomplete response to ursodeox-ycholic acid. J Clin Gastroenterol 2005;39(2):168–71.

87. Rabahi N, Chretien Y, Gaouar F, et al. Triple therapy with ursodeoxycholic acid, budesonide and mycophenolate mofetil in patients with features of severe pri-mary biliary cirrhosis not responding to ursodeoxycholic acid alone. Gastroen-terol Clin Biol 2010;34(4–5):283–7.

88. Gong Y, Christensen E, Gluud C. Azathioprine for primary biliary cirrhosis. Cochrane Database Syst Rev 2007;(3):CD006000.

89. Heathcote J, Ross A, Sherlock S. A prospective controlled trial of azathioprine in primary biliary cirrhosis. Gastroenterology 1976;70(5 PT.1):656–60.

90. Christensen E, Altman DG, Neuberger J, et al. Updating prognosis in primary biliary cirrhosis using a time-dependent Cox regression model. PBC1 and PBC2 trial groups. Gastroenterology 1993;105(6):1865–76.
91. Myers RP, Swain MG, Lee SS, et al. B-cell depletion with rituximab in patients with primary biliary cirrhosis refractory to ursodeoxycholic acid. Am J Gastroenterol 2013;108(6):933–41.
92. Tsuda M, Moritoki Y, Lian ZX, et al. Biochemical and immunologic effects of rituximab in patients with primary biliary cirrhosis and an incomplete response to ursodeoxycholic acid. Hepatology 2012;55(2):512–21.
93. Longo M, Crosignani A, Battezzati PM, et al. Hyperlipidaemic state and cardiovascular risk in primary biliary cirrhosis. Gut 2002;51(2):265–9.
94. Stanca CM, Bach N, Allina J, et al. Atorvastatin does not improve liver biochemistries or Mayo Risk Score in primary biliary cirrhosis. Dig Dis Sci 2008;53(7):1988–93.
95. Stojakovic T, Putz-Bankuti C, Fauler G, et al. Atorvastatin in patients with primary biliary cirrhosis and incomplete biochemical response to ursodeoxycholic acid. Hepatology 2007;46(3):776–84.
96. Ritzel U, Leonhardt U, Nather M, et al. Simvastatin in primary biliary cirrhosis: effects on serum lipids and distinct disease markers. J Hepatol 2002;36(4):454–8.
97. Abu Rajab M, Kaplan MM. Statins in primary biliary cirrhosis: are they safe? Dig Dis Sci 2010;55(7):2086–8.
98. Cash WJ, O'Neill S, O'Donnell ME, et al. Randomized controlled trial assessing the effect of simvastatin in primary biliary cirrhosis. Liver Int 2013;33(8):1166–74.
99. Spengler U, Pape GR, Hoffmann RM, et al. Differential expression of MHC class II subregion products on bile duct epithelial cells and hepatocytes in patients with primary biliary cirrhosis. Hepatology 1988;8(3):459–62.
100. Gores GJ, Moore SB, Fisher LD, et al. Primary biliary cirrhosis: associations with class II major histocompatibility complex antigens. Hepatology 1987;7(5):889–92.
101. Kwak B, Mulhaupt F, Myit S, et al. Statins as a newly recognized type of immunomodulator. Nat Med 2000;6(12):1399–402.
102. Kamisako T, Adachi Y. Marked improvement in cholestasis and hypercholesterolemia with simvastatin in a patient with primary biliary cirrhosis. Am J Gastroenterol 1995;90(7):1187–8.
103. Kurihara T, Akimoto M, Abe K, et al. Experimental use of pravastatin in patients with primary biliary cirrhosis associated with hypercholesterolemia. Clin Ther 1993;15(5):890–8.
104. Gong Y, Gluud C. Colchicine for primary biliary cirrhosis. Cochrane Database Syst Rev 2004;(2):CD004481.
105. Raszeja-Wyszomirska J, Miazgowski T. Osteoporosis in primary biliary cirrhosis of the liver. Prz Gastroenterol 2014;9(2):82–7.
106. Guanabens N, Pares A, Marinoso L, et al. Factors influencing the development of metabolic bone disease in primary biliary cirrhosis. Am J Gastroenterol 1990;85(10):1356–62.
107. Pares A, Guanabens N. Osteoporosis in primary biliary cirrhosis: pathogenesis and treatment. Clin Liver Dis 2008;12(2):407–24, x.
108. Musialik J, Petelenz M, Gonciarz Z. Effects of alendronate on bone mass in patients with primary biliary cirrhosis and osteoporosis: preliminary results after one year. Scand J Gastroenterol 2005;40(7):873–4.

109. Zein CO, Jorgensen RA, Clarke B, et al. Alendronate improves bone mineral density in primary biliary cirrhosis: a randomized placebo-controlled trial. Hepatology 2005;42(4):762–71.
110. Levy C, Harnois DM, Angulo P, et al. Raloxifene improves bone mass in osteopenic women with primary biliary cirrhosis: results of a pilot study. Liver Int 2005; 25(1):117–21.
111. Poupon RE, Lindor KD, Cauch-Dudek K, et al. Combined analysis of randomized controlled trials of ursodeoxycholic acid in primary biliary cirrhosis. Gastroenterology 1997;113(3):884–90.

Work in Progress
Drugs in Development

Gwilym J. Webb, BMBCh, MA, MRCP, Gideon M. Hirschfield, FRCP, PhD*

KEYWORDS

- Primary biliary cirrhosis • Unmet need • Novel therapies • Immunomodulators

KEY POINTS

- A proportion of patients with primary biliary cholangitis are unresponsive to, or intolerant of, ursodeoxycholic acid and obeticholic acid; these patients need alternative therapies.
- The recently approved obeticholic acid acts through the farnesoid X receptor. Other compounds exploiting the pathway and one of its key mediators, fibroblast growth factor 19, are under development.
- The peroxisome proliferator-activated receptors family of receptors modulate immune responses, bile acid metabolism, and fibrosis, and may have beneficial effects in primary biliary cholangitis.
- Drugs that inhibit the reabsorption of bile acids in the ileum have been shown to have marked short-term efficacy in treating pruritus.
- Immunomodulatory agents such as those blocking CD40-CD40L interactions, sphingosine-1-phosphate signaling and CX3CL-mediated leukocyte trafficking are under active investigation.

INTRODUCTION

Primary biliary cholangitis (PBC) is an uncommon chronic autoimmune disease of uncertain etiology where there is progressive destruction of small bile duct epithelial cells (**Fig. 1**).[1] The disease is closely associated with the development of autoantibodies including antimitochondrial-specific antinuclear antibodies. With time, PBC results in damage and the disappearance of small bile ducts, leading to intrahepatic

Disclosure Statement: Dr G.J. Webb has received financial support for the epidemiologic study of primary biliary cholangitis from Intercept Pharmaceuticals. Dr G.M. Hirschfield has acted as consultant to Cymabay, GSK, Intercept, Falk, and Novartis. This paper presents independent research funded by the NIHR Birmingham Biomedical Research Centre at the University Hospitals Birmingham NHS Foundation Trust and the University of Birmingham. The views expressed are those of the author(s) and not necessarily those of the NHS, the NIHR or the Department of Health.
National Institute for Health Research (NIHR) Birmingham Biomedical Research Centre, Institute of Immunology and Immunotherapy, University of Birmingham, Birmingham B15 2TT, UK
* Corresponding author.
E-mail address: g.hirschfield@bham.ac.uk

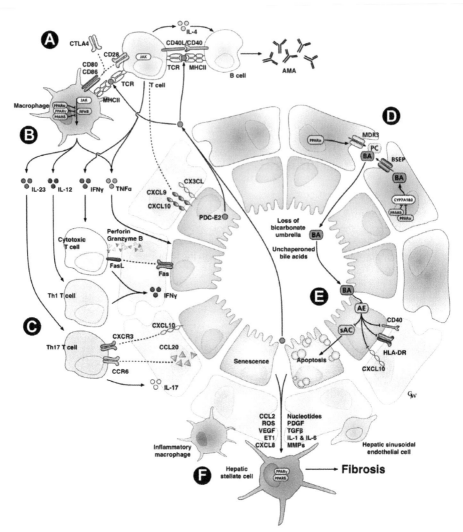

Fig. 1. Selected pathogenic mechanisms in primary biliary cholangitis. (A) Antimitochondrial antibodies are produced through interactions of T and B cells that are specific to PDC-E2. B-Cell activation is promoted by costimulatory molecules including CD40/CD40 L. T-cell activation is both through the TCR and through secondary costimulation through CD28, the latter is regulated by T-cell–expressed or exogenous CTLA4. (B) Immune cell activation is in part mediated by JAK-STAT and NF-κB signaling; PPAR ligation may reduce NF-κB activation. (C) Activated T cells (positioned by CXCL9, CXCL10 and CX3CL) produce cytokines including IFN-γ, TNF-α, and interleukin (IL)-4. With disease progression, cytotoxic and Th1 dominant inflammatory infiltrate shifts toward an increase in Th17-positive cells. Cytotoxic T cells induce apoptosis or senescence through FasL–Fas interactions and the secretion of perforins and granzyme B; both cytotoxic T cells and Th1 cells produce cytotoxic IFN-γ; IL-17–secreting Th17 cells appear later and are positioned by CXCR3–CXCL10 and CCR6-CCL20. (D) Enzymes including CYP7A1&2 convert cholesterol to BAs, which are exported by bile salt exporter pumps. BA production is reduced by ligation of FGFR4, PPAR-α or PPAR-δ. See also **Fig. 2**. In health, BA are chaperoned by phosphatidylcholine and exported by MDR3. (E) In primary biliary cholangitis, impaired activity of the apical AE2 and bicarbonate secretion lead to unchaperoned BA directly interfering with the BEC membrane. BEC are

cholestasis, progressive fibrosis, and ultimately decompensated liver disease or hepatocellular carcinoma. As well as causing progressive fibrosis, the disease is also associated with a significant incidence of debilitating pruritus and fatigue.[2]

Therapy with ursodeoxycholic acid (UDCA) in PBC has been associated with delays in progression of fibrosis[3,4] and the development of varices,[5] and recent years have seen a decrease in the requirements for transplantation in PBC in comparison with other autoimmune liver diseases (please see Kimberly A. Wong and colleagues' article, "Current Treatment Options for Primary Biliary Cholangitis," in this issue.)[6] Cohort studies have demonstrated excellent prognosis in those who show biochemical response to UDCA.[7,8] Although metaanalyses have differed as to their conclusion on the overall benefit on survival of UDCA in PBC,[9–12] therapy has become the standard of care.[13,14] However, up to one-half of those diagnosed before 50 years of age do not achieve sufficient UDCA response,[15] and UDCA is ineffective for fatigue and pruritus.[16,17]

Recently, there has been considerable work in trying to fill the gap in therapy for PBC for those unresponsive or intolerant to UDCA—and now obeticholic acid (OCA)—and in those with symptoms of fatigue and pruritus. Herein we aim to summarize the current pipeline of drugs undergoing evaluation and in development for the therapy of PBC.

OBETICHOLIC ACID

Recently, the semisynthetic bile acid OCA (also known as INT-747 and 6α-ethyl-chenodeoxycholic acid; Ocaliva, Intercept Pharmaceuticals) has shown efficacy at improving biochemical surrogate markers of clinical endpoints of death and hepatic decompensation—chiefly in the form of serum alkaline phosphatase reduction—in patients with PBC.[18,19] OCA is now conditionally approved for therapy in those with either insufficient response to or intolerance of UDCA. OCA has also demonstrated biochemical efficacy as monotherapy.[20] There are ongoing efforts in the form of a phase IV clinical trial to establish clinical endpoints of efficacy (NCT02308111).

Despite the established role of UDCA and the promise of OCA, further improvements in therapy are necessary to prevent progressive liver disease: In the POISE trial

---

then vulnerable to the prosenescent and proapoptotic effects of BA; unchaperoned BA further inhibit the activity of AE. This further weakens the bicarbonate umbrella, induces the expression of molecules that promote the immune response (CD40, HLA-DR, and CXCL10), and promotes apoptosis (via soluble adenylate cyclase). (F) Both senescent and apoptotic cells secrete mediators that activate hepatic stellate cells, perpetuate inflammation, and promote fibrosis and further biliary stasis. Hepatic sinusoidal endothelial cells, proinflammatory macrophages, and other cell types also contribute. BEC death releases further PDC-E2. AE, anion exchanger; AMA, antimitochondrial antibodies; BA, bile acids; BEC, biliary epithelial cell; BSEP, bile salt exporter pump; CCL, CC chemokine ligand; CD, cluster of differentiation; CTLA4, cytotoxic T lymphocyte antigen-4; CXCL, chemokine (C-X-C motif) ligand; CYP7A1&2, cholesterol 7-alpha-hydroxylases A1 & A2; ET1, endothelin1; Fas/FasL, CD95/CD95 ligand; FGFR, fibroblast-like growth factor receptor; HLA-DR, human leukocyte antigen–antigen D related MHC II subclass; IFN-γ, interferon-gamma; IL, interleukin; JAK, Janus kinase; MDR3, multidrug resistance protein 3; MMP, matrix metalloproteinase; NF-κB, nuclear factor kappa-light-chain-enhancer of activated B cells; PC, phosphatidylcholines; PDC-E2, pyruvate dehydrogenase complex E2 subunit; PDGF, platelet-derived growth factor; PPAR-α/γ/δ, peroxisome proliferator-activated receptors alpha/gamma/delta; ROS, reactive oxygen species; sAC, soluble adenylate cyclase; TCR, T-cell receptor; TGF-β, transforming growth factor beta; Th1/Th17, T helper type 1 and type 17 cells; TNF-α, tumor necrosis factor-alpha; VEGF, vascular endothelial growth factor.

of OCA, one-half of UDCA nonresponders also did not respond to OCA, as defined by a dichotomous primary endpoint.[18] The durability of biochemical response in OCA seems to be good based on some long-term safety data, but continues to be important to confirm, as does confirmation that OCA-induced biochemical response relates to clinically significant endpoints. This issue of relating short-term surrogate outcomes with longer term outcomes in diseases with a long time-course is a considerable challenge not restricted to OCA21, as regards OCA, a phase IV study is in progress that aims to address OCA's role in those with liver disease that is already advanced at drug initiation and also in relation to longer term clinical endpoints such as death, hepatic decompensation, or a requirement for transplantation (NCT02308111). In addition, a tendency toward hyperlipidemia was noted during a trial of OCA in nonalcoholic steatohepatitis, and whether this could impact cardiovascular risk, and how to manage this clinically, is an ongoing area of research.[21] Furthermore the OCA-induced burden of pruritus, a dose-dependent effect, is something that in real-world practice will need further attention.[19] Importantly, neither UDCA nor OCA are effective for fatigue and neither is proven after transplantation. Long-term safety needs to be better appreciated for OCA in the context of very advanced liver disease (where dose adjustment is needed) and for any therapy that potentially causes long-term changes in fibroblast growth factor (FGF)19 levels, there must be recognition of association with hepatocellular carcinoma in some animal models.[22]

BILE ACIDS AND THEIR DERIVATIVES
Farnesoid X Receptor Agonists

The primary function of the drug OCA is as a potent agonist of the farnesoid X receptor (FXR; **Fig. 2**). Agonism via FXR has a number of effects considered valuable in both PBC and in other liver diseases. The effects of FXR ligation are mediated by alteration of transcription by targeting promoter regions both directly and in combination with retinoic acid receptor-α (RXR).[23–25] Within the liver, FXR agonism tends to reduce synthesis of bile acids from cholesterol by CYP7A1 and CYP7A2. Other reported actions include modulation of triglyceride synthesis, alteration of hepatocyte and cholangiocyte fluid efflux, and reduction of blue acid uptake. FXR ligation also reduces enterocyte bile acid reuptake. OCA is derived from the natural chenodeoxycholic acid by the addition of an ethyl group greatly increasing its action through FXR; UDCA, an epimer of chenodeoxycholic acid, has no significant FXR agonist activity.[25,26]

Non-OCA FXR agonists are under active investigation in both PBC and in other areas of liver disease.[27] Given the efficacy of OCA in PBC, the results of trials in other liver diseases will be of interest to those managing PBC. Active work includes the synthetic steroidal EYP001a (Enyo Pharma; NCT03272009) in combination with entecavir in chronic hepatitis B; the synthetic nonsteroidal, non–bile acid LJN452 (also known as tropifexor, Novartis; NCT02855164 & NCT02516605), which is under active investigation in both nonalcoholic steatohepatitis and PBC[28]; and the nonsteroidal GS9674 (Gilead; previously PX-104, Phenex pharmaceuticals; NCT02943447, NCT02781584 & NCT01999101). The older GW4064, which demonstrated efficacy in animal models of cholestasis, is no longer being pursued in human trials.[29]

Fibroblast Growth Factor 19 Analogues

The signaling molecule FGF19 is primarily produced by ileal enterocytes in response to bile acid exposure (see **Fig. 2**).[30] Its myriad actions include suppression of bile acid synthesis by cholesterol-7α-hydroxylase via FGFR4 and the coreceptor β-Klotho. Correspondingly, either deficiency in the murine homologue of FGF19—FGF15—or

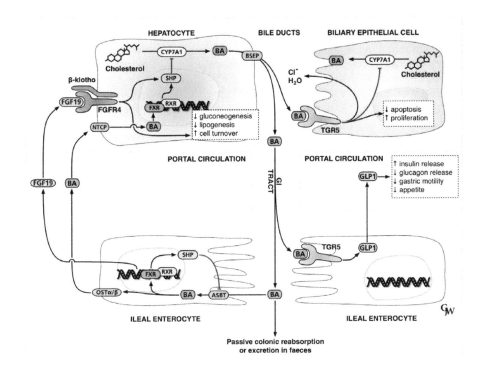

Fig. 2. FXR and TGR ligation by bile acids. BA are synthesized from cholesterol by enzymes including CYP7A1. They are secreted into the biliary ductules by BSEP. Bile acids ligate TGR5 receptors on the apical surface of BEC, causing feedback suppression of further bile acid synthesis, increased ductular chloride and water excretion, and a decrease in BEC apoptosis. Bile acids enter the small bowel lumen in the duodenum via the bile ducts then pass to the ileum. Bile acids may ligate ileal TGR5 receptors releasing GLP1 into the systemic circulation via the portal vein. This tends to increase insulin release, decrease glucagon metabolism, reduce gastric motility and reduce appetite. The majority of bile acids that enter the ileum are actively imported into ileal enterocytes from the lumen by the action of ASBT. Within the enterocyte, bile acids ligate the nuclear FXR, which partly as a monomer and partly as a dimer with RXR induces the activity of SHP, which in turns reduces further uptake of bile acids by ASBT. BA also enter the portal circulation from enterocytes via the OSTα/β transporter. Ligation of FXR causes synthesis and release of FGF19 into the portal circulation. Circulating BA are taken up into the hepatocyte via the Na/taurocholate cotransporting polypeptide (NTCP) transporter, where they ligate FXR. Together with RXR, this downregulates further the synthesis of bile acids via SHP. FGF19 ligates FGFR4 in a signaling complex stabilized by β-Klotho. This induces SHP and downregulates both BA synthesis and gluconeogenesis, reduces lipogenesis and increases cell turnover. ASBT, apical sodium bile acid transporter; BA, bile acids; BEC, biliary epithelial cells; BSEP, bile salt export pump; FXR, farnesoid X-receptor; GLP1, glucagon-like peptide 1; OSTα/β, basolateral bile acid efflux transporters; RXR, retinoic acid receptor-α; SHP, small heterodimeric protein; TGR5, transmembrane G protein-coupled receptor 5. Arrowed lines denote a positive effect, red barred lines denote a negative effect.

in of its receptor FGFR4 results in overexpression of cholesterol-7α-hydroxylase and increased bile acid turnover together with impaired gallbladder filling.[31]

NGM282 is a subcutaneously administered synthetic analogue of FGF19. It has been reported as being nonmitogenic and, therefore, thought not to be associated with neoplastic risk.[32] In contrast with OCA, it does not seem to cause pruritus, although it does cause diarrhea in some 25% of recipients.[33] The diarrhea is thought to be a smooth muscle stimulant action rather than bile acid related.[34] NGM282 has efficacy in ameliorating liver injury in animal models of chemical and bile duct ligation induced cholestasis.[35] In a 28-day trial in UDCA nonresponsive patients with PBC, NGM282 was associated with biochemical improvements and evidence of reduced bile acid synthesis.[36] An extended trial has completed but not yet reported (NCT02135536).

Transmembrane G-Protein Receptor 5 Receptor Agonists

Transmembrane-G-protein-receptor-5 receptors (TGR5; also known as Takeda-G-protein-receptor-5 or GPBAR1) represent an alternative and complimentary bile acid signaling pathway to the FXR pathway. Sensing by TGR5, which is predominantly found in the small intestine and colon, releases glucagon-like peptide-1. TGR5 receptors on pancreatic β cells tend to augment insulin release, whereas its action on a variety of immune cells including Kupffer cells, macrophages, monocytes, and macrophages tends to decrease activation.[25,37,38] Biliary epithelial cell cilia also express TGR5, the ligation of which may negatively regulate bile acid production and augment water and chloride export[39]; and activity through TGR5 via lysophosphatidic acid in skin has recently been associated with bile acid mediated pruritus.[40,41] The action of TGR5 seems to negatively regulate hepatic inflammation in a mouse model of lipopolysaccharide-induced hepatitis[42] through a pure TGR5 agonist (INT-777, Intercept) was not effective in ameliorating MDR2/*ABCB4* deficiency cholangitis.[43] TGR5 agonists have been proposed as targets for the therapy of PBC, but no trials of pure TGR5 modulators are currently recruiting. Combination therapy of FXR agonists and TGR5 agonists (such as INT-767, Intercept) have shown some promise in preclinical studies in MDR2/*ABCB4*–deficient cholangiopathic mice.[43]

PEROXISOME PROLIFERATOR-ACTIVATED RECEPTOR AGONISTS

The family of peroxisome proliferator-activated receptors (PPARs) represents a group of 3 nuclear receptor isoforms encoded by separate genes and known as PPAR-α, PPAR-γ, and PPAR-δ, respectively.[44] All are ligated by unsaturated fatty acids, but each has a differing repertoire of other ligands. They have modulatory roles in inflammation, adipocyte function, glucose and lipid metabolism, and energy homeostasis.[45] Aspects of PPAR function of particular interest in liver disease include PPAR-α, PPAR-γ, and PPAR-δ all reducing effector cytokine production by intrahepatic macrophages, including Kupffer cells, an action of the α and δ forms to promote lipoprotein metabolism and fatty acid oxidation with a tendency to reduce steatosis and oxidative stress, a reduction in the fibrogenic capacity of hepatic stellate cells through PPAR-α and PPAR-γ, an α and γ form regulatory effect on bile acid reabsorption at the enterocyte, a prophosphatidylcholine excretion effect of PPAR-α in the hepatocyte, and finally PPAR-α and -γ exert a negative regulatory effect on hepatocyte bile acid synthesis by reducing cholesterol 7-alpha-hydroxylases A1 and A2 activity.[45]

Fibrates, including fenofibrate and bezafibrate, are agonists of PPAR-α. Fibrates have had a long but inconclusive history in the management of PBC. Both fenofibrate[46] and bezafibrate[47] have been recorded as effecting marked biochemical improvement in patients with PBC, both in UDCA responders and nonresponders, and in monotherapy or in combination with UDCA. However, until recently, controlled trials have been lacking. In mid 2017, a French pan-national randomized placebo-controlled study (BEZURSO) reported the addition of bezafibrate to UDCA in those without biochemical response to baseline therapy.[48] With 100 patients randomized and 2 years of follow-up, marked ameliorations in liver biochemistry, pruritus scores, and liver stiffness as assessed by transient elastography were recorded. The study is yet to be reported other than in abstract form. A complementary controlled trial of fenofibrate is underway in China (NCT02965911). Notably, the cost for the doses of bezafibrate and fenofibrate used approximates to $150 per year.

Seladelpar is a specific PPAR-δ agonist (also MBX-8025, Cymabay Therapeutics). In late 2017, a trial of placebo-controlled study of 41 patients with UDCA nonresponsive PBC who were given the drug was stopped earlier than planned because 3 patients developed significant but self-limiting increases in serum transaminase activities.[49] The majority of patients who received seladelpar, however, had significant decreases in serum alkaline phosphatase activity with all 5 patients who received the intended 12-week course demonstrating reversion to normal levels. Trials of lower doses in patients with PBC are underway (NCT02955602 and NCT03301506)

Elafibranor (GFT505; Genfit) represents a dual PPAR-α and PPAR-γ agonist with proven antifibrotic activity in animal models.[50] In a study of human patients with nonalcoholic steatohepatitis, there was improvement and even resolution of steatosis in a post hoc analyzed subgroup of patients with mild to moderate nonalcoholic steatohepatitis in a study with repeated liver biopsy based assessment.[51] A study of elafibranor in PBC is ongoing (NCT03124108).

IMMUNOLOGIC AGENTS
Ustekinumab

Genome-wide association studies in PBC have highlighted several variants in the IL-12–Tyk2–STAT4–Th1 pathway as being associated with increased risk of developing the disease.[52] IL-12 is produced by activated antigen-presenting cells and promotes Th1 type/interferon-γ producing polarization of CD4$^+$ T cells. This observation corresponds with pathologic findings suggesting an IL-12–rich, interferon-γ–rich intrahepatic environment in early PBC.[53,54] In addition, deletion of the IL-12 p40 subunit (which is also shared with IL-23) in the dnTGFβII mouse model of antimitochondrial antibody-positive cholangitis led to disease amelioration.[55] These findings led to an open-label study of the anti–IL-12/IL-23 agent ustekinumab, which has established efficacy in the therapy of psoriasis. Although therapy was associated with a modest overall decrease in serum alkaline phosphatase activity in a cohort of 20 patients, none attained improvement in liver biochemistry equating to UDCA biochemical response.[56] Further trials of ustekinumab in PBC are not currently open.

CX3CL/Fractalkine Blockade

The interaction between CX3CL or fractalkine and its receptor CX3CR1 have been suggested to mediate a proportion of leukocyte trafficking to intrahepatic bile ducts.[57] Biliary epithelial cells from PBC livers express CX3CL at higher levels than non-PBC diseased controls and normal liver some lymphocyte trafficking to intrahepatic bile ducts.[58] A phase II study is currently recruiting in Japan investigating the potential utility for E6011 (Eisai Inc./EA Pharma Co. Ltd.) in UDCA nonresponsive PBC. The drug, which is administered intravenously, has recently been shown to be well-tolerated in patients with rheumatoid arthritis.[59]

CD40/CD40L Blockade

Interactions between CD4$^+$ helper T cells and B cells are required to drive the specific antibody response seen in PBC. One driver of this interaction is interactions between

CD40 on B cells and CD40L on T cells. Work has suggested increased demethylation of the CD40L promotor region in patients with PBC as compared with healthy controls, and that this finding correlated with serum IgM concentrations.[60] Blockade of CD40 ligand in the dnTGFβRII mouse model of cholangitis with antimitochondrial antibodies.[61] These findings have led to a combined phase I/phase II trial of the CD40 antagonist FFP104 in patients with UDCA nonresponsive PBC. The trial is yet to report but closed early to recruitment.

Abatacept

The immunosuppressive agent abatacept (CTLA4Ig; Orencia, Bristol-Myers-Squibb) is a fusion protein of the Fc region of IgG1 with the extracellular domain of CTLA4 and is currently licensed for the therapy of rheumatoid arthritis. In health, CTLA4 is induced on activated effector T cells and constitutively expressed on regulatory T cells. CTLA4 binds the signaling molecules CD80 and CD86, which are expressed by antigen-presenting cells and provide costimulatory signals through the T-cell tumor necrosis factor family receptor CD28. Cells that receive T-cell receptor signals without CD28 signals typically become anergic on activation whereas conversely uncontrolled signaling through CD28—for example, in CTLA4 deficiency—is associated with multisystem autoimmunity.[62] Single nucleotide variants in CTLA4 have been proposed—but not confirmed—as conferring disease risk in PBC.[52,63] In addition, adjuvant-boosted xenobiotic immunized murine model of cholangitis with antimitochondrial antibodies, blockade of T-cell costimulation with CTLA4Ig showed efficacy.[64] A trial of abatacept in PBC is scheduled to complete by the end of 2017 (NCT02078882); results in abstract form are, however, negative to date.

Sphingosine-1-Phosphate Signaling

Sphingosine-1-phosphate (S1P) is a phosphorylated lysosphingolipid derived from sphingosine by the action of sphingosine phosphatase as part of the sphingolipid metabolic pathway.[65] S1P has been shown to be active in modulation of gene expression by exerting actions on histone acetylation primarily via a family of G-protein–coupled receptors: numbered S1PR15. Agonists of S1P receptors are associated with modulation of immune-mediated processes including both innate and adaptive responses, and the agent figolimod, which is primarily active through the S1P receptor 1, has been shown to be efficacious in multiple sclerosis.[66] There has been some concern that activity through S1P receptors 2 and 3 may be associated with cardiorespiratory side effects and so specific agents have been developed. The novel agent etrasimod (Arena Pharmaceuticals) is selectively active through S1P receptors 1, 4, and 5, seems to be efficacious in a mouse model of colitis, and relatively safe in healthy volunteers.[67] A trial of its efficacy in patients with PBC and inadequate response to UDCA is underway (NCT03155932).

Janus Kinase Inhibitors

The Janus kinases (JAK) are integral signaling molecules in the JAK-signal transducer and activator of transcription pathway that mediates the cellular effects of a number of effector cytokines and hormones.[68] Inhibition of the pathway has shown promise in a number of extrahepatic autoimmune diseases, including rheumatoid arthritis,[69] ulcerative colitis,[70] and psoriasis.[71] In PBC, signaling through several pathways involving JAK-transducer and activator of transcription—including the IL-12 pathway—seems to be relevant to disease pathogenesis.[52] Several orally active JAK inhibitors are available and well-tolerated, and they represent a potential avenue of exploration in PBC.

PRURITUS

Pruritus is frequent and distressing in PBC. It affects more than one-half of patients during their disease course and is associated with a worsened prognosis.[72] The precise mechanism of pruritus in cholestatic liver disease remains the source of some debate: proposed mechanisms include excessive retention of endogenous opioids, direct actions by retained circulating bile acids (including via the TGR5 system), and the relatively recent association of degree of pruritus and serum activities of lysophosphatidic acid, a neuronal activator that is pruritogenic in mice and formed by the action of the enzyme autotaxin.[73]

The management of pruritus is discussed in more details (see Andres F. Carrion and colleagues' article, "Understanding and Treating Pruritus in Primary Biliary Cholangitis," in this issue) and has seen significant advancements recently with reports of the successful use of bile acid reuptake inhibitors and reports that fibrates, as PPAR-α agonists, are efficacious in pruritus.[48]

Bile Acid Reuptake Inhibitors

In health, around 95% of circulating bile acids are reabsorbed in the terminal ileum, primarily through active uptake by the apical sodium-bile acid transporter (ASBT; also ileal bile acid transport; *SLC10A2*; see **Fig. 2**). The ileum is the major site of reabsorption of bile acids, although after bacterial deconjugation and 7α-dehydroxylation, a proportion are reabsorbed in the colon.[25] A range of compounds that inhibit ileal reabsorption of bile acids have been developed by several organizations: SC-425 (Shire), A4250 (Albireo Pharma), lopixibat (formerly LUM001 and also known as maralixibat; Lumena), and GSK2330672(GlaxoSmithKline). Each of these agents is minimally orally absorbed. Although lopixibat was effective in reducing serum bile acids in PBC, there were no significant changes in patient-reported pruritus scores over a 12-week period. GSK2330672, however, showed efficacy in a cross-over study of refractory pruritus, but without evidence of improved biochemistry although reduced serum FGF19 levels.[74] Two areas of concern with ASBT inhibitors include the side effect of diarrhea and a theoretic procarcinogenic effect in the colon.[75] At the time of writing, a follow-up dose-finding study of GSK 2330672 is recruiting (NCT02966834).

OTHER AREAS OF PRIMARY BILIARY CHOLANGITIS CARE REQUIRING IMPROVED THERAPY

Some areas of PBC therapy that require further investigation to broaden therapeutic options. First, antimitochondrial antibodies may be detected incidentally in patients with no evidence of liver disease. These individuals are at significantly greater risk of subsequent development of PBC, especially when AMA is found in the absence of other significant diagnoses.[76,77] It remains unclear how to best treat them.

Second, recurrence of PBC after liver transplantation is well-reported.[78] Reports from cohort studies suggest that ongoing therapy with UDCA is protective against development of recurrent disease.[79,80] However, controlled studies have not been undertaken and the need for protocol biopsies to confidently identify recurrent disease coupled with the declining frequency of transplantation for PBC make this a difficult area to study.[6] A further area of uncertainty is the optimal immunosuppression regime after transplantation; there is an unconfirmed suggestion that recurrence may be more frequent with tacrolimus-based as opposed to cyclosporine-based regimes, although prospective studies are lacking.[81]

Third, fatigue in PBC is a frequent symptom, but is challenging to treat. It is a major management issue identified by patients, is not affected by UDCA administration and seems to portend a worse prognosis.[16,17] To date, although initially promising, both modafinil[82] and rituximab[83] have been shown to lack efficacy and improved therapies are needed.

SPECULATIVE FUTURE THERAPEUTIC DEVELOPMENTS

The frequent nature of pruritus as an adverse effect with OCA and the recent success of inhibitors of bile acid reuptake in the amelioration of pruritus in PBC raise the potential for future combination therapy with these agents: the logical possibility of coadministration of an FXR agonist and an ASBT inhibitor to control the pruritus and increases in serum FGF19 seen in the former, while simultaneously controlling the diarrhea and reducing the increased colonic bile acid exposure seen with latter has not yet been explored. Further, the current paradigm of treatment is additional therapy with a lack of biochemical response. Sequential combination of second-line therapies, for example, combining PPAR and FXR agonists may become a therapeutic paradigm for challenging cases.

The marked and consistent association of PBC with a specific antigen response raises the potential of antigen specific peptide therapy mediated induction of tolerance to the targets of antimitochondrial antibody,[84] or the prospect of boosting antigen-specific regulatory T-cell function (eg, NCT01988506). Further, engineering and then infusing T cells with a receptor specific to the disease-mediating population is a mechanism that has shown promise in a mouse model of the autoimmune skin disease pemphigus vulgaris.[85]

The microbiome of patients with PBC is underexplored. However, disease amelioration is associated with reversions of abnormalities that have been identified in gut flora.[86,87] Recently, it has been shown that in immunotherapy, the gut microbiome is a major determinant of immune response.[88] Manipulation of the microbiome for therapeutic purposes is an area with future potential.

For the management of pruritus, an area of particular focus is the targeting of the production of lysophosphatidic acid—a hypothesized molecular mediator of pruritus. Inhibitors of autotaxin are in development but as yet have not entered trials.[89]

SUMMARY

The management of PBC was revolutionized more than 20 years ago by the widespread introduction of UDCA, which now forms the standard of care. The therapeutic armamentarium has since been augmented by the FXR agonist OCA, which promises to allow a further tranche of patients to achieve biochemical response. However, despite these therapies, significant numbers of patients still do not achieve biochemical response or are intolerant of therapy. Happily, a range of different options seem to be on the horizon: non-OCA FXR agonists or the related FGF19 analogues, which have similar actions but induce less pruritus; PPAR agonists both including long-established fibrates acting through PPAR-α and newer agents active through other subsets of PPAR receptors; and inhibitors of the action of S1P are among agents showing promise. In addition, the management of pruritus in PBC may be on the cusp of a major change, with reports of promising early results with bile acid reuptake inhibitors. No single agent will be universally effective and the individualization of therapy and intelligent therapeutic combination is likely to be required in the future.

REFERENCES

1. Hirschfield GM, Gershwin ME. The immunobiology and pathophysiology of primary biliary cirrhosis. Annu Rev Pathol 2013;8:303–30.

2. Carey EJ, Ali AH, Lindor KD. Primary biliary cirrhosis. Lancet 2015;386:1565–75.
3. Corpechot C, Carrat F, Bonnand AM, et al. The effect of ursodeoxycholic acid therapy on liver fibrosis progression in primary biliary cirrhosis. Hepatology 2000;32:1196–9.
4. Poupon RE, Lindor KD, Parés A, et al. Combined analysis of the effect of treatment with ursodeoxycholic acid on histologic progression in primary biliary cirrhosis. J Hepatol 2003;39:12–6.
5. Lindor KD, Jorgensen RA, Therneau TM, et al. Ursodeoxycholic acid delays the onset of esophageal varices in primary biliary cirrhosis. Mayo Clinic Proc 1997;72:1137–40.
6. Webb GJ, Rana A, Hodson J, et al. Twenty-year comparative analysis of patients with autoimmune liver diseases on transplant waitlists. Clin Gastroenterol Hepatol 2018;16(2):278–87.e7.
7. Pares A, Caballeria L, Rodes J. Excellent long-term survival in patients with primary biliary cirrhosis and biochemical response to ursodeoxycholic acid. Gastroenterology 2006;130:715–20.
8. Kuiper EM, Hansen BE, de Vries RA, et al. Improved prognosis of patients with primary biliary cirrhosis that have a biochemical response to ursodeoxycholic acid. Gastroenterology 2009;136:1281–7.
9. Shi J, Wu C, Lin Y, et al. Long-term effects of mid-dose ursodeoxycholic acid in primary biliary cirrhosis: a meta-analysis of randomized controlled trials. Am J Gastroenterol 2006;101:1529–38.
10. Gong Y, Huang ZB, Christensen E, et al. Ursodeoxycholic acid for primary biliary cirrhosis. Cochrane Database Syst Rev 2008;(3):CD000551.
11. Saffioti F, Gurusamy KS, Eusebi LH, et al. Pharmacological interventions for primary biliary cholangitis: an attempted network meta-analysis. Cochrane Database Syst Rev 2017;(3):CD011648.
12. Rudic JS, Poropat G, Krstic MN, et al. Ursodeoxycholic acid for primary biliary cirrhosis. Cochrane Database Syst Rev 2012;(12):CD000551.
13. Lindor KD, Gershwin ME, Poupon R, et al. Primary biliary cirrhosis. Hepatology 2009;50:291–308.
14. Hirschfield GM, Beuers U, Corpechot C, et al. EASL clinical practice guidelines: the diagnosis and management of patients with primary biliary cholangitis. J Hepatol 2017;67:145–72.
15. Carbone M, Mells GF, Pells G, et al. Sex and age are determinants of the clinical phenotype of primary biliary cirrhosis and response to ursodeoxycholic acid. Gastroenterology 2013;144:560–9.e7 [quiz: e513–64].
16. Jones DE, Al-Rifai A, Frith J, et al. The independent effects of fatigue and UDCA therapy on mortality in primary biliary cirrhosis: results of a 9 year follow-up. J Hepatol 2010;53:911–7.
17. Quarneti C, Muratori P, Lalanne C, et al. Fatigue and pruritus at onset identify a more aggressive subset of primary biliary cirrhosis. Liver Int 2015;35:636–41.
18. Nevens F, Andreone P, Mazzella G, et al. A placebo-controlled trial of obeticholic acid in primary biliary cholangitis. N Engl J Med 2016;375:631–43.
19. Hirschfield GM, Mason A, Luketic V, et al. Efficacy of obeticholic acid in patients with primary biliary cirrhosis and inadequate response to ursodeoxycholic acid. Gastroenterology 2015;148:751–61.e8.
20. Kowdley KV, Luketic V, Chapman R, et al. A randomized trial of obeticholic acid monotherapy in patients with primary biliary cholangitis. Hepatology 2017. [Epub ahead of print].

21. Neuschwander-Tetri BA, Loomba R, Sanyal AJ, et al. Farnesoid X nuclear receptor ligand obeticholic acid for non-cirrhotic, non-alcoholic steatohepatitis (FLINT): a multicentre, randomised, placebo-controlled trial. Lancet 2015;385:956–65.

22. Schaap FG, Jansen PLM, Olde Damink SWM. Chronic elevation of plasma FGF19 in long-term FXR agonist therapy, a happy marriage or cause for oncologic concern? Hepatology 2018;67(2):782–4.

23. Makishima M, Okamoto AY, Repa JJ, et al. Identification of a nuclear receptor for bile acids. Science 1999;284:1362–5.

24. Parks DJ, Blanchard SG, Bledsoe RK, et al. Bile acids: natural ligands for an orphan nuclear receptor. Science 1999;284:1365–8.

25. Schaap FG, Trauner M, Jansen PL. Bile acid receptors as targets for drug development. Nat Rev Gastroenterol Hepatol 2014;11:55–67.

26. Halilbasic E, Claudel T, Trauner M. Bile acid transporters and regulatory nuclear receptors in the liver and beyond. J Hepatol 2013;58:155–68.

27. Verbeke L, Farre R, Trebicka J, et al. Obeticholic acid, a farnesoid X receptor agonist, improves portal hypertension by two distinct pathways in cirrhotic rats. Hepatology 2014;59:2286–98.

28. Tully DC, Rucker PV, Chianelli D, et al. Discovery of tropifexor (LJN452), a highly potent non-bile acid FXR agonist for the treatment of cholestatic liver diseases and Nonalcoholic Steatohepatitis (NASH). J Med Chem 2017;60(24):9960–73.

29. Liu Y, Binz J, Numerick MJ, et al. Hepatoprotection by the farnesoid X receptor agonist GW4064 in rat models of intra- and extrahepatic cholestasis. J Clin Invest 2003;112:1678–87.

30. Zhang JH, Nolan JD, Kennie SL, et al. Potent stimulation of fibroblast growth factor 19 expression in the human ileum by bile acids. Am J Physiol Gastrointest Liver Physiol 2013;304:G940–8.

31. Fukumoto S. Actions and mode of actions of FGF19 subfamily members. Endocr J 2008;55:23–31.

32. Ling L, Phung V, Wang X, et al. NGM282, a Potent Inhibitor of CYP7A1, Prevents FGF19-Mediated HCC Tumor Development in db/db and rasH2 Mice. Hepatology 2014;60:216A–7A.

33. Mayo MJ, Wigg AJ, Hudgens S, et al. Impact of NGM282 on the incidence and severity of pruritus in primary biliary cirrhosis patients and correlations with liver chemistries and serum bile acids. Hepatology 2015;62:520A–1A.

34. Oduyebo I, Nelson AD, Khemani D, et al. NGM282, variant of FGF19, is a gastric and colonic prokinetic and stimulates bowel function in patients with functional constipation: phase 1B, two-dose, placebo controlled study. Gastroenterology 2017;152:S1315.

35. Luo J, Ko B, To C, et al. Hepatoprotective effects of NGM282 compared to obeticholic acid and bezafibrate in mouse models of cholestasis. J Hepatol 2014;60: S531.

36. Mayo MJ, Wigg AJ, Roberts SK, et al. NGM282, a novel variant of FGF-19, demonstrates biologic activity in primary biliary cirrhosis patients with an incomplete response to ursodeoxycholic acid: results of a phase 2 multicenter, randomized, double blinded, placebo controlled trial. Hepatology 2015;62:263A–4A.

37. van Nierop FS, Scheltema MJ, Eggink HM, et al. Clinical relevance of the bile acid receptor TGR5 in metabolism. Lancet Diabetes Endocrinol 2017;5:224–33.

38. Pols TW, Noriega LG, Nomura M, et al. The bile acid membrane receptor TGR5 as an emerging target in metabolism and inflammation. J Hepatol 2011;54:1263–72.

39. Keitel V, Ullmer C, Haussinger D. The membrane-bound bile acid receptor TGR5 (Gpbar-1) is localized in the primary cilium of cholangiocytes. Biol Chem 2010; 391:785–9.
40. Alemi F, Kwon E, Poole DP, et al. The TGR5 receptor mediates bile acid-induced itch and analgesia. J Clin Invest 2013;123:1513–30.
41. Lieu T, Jayaweera G, Zhao P, et al. The bile acid receptor TGR5 activates the TRPA1 channel to induce itch in mice. Gastroenterology 2014;147:1417–28.
42. Wang YD, Chen WD, Yu D, et al. The G-protein-coupled bile acid receptor, Gpbar1 (TGR5), negatively regulates hepatic inflammatory response through antagonizing nuclear factor kappa light-chain enhancer of activated B cells (NF-kappaB) in mice. Hepatology 2011;54:1421–32.
43. Baghdasaryan A, Claudel T, Gumhold J, et al. Dual farnesoid X receptor/TGR5 agonist INT-767 reduces liver injury in the Mdr2-/- (Abcb4-/-) mouse cholangiopathy model by promoting biliary HCO(-)(3) output. Hepatology 2011;54:1303–12.
44. Berger J, Moller DE. The mechanisms of action of PPARs. Annu Rev Med 2002; 53:409–35.
45. Gross B, Pawlak M, Lefebvre P, et al. PPARs in obesity-induced T2DM, dyslipidaemia and NAFLD. Nat Rev Endocrinol 2017;13:36–49.
46. Levy C, Peter JA, Nelson DR, et al. Pilot study: fenofibrate for patients with primary biliary cirrhosis and an incomplete response to ursodeoxycholic acid. Aliment Pharmacol Ther 2011;33:235–42.
47. Reig A, Sese P, Pares A. Effects of bezafibrate on outcome and pruritus in primary biliary cholangitis with suboptimal ursodeoxycholic acid response. Am J Gastroenterol 2018;113(1):49–55.
48. Corpechot C, Chazouillères O, Rousseau A, et al. 2-year multicenter, double-blind, randomized, placebo-controlled study of bezafibrate for the treatment of primary biliary cholangitis in patients with inadequate biochemical response to ursodeoxycholic acid therapy (Bezurso). J Hepatol 2017;66:S89.
49. Jones D, Boudes PF, Swain MG, et al. Seladelpar (MBX-8025), a selective PPAR-delta agonist, in patients with primary biliary cholangitis with an inadequate response to ursodeoxycholic acid: a double-blind, randomised, placebo-controlled, phase 2, proof-of-concept study. Lancet Gastroenterol Hepatol 2017;2:716–26.
50. Staels B, Rubenstrunk A, Noel B, et al. Hepatoprotective effects of the dual peroxisome proliferator-activated receptor alpha/delta agonist, GFT505, in rodent models of nonalcoholic fatty liver disease/nonalcoholic steatohepatitis. Hepatology 2013;58:1941–52.
51. Ratziu V, Harrison SA, Francque S, et al. Elafibranor, an agonist of the peroxisome proliferator-activated receptor-alpha and -delta, induces resolution of nonalcoholic steatohepatitis without fibrosis worsening. Gastroenterology 2016;150:1147–59.e5.
52. Webb GJ, Siminovitch KA, Hirschfield GM. The immunogenetics of primary biliary cirrhosis: a comprehensive review. J Autoimmun 2015;64:42–52.
53. Yang C-Y, Ma X, Tsuneyama K, et al. IL-12/Th1 and IL-23/Th17 biliary microenvironment in primary biliary cirrhosis: implications for therapy. Hepatology 2014; 59(5):1944–53.
54. Nagano T, Yamamoto K, Matsumoto S, et al. Cytokine profile in the liver of primary biliary cirrhosis. J Clin Immunol 1999;19:422–7.
55. Yoshida K, Yang GX, Zhang W, et al. Deletion of interleukin-12p40 suppresses autoimmune cholangitis in dominant negative transforming growth factor β receptor type II mice. Hepatology 2009;50:1494–500.

56. Hirschfield GM, Gershwin ME, Strauss R, et al. Ustekinumab for patients with primary biliary cholangitis who have an inadequate response to ursodeoxycholic acid: a proof-of-concept study. Hepatology 2016;64:189–99.
57. Efsen E, Grappone C, DeFranco RM, et al. Up-regulated expression of fractalkine and its receptor CX3CR1 during liver injury in humans. J Hepatol 2002;37:39–47.
58. Shimoda S, Harada K, Niiro H, et al. CX3CL1 (fractalkine): a signpost for biliary inflammation in primary biliary cirrhosis. Hepatology 2010;51:567–75.
59. Tanaka Y, Takeuchi T, Umehara H, et al. Safety, pharmacokinetics, and efficacy of E6011, an antifractalkine monoclonal antibody, in a first-in-patient phase 1/2 study on rheumatoid arthritis. Mod Rheumatol 2018;28(1):58–65.
60. Lleo A, Zhang W, Zhao M, et al. DNA methylation profiling of the X chromosome reveals an aberrant demethylation on CXCR3 promoter in primary biliary cirrhosis. Clin Epigenetics 2015;7:61.
61. Tanaka H, Yang GX, Iwakoshi N, et al. Anti-CD40 ligand monoclonal antibody delays the progression of murine autoimmune cholangitis. Clin Exp Immunol 2013; 174(3):364–71.
62. Tivol EA, Borriello F, Schweitzer AN, et al. Loss of CTLA-4 leads to massive lymphoproliferation and fatal multiorgan tissue destruction, revealing a critical negative regulatory role of CTLA-4. Immunity 1995;3:541–7.
63. Qiu F, Tang R, Zuo X, et al. A genome-wide association study identifies six novel risk loci for primary biliary cholangitis. Nat Commun 2017;8:14828.
64. Dhirapong A, Yang GX, Nadler S, et al. Therapeutic effect of cytotoxic T lymphocyte antigen 4/immunoglobulin on a murine model of primary biliary cirrhosis. Hepatology 2013;57:708–15.
65. Orr Gandy KA, Obeid LM. Targeting the sphingosine kinase/sphingosine 1-phosphate pathway in disease: review of sphingosine kinase inhibitors. Biochim Biophys Acta 2013;1831:157–66.
66. Kappos L, Radue EW, O'Connor P, et al. A placebo-controlled trial of oral fingolimod in relapsing multiple sclerosis. N Engl J Med 2010;362:387–401.
67. Peyrin-Biroulet L, Christopher R, Trokan L, et al. Safety, pharmacokinetics and pharmacodynamics of etrasimod (APD334), an oral, selective S1P receptor modulator, after single dose escalation in healthy volunteers. 2016. Available at: https://www.ecco-ibd.eu/publications/congress-abstract-s/abstracts-2017/item/p369-safety-and-lymphocyte-lowering-properties-of-etrasimod-apd334-an-oral-potent-next-generation-selective-s1p-receptor-modulator-after-dose-escalation-in-healthy-volunteers-2.html. Accessed April 18, 2018.
68. O'Shea JJ, Plenge R. JAK and STAT signaling molecules in immunoregulation and immune-mediated disease. Immunity 2012;36:542–50.
69. Fleischmann R, Kremer J, Cush J, et al. Placebo-controlled trial of tofacitinib monotherapy in rheumatoid arthritis. N Engl J Med 2012;367:495–507.
70. Sandborn WJ, Ghosh S, Panes J, et al. Tofacitinib, an oral Janus kinase inhibitor, in active ulcerative colitis. N Engl J Med 2012;367:616–24.
71. Papp KA, Menter A, Strober B, et al. Efficacy and safety of tofacitinib, an oral Janus kinase inhibitor, in the treatment of psoriasis: a Phase 2b randomized placebo-controlled dose-ranging study. Br J Dermatol 2012;167:668–77.
72. Kremer AE, Namer B, Bolier R, et al. Pathogenesis and management of pruritus in PBC and PSC. Dig Dis 2015;33(Suppl 2):164–75.
73. Kremer AE, van Dijk R, Leckie P, et al. Serum autotaxin is increased in pruritus of cholestasis, but not of other origin, and responds to therapeutic interventions. Hepatology 2012;56:1391–400.

74. Hegade VS, Kendrick SF, Dobbins RL, et al. Effect of ileal bile acid transporter inhibitor GSK2330672 on pruritus in primary biliary cholangitis: a double-blind, randomised, placebo-controlled, crossover, phase 2a study. Lancet 2017;389: 1114–23.
75. Bernstein H, Bernstein C, Payne CM, et al. Bile acids as carcinogens in human gastrointestinal cancers. Mutat Res 2005;589:47–65.
76. Kisand KE, Metsküla K, Kisand KV, et al. The follow-up of asymptomatic persons with antibodies to pyruvate dehydrogenase in adult population samples. J Gastroenterol 2001;36:248–54.
77. Dahlqvist G, Gaouar F, Carrat F, et al. Large-scale characterization study of patients with antimitochondrial antibodies but nonestablished primary biliary cholangitis. Hepatology 2017;65:152–63.
78. Neuberger J, Portmann B, Macdougall BR, et al. Recurrence of primary biliary cirrhosis after liver transplantation. N Engl J Med 1982;306:1–4.
79. Bosch A, Dumortier J, Maucort-Boulch D, et al. Preventive administration of UDCA after liver transplantation for primary biliary cirrhosis is associated with a lower risk of disease recurrence. J Hepatol 2015;63:1449–58.
80. Charatcharoenwitthaya P, Pimentel S, Talwalkar JA, et al. Long-term survival and impact of ursodeoxycholic acid treatment for recurrent primary biliary cirrhosis after liver transplantation. Liver Transplant 2007;13:1236–45.
81. Carbone M, Mells GF, Alexander GJ, et al. Calcineurin inhibitors and the IL12A locus influence risk of recurrent primary biliary cirrhosis after liver transplantation. Am J Transplant 2013;13:1110–1.
82. Silveira MG, Gossard AA, Stahler AC, et al. A randomized, placebo-controlled clinical trial of efficacy and safety: modafinil in the treatment of fatigue in patients with primary biliary cirrhosis. Am J Ther 2017;24:e167–76.
83. Jopson L, Newton JL, Palmer J, et al. LBP-506-B-cell depleting therapy (rituximab) as a treatment for fatigue in primary biliary cholangitis: a randomised controlled trial (RITPBC). J Hepatol 2017;66:S96.
84. Clemente-Casares X, Blanco J, Ambalavanan P, et al. Expanding antigen-specific regulatory networks to treat autoimmunity. Nature 2016;530:434–40.
85. Ellebrecht CT, Bhoj VG, Nace A, et al. Reengineering chimeric antigen receptor T cells for targeted therapy of autoimmune disease. Science 2016;353:179–84.
86. Li F, Jiang C, Krausz KW, et al. Microbiome remodelling leads to inhibition of intestinal farnesoid X receptor signalling and decreased obesity. Nat Commun 2013;4:2384.
87. Tang R, Wei Y, Li Y, et al. Gut microbial profile is altered in primary biliary cholangitis and partially restored after UDCA therapy. Gut 2018;67(3):534–41.
88. Gopalakrishnan V, Spencer CN, Nezi L, et al. Gut microbiome modulates response to anti-PD-1 immunotherapy in melanoma patients. Science 2018; 359(6371):97–103.
89. Albers HM, Dong A, van Meeteren LA, et al. Boronic acid-based inhibitor of autotaxin reveals rapid turnover of LPA in the circulation. Proc Natl Acad Sci U S A 2010;107:7257–62.

Understanding and Treating Pruritus in Primary Biliary Cholangitis

Andres F. Carrion, MD[a],*, Jordan D. Rosen, BS[b], Cynthia Levy, MD[c]

KEYWORDS

- Cholestasis • Itch • Refractory • Intractable • Therapy

KEY POINTS

- Pruritus is reported by up to 80% of patients with primary biliary cholangitis (PBC) during long-term follow-up.
- Pathophysiological mechanisms of pruritus in PBC include the accumulation of pruritogenic bile acids and bile salts, modulation of itch pathways through autotaxin-lysophosphatidic acid, an imbalance between different types of receptors for endogenous opioids, and modulation of the perception of pruritus by serotonin and substance P.
- Bile acid–binding resins such as cholestyramine are first-line therapy. Rifampin has a large body of evidence supporting its efficacy as a second-line agent but it must be used cautiously due to risk of hepatotoxicity and multiple drug–drug interactions.
- Opioid antagonists and sertraline are useful alternatives.
- Invasive therapeutic strategies for patients with debilitating pruritus include plasmapheresis, nasobiliary drainage, and filtration using the molecular adsorbent recirculating system where available.

Primary biliary cholangitis (PBC) is the most common chronic cholestatic liver disease in adults in the United States and is characterized by inflammation targeting cholangiocytes of the interlobular and septal bile ducts.[1] Although most patients currently diagnosed with PBC are asymptomatic (60%), fatigue and pruritus are the most common symptoms reported over long-term follow-up. For instance, pruritus is only present in 19% of patients at the time of initial diagnosis of PBC but is reported by up to 80% of those followed up for 10 years after establishing the diagnosis.[2] The reported

The authors have nothing to disclose.
[a] Division of Gastroenterology and Hepatology, Texas Tech University Health Sciences Center, 4800 Alberta Avenue, El Paso, TX 79905, USA; [b] Department of Dermatology and Cutaneous Surgery, Miami Itch Center, University of Miami Miller School of Medicine, Miami, FL, USA; [c] Division of Hepatology, Schiff Center for Liver Diseases, University of Miami Miller School of Medicine, Miami, FL, USA
* Corresponding author. 4800 Alberta Avenue, El Paso, TX 79905.
E-mail address: a.carrion@ttuhsc.edu

Clin Liver Dis 22 (2018) 517–532
https://doi.org/10.1016/j.cld.2018.03.005
1089-3261/18/© 2018 Elsevier Inc. All rights reserved.

risk of developing pruritus in patients with untreated PBC without this symptom is 27% per year; however, the natural history of pruritus in PBC is highly variable and improvement or resolution may also occur in up to 23% of patients per year.[3]

Pruritus in PBC is characteristically generalized and intermittent; however, in some patients it may be persistent and occasionally even debilitating. It is usually more severe in the limbs, particularly in soles of feet and palms of hands; it is exacerbated by heat, pressure, or contact to wool. Similar to fatigue, the severity of pruritus does not correlate with histologic progression of PBC and may actually improve during advanced stages in certain patients. Circadian variation of the severity of pruritus is frequently reported, with worsening of this symptom in the late evenings and at night.[4]

PATHOPHYSIOLOGY OF PRURITUS IN PRIMARY BILIARY CHOLANGITIS

A brief review of the pathophysiology of pruritus in PBC is necessary to better understand currently available and investigational therapeutic options (**Table 1**). Transduction of an itch into neural signals begins with activation of a peripheral receptor. There are 2 major classes of peripheral itch receptors: transient receptor potential (TRP) and G protein-coupled receptors. Itch receptors can be found on unmyelinated peripheral neurons known as C-fibers, which can be subdivided into mechanoinsensitive histamine-responsive and mechanosensitive histamine-unresponsive subtypes. The ascending pruritic neural pathway can be summarized as follows: sensory itch signals

Table 1
Mechanisms of action of various therapeutic interventions for pruritus in pruritus in primary biliary cholangitis

Mechanism of Action	Agents	Comments
Interference with enterohepatic circulation of bile acids	Cholestyramine	First-line therapy
	Colesevelam	Not recommended for patients who previously failed cholestyramine
	Colestipol	No data on PBC
	Maralixibat	Investigational
	GSK2330672	Investigational
	Nasobiliary drainage	Invasive
PXR agonist, decreases LPA and autotaxin levels	Rifampin	Important drug–drug interactions
Endogenous opioid antagonists	Naltrexone	Possible opioid withdrawal symptoms
	Naloxone	Intravenous
	Nalfurafine hydrochloride	Available in Japan
Modulation of serotonin	Sertraline	Short-lasting effect
	Ondansetron	Short-lasting effect
Activation of PPAR-α	Bezafibrate	May also lead to normalization of alkaline phosphatase, although independently of its effect on pruritus
	Fenofibrate	
Substance P or NK-1 modulation	Aprepitant	Not enough data on PBC
Modulation of nonspecific nociceptive pathways	Dronabinol	Only 1 small case series reported efficacy

Abbreviations: LPA, lysophosphatidic acid; NK-1, neurokinin-1; PPAR, peroxisome proliferator-activated receptor; PXR, pregnane X receptor.

transmitted through these fibers traverse the dorsal root ganglia and synapse on second order neurons in the dorsal horn of the spinal cord. These secondary neurons cross to the contralateral side to project through the spinothalamic tract to the ventromedial nucleus of the thalamus and end at the primary sensory cortex, supplementary motor area, anterior cingulate cortex, and inferior parietal lobe (**Fig. 1**).[4] Itch receptors can be activated by a vast array of exogenous and endogenous mediators (see following discussion).

Bile Acids and Bile Salts

One of the initial theories about the pathophysiology of pruritus in PBC was centered on elevated plasma levels of pruritogenic bile acids and their accumulation in the skin. This hypothesis has been supported by studies demonstrating that direct injection of bile acids into the skin induces pruritus. However, the exact role of bile acids and bile salts in this context remains incompletely understood because some patients with PBC have no pruritus despite elevated levels of serum bile acids and there is a lack of correlation between concentrations of serum bile acids and the severity of pruritus. Data from recent animal studies provide important insights about specific signaling pathways associated with these molecules. Bile acids regulate multiple cell types by activating nuclear and plasma membrane receptors such as the farnesoid X receptor and the TGR5 receptor; the latter is expressed in neurons of the dorsal root ganglia and spinal cord. Studies in mice have demonstrated that bile acids activate TGR5 and Mas-related G protein-coupled receptors (Mrgprs), two important receptors in neural pathways that transmit itch. Both TGR5 and Mrgprs sensitize TRP ankyrin 1 (TRPA1) on sensory neurons, stimulating the release of neuropeptides that transmit itch sensation in the spinal cord.[5,6]

Lysophosphatidic Acid

In recent years, lysophosphatidic acid (LPA) has emerged as the most important mediator involved in PBC and cholestatic itch. LPA is a bioactive signaling phospholipid synthesized from lysophosphatidylcholine by the enzyme autotaxin, also known as lysophospholipase D.[4] A series of LPA receptors have been reported; however, these receptors have not yet been linked to pruritic pathways. LPA can also bind and activate the TRP vanilloid 1 (TRPV1), a capsaicin receptor that plays an important role in sensory transmission of itch and pain. Intradermal injection of LPA causes a dose-dependent scratching behavior in mice and induces pruritus in humans.[7] In patients with cholestasis and pruritus, autotaxin activity is significantly higher than in those with cholestasis without pruritus and autotaxin levels correlate with the severity of pruritus.[8] Furthermore, response to therapeutic interventions for pruritus (ie, bile acid–binding resins or rifampin) is associated with decreased serum autotaxin activity, thus supporting the role of autotaxin-LPA in the pathogenesis of pruritus in cholestasis.[9] Future research should focus on identifying factors associated with increased levels of autotaxin in PBC, and the exact receptors and pathways by which LPA induces pruritus.

Endogenous Opioids

Although pain and itch are often thought of as independent sensory pathways, the two are in fact interlinked. A series of inhibitory interneurons within the dorsal horn of the spinal cord presumably connect these two sensory pathways. The pruritic effects of opioids vary depending on the activity of opioid receptor subtypes. Endogenous opioids can activate mu-opioid receptors (MORs) to induce itch, whereas activation of kappa-opioid receptors (KORs) inhibit itch.[10] An imbalance between MOR

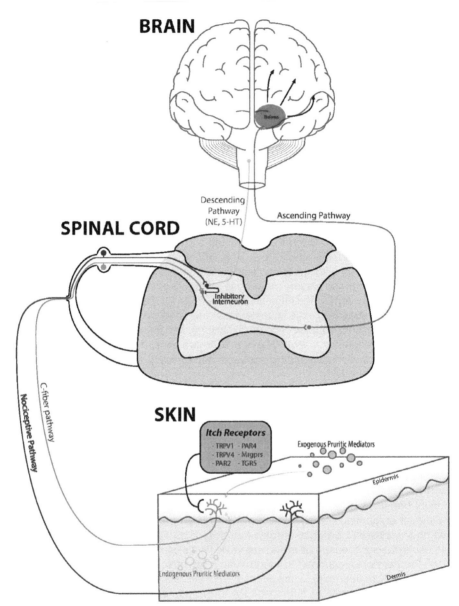

Fig. 1. Overview of the neural pathways of pruritus in PBC. In the epidermis of the skin, pruritic stimuli are transduced into neural signals by itch receptors located on C-fibers. Signals are transmitted on C-fibers from the skin to the dorsal horn of the spinal cord, where they synapse and activate secondary neurons. Secondary neurons decussate and synapse on other neurons, which ascend through the spinothalamic tract and eventually project to the thalamus. Activation of the descending or nociceptive pathway may activate inhibitory interneurons located in the dorsal horn of the spinal cord, inhibiting ascending transmission of pruritic neural signaling. 5-HT, 5-hydroxytryptamine; Mrgprs, Mas-related G protein-coupled receptors; PAR, proliferator-activated receptor; TRPV transient receptor potential vanilloid.

(overexpressed) and KOR (down-regulated) has been suggested in diseases associated with pruritus such as end-stage renal disease and cholestasis. As PBC progresses, hepatic clearance of endogenous opioids (methionine-enkephalin, leucine-enkephalin) declines with consequent increased levels. However, the severity of pruritus in PBC does not correlate with endogenous opioid levels. A recent publication examined two MORs: MOR1, which can induce analgesia independent of pruritus; and MOR1D, which is associated with analgesia and pruritus. The difference in opioid-induced pruritus between the two may stem from the association of MOR1D with gastrin-related protein receptor, an important molecular receptor involved in itch pathways in the central nervous system. It is unclear which MOR subtype is involved in pruritus in PBC; however, possible uncoupling of analgesia and pruritus through this mechanism could yield novel therapeutic options.[11]

Serotonin

Serotonin may be involved in both central regulation and the primary afferent response of pruritic stimuli. Inhibitory itch interneurons located in the spinal cord can be modulated centrally by descending serotonergic itch pathways originating in the medulla.[12] In the periphery, itch occurs with injection of serotonin into the skin of mice; however, its role in itch in humans remains unclear.[13] Furthermore, serotonin has been linked to TRPV4 found on C fibers.[14] Selective serotonin reuptake inhibitors have been shown to cause a mild reduction in pruritus of PBC; however, the concentration of serotonin has not been found to correlate with the severity of pruritus in PBC (see later discussion).[15]

Substance P

Primary afferent neurons release the neuropeptide substance P into the spinal cord in response to adverse stimuli such as itch, where it acts through the neurokinin-1 (NK-1) receptor and, possibly, Mrgprs.[16] In a study, subjects with chronic liver disease who also suffer from pruritus had concentrations of substance P twelve times higher than that of subjects not suffering from pruritus.[17] However, in primates, a model believed to respond to pruritogens similarly to humans, intraspinal administration of substance P was not found to correlate with itch.[18,19]

Nitric Oxide

The role of nitric oxide (NO) in pruritus in patients with PBC is heavily contested. NO is produced by NO synthase (NOS) from L-arginine. A variety of cellular processes, including the C-fiber itch pathway, involve NO. Interestingly, the pruritic effects of substance P can be blocked with pretreatment with NOS inhibitors.[20] Furthermore, NO has been implicated in the pathophysiology of many nonpruritic manifestations of cholestatic diseases (ie, cardiac complications).[21] That being said, the ubiquity and nonspecific association of NO with inflammation lowers the likelihood of NO playing an active role in pruritus experienced by patients with PBC.

TREATMENT OF PRURITUS IN PRIMARY BILIARY CHOLANGITIS

Pruritus is a characteristic symptom of PBC that adversely affects patients' quality of life; thus, it deserves an aggressive and systematic therapeutic approach that can be individualized (**Fig. 2**).[22] Treatment of PBC with ursodeoxycholic acid (UDCA) has not been conclusively associated with improvement or worsening of pruritus in PBC; in contrast, obeticholic acid (OCA) is associated with dose-dependent increases in the incidence and exacerbation of pruritus.[23–25]

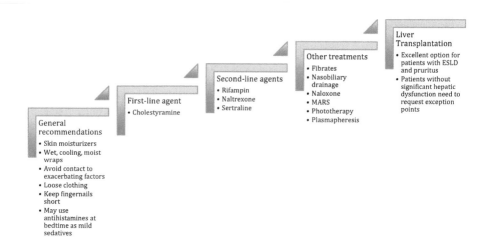

Fig. 2. Stepwise approach to treatment of pruritus in PBC. ESLD, end-stage liver disease; MARS, molecular adsorbent recirculation system.

General Recommendations

The use of skin moisturizers or other topical interventions, such as wet, cooling, or moist wraps, as well as topical agents, such as camphor or menthol, are of unproven efficacy in improving pruritus in PBC. However, most clinicians recommend these interventions as front-line therapies mainly because of easy access, affordability, and lack of significant adverse events (AEs) in an overwhelming number of cases. In addition, the authors recommend using loose clothing, avoiding wool, and trimming fingernails to minimize excoriations. Most patients derive some benefit from these interventions.

Antihistamine agents are also commonly prescribed, although their efficacy in PBC remains controversial.[26] Most of the benefit achieved by antihistamine agents is thought to be related to their sedative effects rather than control of itch; thus, use of these agents should be reserved for patients with significant nocturnal pruritus.[27] Exacerbation of sicca symptoms, commonly present in patients with PBC, is an expected side effect of antihistamine agents and may limit their use. Additionally, impaired metabolism of some of these agents in the setting of hepatic dysfunction may significantly impair drug elimination and increase their half-life.[28,29]

First-Line Pharmacotherapy

Bile acid–binding resins

Bile acid–binding resins are currently endorsed by guidelines as first-line therapy for pruritus in PBC based on extensive clinical experience and a favorable safety profile.[30,31] Bile acid–binding resins currently available in the United States include cholestyramine, colestipol, and colesevelam; however, cholestyramine is the only one licensed for treatment of pruritus in cholestasis. Pruritus usually improves within 4 to 11 days. Importantly, bile acid–binding resins may reduce absorption of other medications, thus other drugs should not be administered within the window of 2 to 4 hours before or after. This is especially important when timing the administration of UDCA and/or OCA to avoid a negative impact on their efficacy.

Cholestyramine is a nonabsorbable anion exchange resin licensed for the treatment of hypercholesterolemia and cholestatic pruritus. This agent was first reported to treat pruritus in PBC more than half century ago, and its efficacy and safety have been corroborated by subsequent trials, although rigorously designed and well-conducted randomized trials are lacking.[32–34] The recommended dose of cholestyramine for treatment of pruritus in PBC is 4 g orally up to 4 times a day (maximum 16 g/day). To help minimize side effects, particularly gastrointestinal effects such as nausea, bloating, and/or constipation, the authors recommend starting therapy at lower doses (ie, 2 g orally up to 4 times a day) and progressively increasing the dose over subsequent days or weeks as tolerated and as needed. A bedtime dose may help patients sleep through the night and reduce complaints about side effects. In addition to side effects, poor compliance with this agent may also be due to its taste, which can sometimes be masked by mixing it with flavored juices.[31]

Colesevelam has significantly higher bile acid–binding capacity and a more favorable side effect profile than cholestyramine; however, this agent is only licensed in the United States for treatment of hypercholesterolemia and type 2 diabetes mellitus; thus, its use for treatment of pruritus is off-label. Results from a randomized, placebo-controlled trial evaluating the efficacy and safety of colesevelam for treatment of refractory pruritus in cholestatic liver diseases (mainly PBC and primary sclerosing cholangitis) demonstrated no significant differences between the groups with respect to reduction in pruritus scores or cutaneous scratch lesions, or improvement in quality of life.[35] Importantly, these negative results might have been due to selection of subjects who previously failed to respond to cholestyramine. The efficacy of colesevelam in patients who are naïve to bile acid–binding resins remains uncertain.

Second-Line Pharmacotherapy

Several agents can be used as second-line therapy for treatment of pruritus in PBC not responding to bile acid–binding resins.

Rifampin

Rifampin (also known as rifampicin) is a heterocyclic antibiotic primarily used for treatment of mycobacterial infections but can be used off-label as a second-line therapy in patients with PBC whose pruritus does not respond to or cannot tolerate bile acid–binding resins.[36,37] This agent was initially studied for treatment of pruritus in PBC almost three decades ago and its efficacy in this setting has been corroborated by subsequent studies and two meta-analyses.[36,38–40]

The mechanism by which rifampin ameliorates pruritus in PBC is largely unknown but may be through enhancement of the mixed function oxidase system, leading to an increase in the rate of bile acid metabolism and excretion, and/or competition for hepatic bile acid uptake. The latter may lead to an increase in serum bilirubin levels in some patients and, in rare cases, severe hepatotoxicity. Rifampin can also activate pregnane X receptor and lead to a decrease in autotaxin levels (the enzyme involved in LPA synthesis).[41]

The recommended starting dose for treatment of pruritus in PBC is 150 mg orally daily or twice daily, which can be cautiously escalated to a maximum of 600 mg/day in divided doses based on clinical need and absence of signs of hepatotoxicity. The average time to effect is approximately 2 days.

Rifampin is associated with minor transient and asymptomatic elevations in serum aminotransferases and bilirubin levels in 10% to 20% of individuals without liver disease treated with this agent for infections. Generally, these abnormalities do not require dose adjustments or discontinuation of this agent. Elevations in serum bilirubin levels (more commonly total and indirect bilirubin) usually occur during the first few days of therapy and are typically followed by a decrease to below baseline in individuals without liver disease. However, marked elevations of the total and direct bilirubin may occur within few weeks of starting therapy in individuals with significant underlying liver disease, particularly cirrhosis, as well as in those with mutations in the hepatic canalicular multidrug resistance-associated protein 2, also known as adenosine triphosphate (ATP)-binding cassette subfamily C member 2 involved in biliary transport.[42] Importantly, most patients who develop hepatotoxicity usually do so during the first 2 months of therapy; thus, close monitoring is advised during this period.[43] Continuation of rifampin therapy after development of elevation of aminotransferases can lead to progressive and severe hepatic dysfunction.[43] Many patients choose not to use rifampin when told about the possibility of hepatotoxicity; however, when used, this drug has an impressive and rapid effect on pruritus.

Rifampin can affect vitamin K metabolism, thus leading to prolongation of the prothrombin time (and the international normalized ratio).[44] Important interactions with numerous other medications may occur in patients taking rifampin, mainly through its effects as a potent inducer of cytochrome P450 (CYP) isoenzymes (particularly CYP3A4), as well as induction of uridine 5'-diphospho-glucuronosyltransferase (UDP)-glucuronosyltransferase 1A (UGT1A) and P-glycoprotein expression.[45] Of note, there are no predicted interactions between rifampin and UDCA or OCA.

Reddish-orange discoloration of urine, tears, and other body secretions is expected during treatment with rifampin and patients and caregivers must be alerted before starting therapy. Additional common side effects occurring in patients treated with rifampin may include gastrointestinal effects such as nausea, vomiting, diarrhea, and abdominal pain. Less common but serious reactions, including hemolytic anemia, leukopenia and agranulocytosis, thrombocytopenia, renal impairment, severe dermatologic reactions, and anaphylaxis, have been reported.[45–47]

Opioid antagonists

Opioid receptor blockers such as naltrexone can offer an additional effective option for treatment of pruritus in PBC.[30,31,45–48] Naloxone is only available in intravenous formulation; thus, its use in PBC is significantly limited, although continuous infusion of this agent results in amelioration of pruritus and can be considered for selected hospitalized patients with pruritus refractory to other pharmacologic agents.[49] Nalmefene is a long-acting oral opioid antagonist not currently available outside research protocols. Scarce data support its efficacy in treating pruritus in PBC.[50,51]

In patients with PBC, blockade of MORs with naltrexone can also ameliorate pruritus.[52,53] The efficacy of naltrexone for control of pruritus in PBC was demonstrated in two small randomized controlled trials.[53,54] Furthermore, an observational series reported that 93% of subjects with pruritus refractory to cholestyramine and/or rifampin had a significant clinical response during treatment with naltrexone.[55] This agent is usually started at a dose of 12.5 to 25 mg orally daily. Progressive dose escalation to a maximum of 50 mg orally daily may be needed based on clinical response.[30,31,56]

Regardless of which opioid antagonist is used, patients with PBC may experience opioid withdrawal symptoms with initiation of therapy, including nausea, adrenergic signs and symptoms, colicky abdominal pain, and anorexia due to high levels of endogenous circulating opioids.[57] These symptoms are usually self-limited and last no longer than 2 to 3 days in most cases.[54] Importantly, patients with underlying chronic painful conditions (ie, postherpetic neuralgia) may experience uncontrolled pain following initiation of therapy with opioid antagonists.[55]

Modulators of serotoninergic pathways

Sertraline is a selective serotonin reuptake inhibitor licensed for several psychiatric indications that has demonstrated efficacy in improving pruritus in PBC in few small studies.[15,58] Importantly, improvement in pruritus associated with this agent seems to be independent of improvement of depression.[58] The recommended dose of sertraline for treatment of pruritus in PBC is 75 to 100 mg orally daily (off-label use). Dose reduction by 50% is recommended for patients with hepatic dysfunction. This agent is usually well tolerated; however, insomnia, diarrhea, and visual hallucinations have been reported as AEs and increased mood stability as a beneficial effect.[58] Serotonin syndrome may occur in patients treated with sertraline and its severity varies widely from benign to life-threating. Classic clinical manifestations include mental status changes, autonomic hyperactivity, and neuromuscular abnormalities. This syndrome may occur at therapeutic doses or with drug overdose, as well as in the setting of drug–drug interactions. Antidepressant discontinuation syndrome has also been described in patients abruptly stopping selective serotonin reuptake inhibitors and manifests clinically with flu-like symptoms, insomnia, nausea, sensory disturbances, and hyperarousal. Serotonin syndrome requires prompt discontinuation of the implicated agent and, occasionally, administration of serotonin antagonists and/or pharmacologic sedation, whereas discontinuation syndrome rapidly improves following reinstitution of the selective serotonin reuptake inhibitor.[59,60]

Ondansetron selectively antagonizes 5-hydroxytryptamine 3 receptors and was evaluated for treatment of pruritus in PBC in few studies following an initial report of a single patient experiencing complete relief from pruritus due to PBC within 30 minutes of administration of 8 mg intravenously, with the effect lasting 4 hours.[61] Subsequent studies, including a randomized placebo-controlled trial, demonstrated a small but significant benefit of ondansetron in improving pruritus in PBC.[62,63]

Modulation of other itch pathways

The antiemetic aprepitant is a substance P or NK-1 antagonist that was studied for the treatment of pruritus in an open-label study including 20 subjects; however, only 1 subject had pruritus due to hepatic causes. Following a median treatment duration of one week with aprepitant 80 mg orally daily, 80% of subjects experienced significant improvement of pruritus.[64] Although aprepitant may have a role in treatment of cholestatic pruritus based on pathophysiologic mechanisms that include release of substance P and its interaction with NK-1 receptors in response to stimuli such as itch, further trials focusing on pruritus in PBC are needed before conclusions about its efficacy in this population can be assumed.

Invasive Therapeutic Strategies for Removal of Pruritogenic Substances

Nasobiliary drainage through endoscopic retrograde cholangiopancreatography (ERCP) alters the enterohepatic circulation by diverting bile and bile salts away from the ileum.[65] The efficacy and safety of this intervention for treatment of refractory pruritus in subjects with cholestatic diseases was assessed in a small retrospective study (12 out of 27 subjects had PBC). Nasobiliary drainage for a median duration of 7 days resulted in reduction of pruritus in 90% and complete resolution of this symptom in 41% of subjects; 33% of subjects were free of pruritus within 24 hours. The median duration of treatment response for subjects with PBC was 13 days. AEs occurred commonly (34%), mainly following ERCP and placement of the nasobiliary drain, with nonsevere post-ERCP pancreatitis being the most common (31%).[66]

Plasmapheresis, also known as therapeutic plasma exchange, entails separation of the blood, exchange of plasma (either with albumin or donor fresh frozen plasma), and return of blood components to the patient through a multilumen central venous catheter. This intervention was studied in 17 subjects with pruritus unresponsive to cholestyramine and rifampin. Improvement of pruritus was noted following plasmapheresis compared with baseline and no significant worsening of pruritus occurred after 30 days; and, although increased pruritus was noted at 90 days of follow-up, scores on the numerical rating scale were still significantly lower compared with baseline. The median number of admissions per subject was 2, with a mean time in between admissions of 9.8 months and 2 to 4 plasmapheresis performed during each admission. The main reported AE was difficulty inserting the central venous catheter in 2 subjects.[67]

In the largest series published to date, the molecular adsorbent recirculating system (MARS) improved pruritus refractory to medical therapies such as bile acid–binding resins, rifampin, or naltrexone in 19 of 20 subjects with PBC treated with an average of 2.2 sessions and 15.7 hours per subject. Overall, pruritus improvement was satisfactory in 75% of treated subjects. The beneficial effects of MARS on pruritus in PBC may be due to marked reductions of circulating bile acids that occur immediately after treatment and persist up to 30 days. In addition, reduction in serum levels of autotaxin were noted and correlated with improvement in itching.[68]

Liver Transplantation

End-stage liver disease due to PBC is currently a relatively uncommon indication for liver transplantation (LT) in the United States, mainly because of early diagnosis and widespread use of UDCA. Whether LT should be considered for patients with less severe hepatic dysfunction but debilitating symptoms such as intractable pruritus remains controversial; however, LT rapidly improves cholestatic pruritus and is associated with increased quality of life. Furthermore, how to include these patients in the current organ allocation system, which follows an urgency-based model by using the model for end-stage liver disease (MELD) score for prioritization, remains an ongoing challenge. Under this organ allocation scheme, patients with PBC and intractable pruritus but without severe hepatic dysfunction have no prospect of undergoing transplantation unless living donor LT is available or exception points are granted by regional review boards. Exception points for intractable pruritus in PBC may be granted on an individual basis by regional review boards; however, this is not a standard indication for exception points. Furthermore, practices related to exception points vary widely from region to region.[69,70]

Investigational Agents and Therapies for Treatment of Pruritus in Primary Biliary Cholangitis

Fibrates

Fibrates are agonists of peroxisome proliferator-activated receptors alpha and recent data suggest a beneficial therapeutic effect on pruritus.[71,72] Bezafibrate improved or completely resolved pruritus in most subjects (25 out of 26) with PBC and pruritus at baseline treated with this agent because of suboptimal biochemical response of PBC to UDCA. Furthermore, discontinuation of bezafibrate following improvement or resolution of pruritus during therapy led to exacerbation or recurrence of this symptom in all subjects (median time 10 weeks) with subsequent improvement or resolution after therapy was resumed. Importantly, the effect of bezafibrate on pruritus seems to be independent of alkaline phosphatase response. AEs during treatment were uncommon and included myalgia without elevation of muscle enzymes and gastrointestinal discomfort.[71]

Phototherapy

Phototherapy with ultraviolet (UV) light B has been studied for more than 3 decades as a therapeutic approach for pruritus refractory to pharmacologic interventions. The initial publication of UV light for treatment of pruritus in PBC reported that 5 out of 6 subjects responded favorably to this therapy.[73] However, to this date, data about the efficacy and safety of UV light therapy for pruritus in PBC remain largely confined to case reports and 1 small case series.[74–76] Because pruritus in PBC follows a specific circadian pattern (worse at night and improved during the daytime), efficacy of bright-light therapy reflected toward the eyes using fluorescent bulbs emitting full-spectrum light (an established therapy for seasonal affective disorder) was assessed in a pilot study but demonstrated nonstatistically significant improvement in pruritus.[77]

Nalfurafine hydrochloride
Nalfurafine hydrochloride is a KOR agonist currently licensed in Japan for treatment of uremic pruritus. This agent was recently evaluated for treatment of pruritus related to chronic liver diseases in a small open-label trial (11 out of 18 subjects had PBC). Complete resolution of pruritus occurred in 7 out of 18 subjects and improvement of this symptom was reported in all subjects treated with nalfurafine hydrochloride 2.5 µg orally daily.[78] Results from a recently published randomized, placebo-controlled trial corroborate the efficacy of this agent for treatment of pruritus in PBC. This trial, in which 60 out of 214 subjects had PBC, evaluated the efficacy and safety of 2 doses of nalfurafine hydrochloride, 2.5 and 5 µg orally daily. Improvement of pruritus was documented in both treatment arms compared with placebo, with no significant differences between the two doses of nalfurafine hydrochloride. When data were analyzed according to the cause of liver disease, only nalfurafine hydrochloride 2.5 µg orally daily showed a significant reduction in pruritus compared with placebo.[79] Reported AEs occurred more commonly in subjects treated with nalfurafine hydrochloride versus placebo, without significant difference between the 2.5 µg and 5 µg doses. The most common AEs were increased serum prolactin levels, urinary frequency, insomnia, somnolence, and constipation.[79]

Delta-9-tetrahydrocannabinol
Delta-9-tetrahydrocannabinol is the active substance in cannabis (marijuana) and the prescription drug dronabinol and has well-established effects on modulation of nociceptive pathways.[80] A small case series reported the use of dronabinol in 3 subjects with refractory pruritus due to PBC at a dose of 5 mg orally thrice daily with complete resolution of pruritus.[81]

Ileal apical sodium bile acid transporter inhibitors
Ileal apical sodium bile acid transporter (ASBT) inhibitors are a new class of agents under investigation for treatment of pruritus in PBC. ASBT is a brush border membrane glycoprotein primarily expressed in the distal ileum and responsible for reabsorption of bile acids and maintenance of the enterohepatic circulation, which is upregulated in cholestatic liver diseases.[82,83] ASBT inhibitors under investigation for treatment of pruritus in PBC include maralixibat and GSK2330672.[84–86]

Maralixibat was recently studied in a phase 2 randomized, placebo-controlled trial (NCT01904058) aimed at evaluating the efficacy (changes from baseline in pruritus) and safety of this agent in subjects with PBC. Similar to bile acid–binding resins, this agent also targets the enterohepatic circulation of bile acids but at a cellular rather than endoluminal (absorptive) level. Recent data demonstrated no significant differences in reduction of pruritus compared with baseline after 13 weeks of treatment with maralixibat compared with placebo. AEs were common in subjects treated with maralixibat, with diarrhea reported in 62% and abdominal pain in 24% of subjects (including 2 subjects who discontinued treatment due to these AEs).[84]

The efficacy and safety of GSK2330672 for treatment of pruritus in PBC was evaluated in a phase 2a randomized placebo-controlled crossover trial. Compared with placebo, GSK2330672 demonstrated significantly greater reductions from baseline in subjects' experience of pruritus as measured by validated scales, as well as greater reductions of conjugated bile acids. The overall frequency of reported AEs was comparable in the GSK2330672 and placebo groups (81%) but diarrhea (33%) and abdominal pain (14%) occurred more commonly in the GSK2330672 group.[86]

SUMMARY

Pruritus is extremely common in PBC and its severity can vary from mild to debilitating. Tricks of the trade used by experienced clinicians for treatment of severe pruritus include emphasizing conservative measures, combining agents with different mechanisms of action and using (albeit rarely) invasive and/or experimental interventions. Therapies that have demonstrated efficacy in case series, observational, or open-label studies should undergo further evaluation in well-designed randomized clinical trials; however, these can be considered on an individual basis for patients with intractable pruritus refractory to other established interventions.

REFERENCES

1. Carey EJ, Ali AH, Lindor KD. Primary biliary cirrhosis. Lancet 2015;386(10003): 1565–75.
2. Prince M, Chetwynd A, Newman W, et al. Survival and symptom progression in a geographically based cohort of patients with primary biliary cirrhosis: follow-up for up to 28 years. Gastroenterology 2002;123(4):1044–51.
3. Talwalkar JA, Souto E, Jorgensen RA, et al. Natural history of pruritus in primary biliary cirrhosis. Clin Gastroenterol Hepatol 2003;1(4):297–302.
4. Beuers U, Kremer AE, Bolier R, et al. Pruritus in cholestasis: facts and fiction. Hepatology 2014;60(1):399–407.
5. Alemi F, Kwon E, Poole DP, et al. The TGR5 receptor mediates bile acid-induced itch and analgesia. J Clin Invest 2013;123(4):1513–30.
6. Lieu T, Jayaweera G, Zhao P, et al. The bile acid receptor TGR5 activates the TRPA1 channel to induce itch in mice. Gastroenterology 2014;147(6):1417–28.
7. Kremer AE, Namer B, Bolier R, et al. Pathogenesis and management of pruritus in PBC and PSC. Dig Dis 2015;33(Suppl 2):164–75.
8. Kittaka H, Uchida K, Fukuta N, et al. Lysophosphatidic acid-induced itch is mediated by signalling of LPA5 receptor, phospholipase D and TRPA1/TRPV1. J Physiol 2017;595(8):2681–98.
9. Kremer AE, van Dijk R, Leckie P, et al. Serum autotaxin is increased in pruritus of cholestasis, but not of other origin, and responds to therapeutic interventions. Hepatology 2012;56(4):1391–400.
10. Tajiri K, Shimizu Y. Recent advances in the management of pruritus in chronic liver diseases. World J Gastroenterol 2017;23(19):3418–26.
11. Liu XY, Liu ZC, Sun YG, et al. Unidirectional cross-activation of GRPR by MOR1D uncouples itch and analgesia induced by opioids. Cell 2011;147(2):447–58.
12. Carstens E, Akiyama T. Central mechanisms of itch. Curr Probl Dermatol 2016;50: 11–7.
13. Yamaguchi T, Nagasawa T, Satoh M, et al. Itch-associated response induced by intradermal serotonin through 5-HT2 receptors in mice. Neurosci Res 1999;35(2): 77–83.
14. Akiyama T, Ivanov M, Nagamine M, et al. Involvement of TRPV4 in serotonin-evoked scratching. J Invest Dermatol 2016;136(1):154–60.

15. Browning J, Combes B, Mayo MJ. Long-term efficacy of sertraline as a treatment for cholestatic pruritus in patients with primary biliary cirrhosis. Am J Gastroenterol 2003;98(12):2736–41.
16. Azimi E, Reddy VB, Pereira PJS, et al. Substance P activates mas-related G protein-coupled receptors to induce itch. J Allergy Clin Immunol 2017;140(2): 447–53.e3.
17. Trivedi M, Bergasa NV. Serum concentrations of substance P in cholestasis. Ann Hepatol 2010;9(2):177–80.
18. Ko MC, Naughton NN. Antinociceptive effects of nociceptin/orphanin FQ administered intrathecally in monkeys. J Pain 2009;10(5):509–16.
19. Ding H, Hayashida K, Suto T, et al. Supraspinal actions of nociceptin/orphanin FQ, morphine and substance P in regulating pain and itch in non-human primates. Br J Pharmacol 2015;172(13):3302–12.
20. Ostadhadi S, Foroutan A, Momeny M, et al. Evidence for the involvement of nitric oxide in cholestasis-induced itch associated response in mice. Biomed Pharmacother 2016;84:1367–74.
21. Nahavandi A, Dehpour AR, Mani AR, et al. The role of nitric oxide in bradycardia of rats with obstructive cholestasis. Eur J Pharmacol 2001;411(1–2):135–41.
22. Mells GF, Pells G, Newton JL, et al. Impact of primary biliary cirrhosis on perceived quality of life: the UK-PBC national study. Hepatology 2013;58(1): 273–83.
23. Carbone M, Mells GF, Pells G, et al. Sex and age are determinants of the clinical phenotype of primary biliary cirrhosis and response to ursodeoxycholic acid. Gastroenterology 2013;144(3):560–9.e7 [quiz: e513–64].
24. Gong Y, Huang Z, Christensen E, et al. Ursodeoxycholic acid for patients with primary biliary cirrhosis: an updated systematic review and meta-analysis of randomized clinical trials using Bayesian approach as sensitivity analyses. Am J Gastroenterol 2007;102(8):1799–807.
25. Nevens F, Andreone P, Mazzella G, et al. A placebo-controlled trial of obeticholic acid in primary biliary cholangitis. N Engl J Med 2016;375(7):631–43.
26. Verma A, Jazrawi RP, Ahmed HA, et al. Prescribing habits in primary biliary cirrhosis: a national survey. Eur J Gastroenterol Hepatol 1999;11(8):817–20.
27. Rishe E, Azarm A, Bergasa NV. Itch in primary biliary cirrhosis: a patients' perspective. Acta Derm Venereol 2008;88(1):34–7.
28. Simons FE, Watson WT, Minuk GY, et al. Cetirizine pharmacokinetics and pharmacodynamics in primary biliary cirrhosis. J Clin Pharmacol 1993;33(10):949–54.
29. Simons FE, Watson WT, Chen XY, et al. The pharmacokinetics and pharmacodynamics of hydroxyzine in patients with primary biliary cirrhosis. J Clin Pharmacol 1989;29(9):809–15.
30. Lindor KD, Gershwin ME, Poupon R, et al. Primary biliary cirrhosis. Hepatology 2009;50(1):291–308.
31. European Association for the Study of the Liver. Electronic address: easloffice@easloffice.eu, European Association for the Study of the Liver. EASL clinical practice guidelines: the diagnosis and management of patients with primary biliary cholangitis. J Hepatol 2017;67(1):145–72.
32. Van Itallie TB, Hashim SA, Crampton RS, et al. The treatment of pruritus and hypercholesteremia of primary biliary cirrhosis with cholestyramine. N Engl J Med 1961;265:469–74.
33. Datta DV, Sherlock S. Cholestyramine for long term relief of the pruritus complicating intrahepatic cholestasis. Gastroenterology 1966;50(3):323–32.

34. Carey JB Jr, Williams G. Relief of the pruritus of jaundice with a bile-acid sequestering resin. JAMA 1961;176:432–5.

35. Kuiper EM, van Erpecum KJ, Beuers U, et al. The potent bile acid sequestrant colesevelam is not effective in cholestatic pruritus: results of a double-blind, randomized, placebo-controlled trial. Hepatology 2010;52(4):1334–40.

36. Ghent CN, Carruthers SG. Treatment of pruritus in primary biliary cirrhosis with rifampin. Results of a double-blind, crossover, randomized trial. Gastroenterology 1988;94(2):488–93.

37. Podesta A, Lopez P, Terg R, et al. Treatment of pruritus of primary biliary cirrhosis with rifampin. Dig Dis Sci 1991;36(2):216–20.

38. Bachs L, Pares A, Elena M, et al. Effects of long-term rifampicin administration in primary biliary cirrhosis. Gastroenterology 1992;102(6):2077–80.

39. Khurana S, Singh P. Rifampin is safe for treatment of pruritus due to chronic cholestasis: a meta-analysis of prospective randomized-controlled trials. Liver Int 2006;26(8):943–8.

40. Tandon P, Rowe BH, Vandermeer B, et al. The efficacy and safety of bile acid binding agents, opioid antagonists, or rifampin in the treatment of cholestasis-associated pruritus. Am J Gastroenterol 2007;102(7):1528–36.

41. Bolier R, Oude Elferink RP, Beuers U. Advances in pathogenesis and treatment of pruritus. Clin Liver Dis 2013;17(2):319–29.

42. Tocchetti GN, Rigalli JP, Arana MR, et al. Modulation of expression and activity of intestinal multidrug resistance-associated protein 2 by xenobiotics. Toxicol Appl Pharmacol 2016;303:45–57.

43. Prince MI, Burt AD, Jones DE. Hepatitis and liver dysfunction with rifampicin therapy for pruritus in primary biliary cirrhosis. Gut 2002;50(3):436–9.

44. Sampaziotis F, Griffiths WJ. Severe coagulopathy caused by rifampicin in patients with primary sclerosing cholangitis and refractory pruritus. Br J Clin Pharmacol 2012;73(5):826–7.

45. Chen J, Raymond K. Roles of rifampicin in drug-drug interactions: underlying molecular mechanisms involving the nuclear pregnane X receptor. Ann Clin Microbiol Antimicrob 2006;5:3.

46. Okano M, Kitano Y, Igarashi T. Toxic epidermal necrolysis due to rifampicin. J Am Acad Dermatol 1987;17(2 Pt 1):303–4.

47. Nyirenda R, Gill GV. Stevens-Johnson syndrome due to rifampicin. Br Med J 1977;2(6096):1189.

48. Jones EA, Bergasa NV. The pruritus of cholestasis. Hepatology 1999;29(4):1003–6.

49. Bergasa NV, Alling DW, Talbot TL, et al. Effects of naloxone infusions in patients with the pruritus of cholestasis. A double-blind, randomized, controlled trial. Ann Intern Med 1995;123(3):161–7.

50. Bergasa NV, Alling DW, Talbot TL, et al. Oral nalmefene therapy reduces scratching activity due to the pruritus of cholestasis: a controlled study. J Am Acad Dermatol 1999;41(3 Pt 1):431–4.

51. Bergasa NV, Schmitt JM, Talbot TL, et al. Open-label trial of oral nalmefene therapy for the pruritus of cholestasis. Hepatology 1998;27(3):679–84.

52. Pongcharoen P, Fleischer AB Jr. An evidence-based review of systemic treatments for itch. Eur J Pain 2016;20(1):24–31.

53. Wolfhagen FH, Sternieri E, Hop WC, et al. Oral naltrexone treatment for cholestatic pruritus: a double-blind, placebo-controlled study. Gastroenterology 1997;113(4):1264–9.

54. Terg R, Coronel E, Sorda J, et al. Efficacy and safety of oral naltrexone treatment for pruritus of cholestasis, a crossover, double blind, placebo-controlled study. J Hepatol 2002;37(6):717–22.
55. McRae CA, Prince MI, Hudson M, et al. Pain as a complication of use of opiate antagonists for symptom control in cholestasis. Gastroenterology 2003;125(2): 591–6.
56. European Association for the Study of the Liver. EASL clinical practice guidelines: management of cholestatic liver diseases. J Hepatol 2009;51(2):237–67.
57. Jones EA, Dekker LR. Florid opioid withdrawal-like reaction precipitated by naltrexone in a patient with chronic cholestasis. Gastroenterology 2000;118(2): 431–2.
58. Mayo MJ, Handem I, Saldana S, et al. Sertraline as a first-line treatment for cholestatic pruritus. Hepatology 2007;45(3):666–74.
59. Shelton RC. The nature of the discontinuation syndrome associated with antidepressant drugs. J Clin Psychiatry 2006;67(Suppl 4):3–7.
60. Wang RZ, Vashistha V, Kaur S, et al. Serotonin syndrome: preventing, recognizing, and treating it. Cleve Clin J Med 2016;83(11):810–7.
61. Schworer H, Ramadori G. Improvement of cholestatic pruritus by ondansetron. Lancet 1993;341(8855):1277.
62. Jones EA, Molenaar HA, Oosting J. Ondansetron and pruritus in chronic liver disease: a controlled study. Hepatogastroenterology 2007;54(76):1196–9.
63. Muller C, Pongratz S, Pidlich J, et al. Treatment of pruritus in chronic liver disease with the 5-hydroxytryptamine receptor type 3 antagonist ondansetron: a randomized, placebo-controlled, double-blind cross-over trial. Eur J Gastroenterol Hepatol 1998;10(10):865–70.
64. Stander S, Siepmann D, Herrgott I, et al. Targeting the neurokinin receptor 1 with aprepitant: a novel antipruritic strategy. PLoS One 2010;5(6):e10968.
65. Hofmann AF, Huet PM. Nasobiliary drainage for cholestatic pruritus. Hepatology 2006;43(5):1170–1.
66. Hegade VS, Krawczyk M, Kremer AE, et al. The safety and efficacy of nasobiliary drainage in the treatment of refractory cholestatic pruritus: a multicentre European study. Aliment Pharmacol Ther 2016;43(2):294–302.
67. Krawczyk M, Liebe R, Wasilewicz M, et al. Plasmapheresis exerts a long-lasting antipruritic effect in severe cholestatic itch. Liver Int 2017;37(5):743–7.
68. Pares A, Herrera M, Aviles J, et al. Treatment of resistant pruritus from cholestasis with albumin dialysis: combined analysis of patients from three centers. J Hepatol 2010;53(2):307–12.
69. Argo CK, Stukenborg GJ, Schmitt TM, et al. Regional variability in symptom-based MELD exceptions: a response to organ shortage? Am J Transplant 2011;11(11):2353–61.
70. Khungar V, Goldberg DS. Liver transplantation for cholestatic liver diseases in adults. Clin Liver Dis 2016;20(1):191–203.
71. Reig A, Sese P, Pares A. Effects of bezafibrate on outcome and pruritus in primary biliary cholangitis with suboptimal ursodeoxycholic acid response. Am J Gastroenterol 2018;113(1):49–55.
72. Corpechot C, Chazouilleres O, Rousseau D, et al. A 2-year multicenter, double-blind, randomized, placebo-controlled study of bezafibrate for the treatment of primary biliary cholangitis in patients with inadequate biochemical response to ursodeoxycholic acid therapy (Bezurso). J Hepatol 2017;66(1):S89.
73. Hanid MA, Levi AJ. Phototherapy for pruritus in primary biliary cirrhosis. Lancet 1980;2(8193):530.

74. Pinheiro NC, Marinho RT, Ramalho F, et al. Refractory pruritus in primary biliary cirrhosis. BMJ Case Rep 2013;2013 [pii:bcr2013200634].

75. Cerio R, Murphy GM, Sladen GE, et al. A combination of phototherapy and cholestyramine for the relief of pruritus in primary biliary cirrhosis. Br J Dermatol 1987; 116(2):265–7.

76. Decock S, Roelandts R, Steenbergen WV, et al. Cholestasis-induced pruritus treated with ultraviolet B phototherapy: an observational case series study. J Hepatol 2012;57(3):637–41.

77. Bergasa NV, Link MJ, Keogh M, et al. Pilot study of bright-light therapy reflected toward the eyes for the pruritus of chronic liver disease. Am J Gastroenterol 2001; 96(5):1563–70.

78. Kamimura K, Yokoo T, Kamimura H, et al. Long-term efficacy and safety of nalfurafine hydrochloride on pruritus in chronic liver disease patients: patient-reported outcome based analyses. PLoS One 2017;12(6):e0178991.

79. Kumada H, Miyakawa H, Muramatsu T, et al. Efficacy of nalfurafine hydrochloride in patients with chronic liver disease with refractory pruritus: a randomized, double-blind trial. Hepatol Res 2017;47(10):972–82.

80. Maione S, Costa B, Di Marzo V. Endocannabinoids: a unique opportunity to develop multitarget analgesics. Pain 2013;154(Suppl 1):S87–93.

81. Neff GW, O'Brien CB, Reddy KR, et al. Preliminary observation with dronabinol in patients with intractable pruritus secondary to cholestatic liver disease. Am J Gastroenterol 2002;97(8):2117–9.

82. Dawson PA, Lan T, Rao A. Bile acid transporters. J Lipid Res 2009;50(12): 2340–57.

83. Lanzini A, De Tavonatti MG, Panarotto B, et al. Intestinal absorption of the bile acid analogue 75Se-homocholic acid-taurine is increased in primary biliary cirrhosis, and reverts to normal during ursodeoxycholic acid administration. Gut 2003;52(9):1371–5.

84. Mayo MJ, Pockros P, Jones D, et al. CLARITY: a phase 2, randomized, double-blind, placebo-controlled study of lopixibat chloride (formerly LUM001) in the treatment of primary biliary cirrhosis associated with itching. J Hepatol 2016; 64(2):S197.

85. Baghdasaryan A, Fuchs CD, Osterreicher CH, et al. Inhibition of intestinal bile acid absorption improves cholestatic liver and bile duct injury in a mouse model of sclerosing cholangitis. J Hepatol 2016;64(3):674–81.

86. Hegade VS, Kendrick SF, Dobbins RL, et al. Effect of ileal bile acid transporter inhibitor GSK2330672 on pruritus in primary biliary cholangitis: a double-blind, randomised, placebo-controlled, crossover, phase 2a study. Lancet 2017; 389(10074):1114–23.

Chronic Complications of Cholestasis

Evaluation and Management

David N. Assis, MD

KEYWORDS

- Primary biliary cholangitis • Cholestasis • Malabsorption
- Fat-soluble vitamin deficiency • Metabolic bone disease • Hyperlipidemia
- Portal hypertension • Hepatocellular carcinoma

KEY POINTS

- Chronic cholestasis increases the risk of fat-soluble vitamin deficiency, most commonly vitamin A and D, particularly in patients with serum bilirubin greater than 2 mg/dL.
- Therapy to prevent osteoporosis and bone fractures should be considered in patients with primary biliary cholangitis (PBC) and a T score less than −1.5.
- Hyperlipidemia is common in PBC; however, coexisting cardiovascular risk should be addressed and the effect of emerging PBC therapies on lipids should be closely monitored.
- Although uncommon, patients with PBC have an increased risk of variceal bleeding from portal hypertension at precirrhotic stages and risk-prediction strategies are indicated.
- The risk of hepatocellular carcinoma is increased in patients with PBC who do not achieve biochemical response to treatment, particularly in men.

INTRODUCTION

Long-term complications of chronic cholestasis not only increase the risk of morbidity and mortality but also have a significant impact on the patient's quality of life. Despite the increasing number of effective therapies for the treatment of primary biliary cholangitis (PBC), cholestatic complications will continue to be present and therefore remain relevant priorities for the discovery and delivery of high-quality care. In addition, the study of new therapies for PBC should include proactive assessment and measurement of their impact on complications of cholestasis. This proactive assessment is important because emerging new therapies for management of cholestasis may or may not impact these manifestations in a beneficial manner.

The author has nothing to disclose.
Department of Medicine, Section of Digestive Diseases, Yale University School of Medicine, 333 Cedar Street, 1080 LMP, New Haven, CT 06510, USA
E-mail address: david.assis@yale.edu

Assis

Complications of chronic cholestasis in patients with PBC include fat-soluble vitamin deficiency, metabolic bone disease, hyperlipidemia, portal hypertension (cirrhotic and precirrhotic), and hepatocellular carcinoma (HCC). The goals of this article are to address these common chronic complications for patients with PBC and to highlight evidence-based best practices for evaluation and effective management of these disorders. Please see Andres F. Carrion and colleagues' article, "Understanding and Treating Pruritus in Primary Biliary Cholangitis," in this issue for detailed information on pruritus.

MALABSORPTION AND FAT-SOLUBLE VITAMIN DEFICIENCY
Definition and Diagnosis

Before the development and subsequent widespread use of ursodeoxycholic acid (UDCA) for treatment of PBC, the natural history of the disease was notable for a significant acceleration in the rate of morbidity and mortality following the onset of symptoms. A key study from the early 1980s highlighted this point, demonstrating that although the 5- and 10-year survival in asymptomatic patients with PBC was comparable to the healthy US population, those who developed any symptoms of disease, including malabsorption, jaundice, or pruritus, had a markedly reduced survival.[1]

Before the existence of any effective therapy for PBC, management primarily focused on the complications of prolonged cholestasis, including steatorrhea, fat-soluble vitamin deficiency, and pruritus.[2] Early studies from the 1960s demonstrated that patients with PBC experienced significant steatorrhea and weight loss, quantified as up to 10 g of fecal fat loss per day after intake of 70 g per day.[3] The steatorrhea was highly associated with decreased availability of bile salts to aid in the absorption of nutrition.

Fortunately, steatorrhea and severe fat-soluble vitamin deficiency have become less common in the past 2 decades. Most patients with clinically measurable fat-soluble vitamin deficiency also have advanced liver disease, especially with prolonged jaundice. One study of 52 patients reported that 17 had measurable deficiency in vitamin A, and one was symptomatic.[4] A larger study from 2001 with nearly 180 patients with PBC stratified the group according to histologic stage of fibrosis.[5] The investigators reported that vitamin A was the most frequently encountered fat-soluble vitamin deficiency (33.5%), followed by deficiencies of vitamin D (13.2%), vitamin K (7.8%), and vitamin E (1.9%). Vitamin A deficiency was associated with the stage of fibrosis (11.1% in stage I and 52.2% in stage IV) in addition to Mayo risk score and total cholesterol level. The only association with vitamin D deficiency occurred with serum albumin levels. The investigators concluded that fat-soluble vitamin deficiency is relatively uncommon in patients with PBC.

However, it is likely that micronutrient deficiency persists in patients with milder degrees of chronic cholestasis. Indeed, despite an appropriate and similar macronutrient diet in both cholestatic patients including PBC and Primary Sclerosing Cholangitis (PSC) and healthy controls, Floreani and colleagues[6] reported significant reductions of both micronutrients and antioxidants specifically in the cholestatic group. Their findings included reduced levels in retinols and α-tocopherols. Furthermore, in the PBC subgroup there was a negative correlation between carotenoids and serum markers of cholestasis, including alkaline phosphatase (ALP) and γ-glutamyl transpeptidase (GGT), albeit at a modest degree ($r = -0.27$, $P<.013$ and $r = -0.26$, $P<.018$, respectively). Interestingly, the investigators did not find a correlation between antioxidant levels and the histologic stage of disease. These findings clearly suggest that reduced micronutrient levels are readily found in cholestatic patients despite an adequate macronutrient diet and correlate with cholestatic markers.

The molecular mechanisms of such findings are not fully clear; however, available data suggest that hepatic stellate cells may have an abnormal vitamin A staining pattern in patients with PBC, characterized by increased quantity of intracellular vitamin A.[7] Therefore, abnormal mobilization of existing intrahepatic vitamin A may partially account for reduced measurable levels in patients with PBC, in addition to concurrent impairment of intestinal absorption due to altered bile itself.

The existence of fat-soluble vitamin deficiency should be suspected particularly in patients with advanced liver disease and ongoing jaundice. Although PBC is not encountered in children, extensive studies focused on the impact of cholestasis on nutrients have been performed in pediatric cholestatic cohorts. These studies suggest that persistent hyperbilirubinemia greater than 2 to 3 mg/dL is strongly associated with fat-soluble vitamin deficiency and may also potentially portend resistance to supplementation in infants.[8,9] Although data from adult patients with PBC suggest that advanced fibrosis is the most relevant risk factor for fat-soluble vitamin deficiency, the data from the pediatric literature highlight the need for vigilance in any patient with prolonged hyperbilirubinemia independent of the stage of fibrosis.

Evaluation and Management

It is important to rule out concurrent medical disorders that could exacerbate malabsorption or fat-soluble vitamin deficiency, and that are more commonly found in some patients with chronic cholestasis, such as celiac disease, intestinal bacterial overgrowth, and pancreatic insufficiency.

All patients with PBC should be screened for vitamin D deficiency with measurement of circulating level of 25-hydroxyvitamin D, the major metabolite of vitamin D. Patients with advanced liver disease should have yearly measurements.[10] Reduced levels of vitamin D should be corrected with supplementation; a dose of 25,000 to 50,000 IU once weekly can be administered.

Measurement of circulating vitamin A levels should be considered in patients with chronic cholestasis from PBC and particularly those with advanced liver disease. If a patient is diagnosed with vitamin A deficiency in the setting of symptoms such as decreased night vision, therapy is indicated with oral therapy with 100,000 IU daily for 3 days followed by 50,000 IU daily for 14 days.[11] Asymptomatic patients with vitamin A deficiency can be treated with 15,000 IU per day or 25,000 to 50,000 IU up to 3 times per week.

Vitamin K deficiency is uncommon in patients with PBC with the exception of prolonged and profound jaundice in advanced liver disease and is characterized by reversible prolongation of prothrombin time. A trial of vitamin K should be administered parenterally in patients with profound jaundice given reduced intestinal absorption.

Vitamin E deficiency is thought to be very uncommon in patients with PBC, although the presence of neurologic abnormalities, such as ataxia, loss of proprioception, or even areflexia, in a patient with prolonged cholestasis should prompt consideration and testing of serum levels. It should be noted that one older study of 26 adults with PBC reported that the ratio of vitamin E to total serum lipid concentration indicated potential relative vitamin E deficiency in up to 27% of patients.[12] Although rigorous evidence on proper dosing is lacking, the finding of vitamin E deficiency, especially in the setting of neurologic impairment, should prompt repletion with parenteral doses and subsequent administration of 400 IU daily.

Regarding the optimal longitudinal screening strategy for fat-soluble vitamin deficiency, guidelines recommend annual measurement of vitamin A, D, E, and K levels in any patient with persistent bilirubin greater than 2 mg/dL (**Box 1**).[10]

Box 1
Repletion of fat-soluble vitamins

- Vitamin A: 25,000 to 50,000 IU 2 to 3 times per week
- Vitamin D: 25,000 to 50,000 IU per week
- Vitamin E: 400 IU daily
- Vitamin K: 10 mg parenterally daily for 3 days

METABOLIC BONE DISEASE
Definition and Diagnosis

Metabolic bone disease from cholestasis, also known as hepatic osteodystrophy, is common in PBC and comprises various distinct conditions, including osteopenia and osteoporosis (defective bone formation) or osteomalacia (defective bone mineralization). The prevalence of mineral bone disease in PBC is thought to be elevated compared with healthy controls, with a prevalence of 30% to 40% in most series.[13–15] One key study reported that older age and severity of PBC were associated with increased risk of osteoporosis, but not menopausal status.[15]

There is significant heterogeneity in the literature regarding case selection and definition of disease, resulting in uncertainty as to the accurate frequency of metabolic bone disease in patients with PBC. Despite this uncertainty, the risk of metabolic disease appears to be related to the overall duration of cholestasis and may progress over time. Indeed, one study from the early 1990s reported that women with PBC have bone loss at twice the rate of healthy women with a mean rate loss of 2% per year.[16]

The pathophysiology of metabolic bone disease in PBC is not fully understood. A study by Janes and colleagues[17] found reduced plasma mitogenic activity of normal human osteoblast-like cells exposed to plasma of jaundiced patients with chronic cholestatic liver disease, suggesting a reduced bone formation due to hyperbilirubinemia. Further research has demonstrated that both lithocholic acid and unconjugated bilirubin can negatively affect osteoblast survival. The effect of lithocholic acid and unconjugated hyperbilirubinemia led to interesting research on the effects of UDCA in the setting of osteoblast dysfunction in PBC. Dubreuil and colleagues[18] demonstrated that UDCA can neutralize the negative effect of bilirubin on osteoblasts and thus increase mineralization by up to 35%. Furthermore, this group subsequently showed that UDCA can reverse the damaging effect of lithocholic acid and bilirubin on osteoblasts, specifically by counteracting their harmful effect on the proapoptotic gene BAX and the antiapoptotic gene BCL2L.[19]

Assessment of the fracture risk is important in patients with PBC who have established or suspected metabolic bone disease. One study from a cohort of 85 patients with PBC in the United Kingdom reported a similar risk of fractures in the PBC group versus controls.[20] However, a large study by Guañabens and colleagues[21] with 185 PBC patients reported a 30.6% prevalence of osteoporosis, which was higher than the prevalence in age- and geographically matched patients (11.2%, $P<.001$), along with a 20% prevalence of overall fractures (vertebral and nonvertebral). Importantly, this cohort of patients with PBC was already taking daily calcium and low-dose vitamin D. The investigators clearly showed that the risk of vertebral fractures was associated with osteoporosis, and furthermore, they suggested that even a lumbar or femoral neck T score less than −1.5 independently increased the risk of vertebral fractures with odds ratios of 8.3 and 6.8, respectively.[21] Therefore, patients with PBC and T scores less than −1.5, measured by dual-energy X-ray absorptiometry (DEXA) imaging, may be considered candidates for strategies to increase bone strength.[22]

Evaluation and Management

All patients with PBC should be assessed for their individual risk of osteoporosis.[10,22] A DEXA imaging study is indicated at the time of disease presentation, and every 2 to 4 years subsequently assuming there is no mineral loss at baseline. Vitamin D serum levels should be measured in all patients. In postmenopausal or perimenopausal women, vitamin D and calcium are recommended for prevention of metabolic bone disease at doses of 1000 IU daily and 1000 to 1500 mg daily, respectively.[10] A classic study of patients with chronic cholestatic liver disease due to PBC demonstrated that intake of vitamin D was significantly associated with serum calcium levels ($r = 0.623$, $P<.02$) and that treatment with vitamin D markedly improved serum calcium absorption.[23]

Recently, a randomized clinical trial in individuals without PBC who took calcium and vitamin D supplements for chemoprevention after the detection of a colonic adenoma revealed a surprisingly small increase in the incidence of serrated polyps of the colon,[24] leading researchers to recommend careful assessment of risks versus benefits of taking these supplements over the long term. These results may lead to understandable inquiries from patients with PBC about how to integrate these findings in the face of recommendations in cholestatic disease. The increased risk of osteoporosis in the setting of malabsorption or advanced liver disease from cholestasis of PBC clearly represents a competing risk. For example, patients with PBC and a T score of < -1.5 have a reported increased risk of fractures, as previously noted, and most likely will benefit from supplementation of calcium and vitamin D. Therefore, the topic of supplementation to prevent or attenuate metabolic bone disease should be openly discussed with the patient so that an informed and individualized decision can be made. Indeed, recent guidelines from the European Society for the Study of the Liver acknowledge the need to individualize the decision.[22]

Additional therapy to improve bone mineral status is indicated for patients with PBC and osteoporosis, most commonly with bisphosphonate drugs. A study from 2003 demonstrated that alendronate was superior to etidronate for improvement in lumbar bone mineral density in a randomized trial of patients with PBC.[25] A subsequent trial by the same group compared alendronate with ibandronate, a monthly administered bisphosphonate, in a randomized trial of 33 women with PBC.[26] They found similar improvement in bone mineral density with both drugs, although the medication adherence to ibandronate was higher.

Another relevant consideration with bisphosphonate therapy is the necessary caution in patients with PBC who have esophageal varices and therefore may be at increased risk of gastritis or esophagitis from nitrogenous (N-containing) oral bisphosphonates.[27] The risk of upper gastrointestinal ulcerations appears to be reduced with risedronate as compared with alendronate.[28] In one study, 4.1% of patients had gastric ulcerations after a 2-week course of risedronate versus 13.2% of patients who used alendronate.[29] Therefore, avoidance of alendronate is advisable in patients with cirrhosis and varices, and parenteral administration of bisphosphonates could be considered in those situations.

Healthy lifestyle choices can also influence the risk of osteoporosis in patients with PBC and should be repeatedly emphasized, specifically the need for regular exercise, avoidance of alcohol, smoking cessation, and good nutrition. Although some patients require the regular use of bile acid resins for treatment of clinically significant pruritus, the use of resins should be minimized when possible to avoid reduction in vitamin D absorption (**Box 2**).

Box 2
Management of metabolic bone disease in primary biliary cholangitis

- DEXA scan at presentation and every 2 to 4 years if baseline is normal
- Regular exercise
- Good nutrition
- Eliminate alcohol intake
- Minimize use of resins
- Calcium: 1000 to 1500 mg/d
- Vitamin D: 800 to 1000 IU/d
- Bisphosphonates in setting of osteoporosis
- Consider therapy also if T score is less than −1.5

HYPERLIPIDEMIA
Definition and Diagnosis

Chronic cholestasis is commonly associated with increased lipid concentrations, with a reported prevalence as high as 80%.[30] A feature of early-stage PBC is the elevation of serum high-density lipoprotein (HDL) cholesterol, and this is partially explained by a decrease in hepatic triglyceride lipase levels.[31] Elevations of serum very-low density lipoprotein and low-density lipoprotein (LDL) are also found early in the disease. However, with disease progression, there is a gradual increase in LDL, a reduction in HDL levels, and the appearance of atypical lipoprotein particles, such as lipoprotein X.[32]

In patients with PBC, these lipid abnormalities are usually not associated with cardiovascular events and therefore traditionally are not considered to be a relevant risk factor. Indeed, a key study by Longo and colleagues[30] analyzed a cohort of 400 patients with PBC for a mean of 6.2 years (with a range of up to 24 years) and observed no increase in cardiovascular disease. Furthermore, a study by Allocca and colleagues[33] did not find an increase in carotid atherosclerotic lesions in patients with PBC and hyperlipidemia. One explanation for this may be that patients with PBC have significantly increased plasma adiponectin levels, a known cardioprotective molecule, compared with patients with hyperlipidemia without cholestasis, such as nonalcoholic steatohepatitis.[34] In addition, Chang and colleagues[35] have proposed that lipoprotein X plays a specific protective role in patients with PBC by preventing oxidation of LDL, thereby reducing atherogenicity and maintaining the integrity of arterial endothelial cells.

Evaluation and Management

Every patient with PBC should have a measurement of fasting lipids as a baseline, and a careful history should be taken to elucidate both personal and family history of cardiovascular disease. Although the presence of hyperlipidemia itself is not typically concerning in patients with PBC, the presence of additional risk factors for cardiovascular outcomes should receive adequate attention and consideration for cholesterol lowering agents.

The use of 3-hydroxy-3-methylglutaryl coenzyme A reductase inhibitors (statins) for cholesterol reduction in patients with PBC is safe and should be considered if clinically indicated, such as in the presence of concurrent metabolic syndrome. In a small study of 6 patients with PBC and hyperlipidemia, simvastatin not only improved total and

LDL cholesterol levels but also reduced serum ALP, GGT, and immunoglobulin M.[36] Two subsequent small, randomized trials of patients with PBC receiving simvastatin versus placebo further demonstrated a beneficial impact on lipids along with a reassuring safety profile.[37,38]

The emerging application of fibrates in the management of PBC in nonresponders or partial responders to UDCA has the additional benefit of lipid reduction. Indeed, several studies report a significant decrease in triglycerides and LDL in patients who have a response to fibrate therapy.[39,40] Such reductions are fully consistent with the mechanism of action for these drugs, and PPARα agonists specifically, which can decrease cholestatic inflammation with and reduce CYP7a1-mediated bile acid synthesis, in addition to their lipid-lower properties.[41]

In contrast, the use of bile acid therapy obeticholic acid (OCA) is associated with alteration in lipid levels because of selective farnesoid X receptor agonism. This alteration in lipids can result in reduced HDL levels in patients with PBC taking OCA.[42,43] The clinical significance of this effect on lipoprotein, and subsequent cardiovascular risk, remains unclear for now, although data from a recent study regarding the effect of OCA on lipoprotein are anticipated (**Box 3**).[44]

PORTAL HYPERTENSION
Definition and Diagnosis

The clinical manifestation of portal hypertension, particularly variceal bleeding, in patients with PBC is usually associated with advanced stages of disease, including decompensated cirrhosis. Therefore, this is generally considered a poor prognostic indicator, which should result in consideration for liver transplantation.[22,45,46] However, a notable subset of patients with PBC will develop portal hypertension and variceal bleeding at precirrhotic stages. These patients may remain compensated for a prolonged period of time, as opposed to the rapid decline typically observed in patients with decompensated cirrhosis. The precirrhotic portal hypertension in these patients may be due to nodular regenerative hyperplasia and subsequent obliteration of portal venules, which has been well described in the setting of PBC.[47] It is not clear to what degree this precirrhotic portal hypertension is linked to the cholestasis of PBC itself. One study reviewing data on 127 patients who previously participated in 2 clinical trials found that 6% of patients with early-stage disease had esophageal varices. However, 95% of patients with PBC and varices had clear markers of advanced disease.[48]

Evaluation and Management

Any patient with PBC and known cirrhosis should receive standard variceal screening with upper endoscopy. In addition, 2 studies have evaluated methods to predict the existence of varices in patients with PBC and the need for endoscopic screening. Levy and colleagues[49] reported that a platelet count less than 140,000 and/or a Mayo risk score of ≥4.5 were strong and independent predictors for the presence

---

Box 3
Management of hyperlipidemia in primary biliary cholangitis

- Treatment of hyperlipidemia in the absence of cardiovascular risk factors is not needed
- Statins are safe and effective for patients with PBC who require therapy
- The emerging use of fibrates for treatment of cholestasis in PBC will also reduce serum lipids
- Obeticholic acid can reduce serum HDL, and lipids should be monitored while on therapy

of varices, with an area under the receiving operating characteristic curve of 0.959. Bressler and colleagues[50] evaluated a cohort of patients with PBC and PSC in comparison to a larger cohort with other chronic liver diseases, reporting that a platelet count less than 200,000, albumin less than 4 g/dL, and bilirubin greater than 1.2 mg/dL were independent predictors of varices specifically for patients with chronic cholestatic liver disease. It is unclear why the threshold platelet count was higher in cholestatic patients compared with other liver diseases (ie, 150,000), but this should further highlight the need for vigilance in patients with PBC who do not yet have signs of advanced liver disease. In addition, recently updated Baveno (VI) guidelines include a liver stiffness by transient elastography of $\geq$20 kPa as a threshold for variceal screening in any patient with chronic liver disease.[51]

Patients with PBC who have any of the above features are candidates for variceal screening, with management as recommended by the Baveno VI guidelines, including consideration for nonselective β-blockers for primary prophylaxis.[51] Patients with PBC often suffer from significant fatigue that could impair the tolerance of β-blockers, and if noted, this should be carefully assessed by the medical provider.

HEPATOCELLULAR CARCINOMA
Definition and Diagnosis

HCC is a well-known complication of cirrhosis regardless of cause. The risk of HCC clearly includes patients with PBC, with an estimated disease-specific incidence rate (IR) of 36 per 1000 person-years. One large study found an overall incidence of 2.4% in a cohort of 667 patients.[52] However, recent data from a large cohort of more than 4500 patients with PBC interestingly suggest that those with earlier stages of disease and treatment nonresponders may also have a higher risk of HCC. Although the overall IR of HCC in the full cohort was 34 per 1000 patient-years, persistent chronic cholestasis despite treatment (biochemical nonresponse) was the single greatest factor predicting future risk of HCC for patients with PBC.[53] Furthermore, the association of biochemical nonresponse with HCC was found both in those with early-stage (IR 4.7) and late-stage disease (IR 11.2). In addition, men who did not achieve biochemical response to treatment were at the highest risk of developing HCC (IR 18.2). These data, therefore, also suggest that new effective therapies for patients who do not respond to first-line therapy with UDCA may have a significant impact on the risk of HCC.

Evaluation and Management

Current recommendations specify that screening for HCC in patients with PBC should be performed only for those with established cirrhosis.[10,22] Screening methods are similar to other advanced liver diseases and should be performed according to established guidelines, which typically comprise ultrasonography with or without serum α-fetoprotein levels every 6 months (**Box 4**).[54]

SUMMARY

The successful development of new therapeutic options for patients with PBC is an undisputed sign of progress, and perhaps in the future PBC will no longer be associated with a risk of refractory, chronic cholestasis. Until then, it is necessary to actively consider the well-known complications of cholestasis and assess their impact in the context of individualized patient care, because they remain associated with significant morbidity. The full effect of emerging treatments for cholestasis on fat-soluble vitamin deficiency, metabolic bone disease, hyperlipidemia, and even HCC risk is not clearly understood. Therefore, researchers should proactively design

---

Box 4
Portal hypertension and hepatocellular carcinoma in primary biliary cholangitis

- Patients with PBC may develop variceal bleeding at precirrhotic stages
- Consider risk-prediction models to estimate risk of variceal development
- Screening and treatment of varices should follow Baveno VI guidelines
- Men who do not achieve biochemical response to treatment have the highest risk of developing hepatocellular carcinoma
- Screening is only recommended for patients with cirrhosis and should follow standard guideline recommendations

---

trials with careful data collection that measure the rates of these complications on a routine basis as part of all new studies. Finally, more extensive and dedicated, research primarily focused on therapies to improve specific complications of chronic cholestasis is needed and will provide meaningful benefits to patients with PBC.

REFERENCES

1. Roll J, Boyer JL, Barry D, et al. The prognostic importance of clinical and histologic features in asymptomatic and symptomatic primary biliary cirrhosis. N Engl J Med 1983;308(1):1–7.
2. Sherlock S. Chronic cholangitides: aetiology, diagnosis, and treatment. Br Med J 1968;3(5617):515–21.
3. Datta DV, Sherlock S. Cholestyramine for long term relief of the pruritus complicating intrahepatic cholestasis. Gastroenterology 1966;50(3):323–32.
4. Kaplan MM, Elta GH, Furie B, et al. Fat-soluble vitamin nutriture in primary biliary cirrhosis. Gastroenterology 1988;95(3):787–92.
5. Phillips JR, Angulo P, Petterson T, et al. Fat-soluble vitamin levels in patients with primary biliary cirrhosis. Am J Gastroenterol 2001;96(9):2745–50.
6. Floreani A, Baragiotta A, Martines D, et al. Plasma antioxidant levels in chronic cholestatic liver diseases. Aliment Pharmacol Ther 2000;14(3):353–8.
7. Nyburg A, Berne B, Nordlinder H, et al. Impaired release of vitamin A from liver in primary biliary cirrhosis. Hepatology 1988;8(1):136–41.
8. Shen YM, Wu JF, Hsu HY, et al. Oral absorbable fat-soluble vitamin formulation in pediatric patients with cholestasis. J Pediatr Gastroenterol Nutr 2012;55(5): 587–91.
9. Schneider BL, Magee JC, Bezerra JA, et al. Efficacy of fat-soluble vitamin supplementation in infants with biliary atresia. Pediatrics 2012;130(3):e607–14.
10. Lindor KD, Gershwin ME, Poupon R, et al, American Association for Study of Liver Diseases. Primary biliary cirrhosis. Hepatology 2009;50(1):291–308.
11. Ludwig J. Idiopathic adult ductopenia: an update. Mayo Clin Proc 1998;73(3): 285–91.
12. Sokol RJ, Kim YS, Hoofnagle JH, et al. Intestinal malabsorption of vitamin E in primary biliary cirrhosis. Gastroenterology 1989;96(2 Pt 1):479–86.
13. Solerio E, Isaia G, Innarella R, et al. Osteoporosis: still a typical complication of primary biliary cirrhosis? Dig Liver Dis 2003;35(5):339–46.
14. Le Gars L, Grandpierre C, Chazouilères O, et al. Bone loss in primary biliary cirrhosis: absence of association with severity of liver disease. Joint Bone Spine 2002;69(2):195–200.

15. Guañabens N, Parés A, Ros I, et al. Severity of cholestasis and advanced histo-logical stage but not menopausal status are the major risk factors for osteopo-rosis in primary biliary cirrhosis. J Hepatol 2005;42(4):573–7.

16. Eastell R, Dickson ER, Hodgson SF, et al. Rates of vertebral bone loss before and after liver transplantation in women with primary biliary cirrhosis. Hepatology 1991;14(2):296–300.

17. Janes CH, Dickson ER, Okazaki R, et al. Role of hyperbilirubinemia in the impair-ment of osteoblast proliferation associated with cholestatic jaundice. J Clin Invest 1995;95(6):2581–6.

18. Dubreuil M, Ruiz-Gaspà S, Guañabens N, et al. Ursodeoxycholic acid increases differentiation and mineralization and neutralizes the damaging effects of bilirubin on osteoblastic cells. Liver Int 2013;33(7):1029–38.

19. Ruiz-Gaspà S, Dubreuil M, Guañabens N, et al. Ursodeoxycholic acid decreases bilirubin-induced osteoblast apoptosis. Eur J Clin Invest 2014;44(12):1206–14.

20. Boulton-Jones JR, Fenn RM, West J, et al. Fracture risk of women with primary biliary cirrhosis: no increase compared with general population controls. Aliment Pharmacol Ther 2004;20(5):551–7.

21. Guañabens N, Cerdá D, Monegal A, et al. Low bone mass and severity of chole-stasis affect fracture risk in patients with primary biliary cirrhosis. Gastroenter-ology 2010;138(7):2348–56.

22. European Association for the Study of the Liver. EASL clinical practice guidelines: the diagnosis and management of patients with primary biliary cholangitis. J Hepatol 2017;67(1):145–72.

23. Bengoa JM, Sitrin MD, Meredith S, et al. Intestinal calcium absorption and vitamin D status in chronic cholestatic liver disease. Hepatology 1984;4(2):261–5.

24. Crockett SD, Barry EL, Mott LA, et al. Calcium and vitamin D supplementation and increased risk of serrated polyps: results from a randomised clinical trial. Gut 2018. https://doi.org/10.1136/gutjnl-2017-315242.

25. Guañabens N, Parés A, Ros I, et al. Alendronate is more effective than etidronate for increasing bone mass in osteopenic patients with primary biliary cirrhosis. Am J Gastroenterol 2003;98(10):2268–74.

26. Guañabens N, Monegal A, Cerdá D, et al. Randomized trial comparing monthly ibandronate and weekly alendronate for osteoporosis in patients with primary biliary cirrhosis. Hepatology 2013;58(6):2070–8.

27. Treeprasertsuk S, Silveira MG, Petz JL, et al. Parenteral bisphosphonates for oste-oporosis in patients with primary biliary cirrhosis. Am J Ther 2011;18(5):375–81.

28. Taggart H, Bolognese MA, Lindsay R, et al. Upper gastrointestinal tract safety of risedronate: a pooled analysis of 9 clinical trials. Mayo Clin Proc 2002;77(3):262–70.

29. Lanza FL, Hunt RH, Thomson AB, et al. Endoscopic comparison of esophageal and gastroduodenal effects of risedronate and alendronate in postmenopausal women. Gastroenterology 2000;119(3):631–8.

30. Longo M, Crosignani A, Battezzati PM, et al. Hyperlipidaemic state and cardio-vascular risk in primary biliary cirrhosis. Gut 2002;51(2):265–9.

31. Hiraoka H, Yamashita S, Mtsuzawa Y, et al. Decrease of hepatic triglyceride lipase levels and increase of cholesteryl ester transfer protein levels in patients with primary biliary cirrhosis: relationship to abnormalities in high-density lipopro-tein. Hepatology 1993;18(1):103–10.

32. Jahn CE, Schaefer EJ, Taam LA, et al. Lipoprotein abnormalities in primary biliary cirrhosis. Association with hepatic lipase inhibition as well as altered cholesterol esterification. Gastroenterology 1985;89(6):1266–78.

33. Allocca M, Crosignani A, Gritti A, et al. Hypercholesterolaemia is not associated with early atherosclerotic lesions in primary biliary cirrhosis. Gut 2006;55(12): 1795–800.
34. Floreani A, Variola A, Niro G, et al. Plasma adiponectin levels in primary biliary cirrhosis: a novel perspective for link between hypercholesterolemia and protection against atherosclerosis. Am J Gastroenterol 2008;103(8):1959–65.
35. Chang PY, Lu SC, Su TC, et al. Lipoprotein-X reduces LDL atherogenicity in primary biliary cirrhosis by preventing LDL oxidation. J Lipid Res 2004;45(11): 2116–22.
36. Ritzel U, Leonhardt U, Nather M, et al. Simvastatin in primary biliary cirrhosis: effects on serum lipids and distinct disease markers. J Hepatol 2002;36(4):454–8.
37. Sjotakovic T, Claudel T, Putz-Bankuti C, et al. Low-dose atorvastatin improves dyslipidemia and vascular function in patients with primary biliary cirrhosis after one year of treatment. Atherosclerosis 2010;209(1):178–83.
38. Cash WJ, O'Neill S, O'Donnell ME, et al. Randomized controlled trial assessing the effect of simvastatin in primary biliary cirrhosis. Liver Int 2013;33(8):1166–74.
39. Reig A, Sesé P, Parés A. Effects of bezafibrate on outcome and pruritus in primary biliary cholangitis with suboptimal ursodeoxycholic acid response. Am J Gastroenterol 2018;113(1):49–55.
40. Corpechot C, Chazouillères O, Rousseau A, et al. A 2-year multicenter, double-blind, randomized, placebo-controlled study of bezafibrate for the treatment of primary biliary cholangitis in patients with inadequate response to ursodeoxycholic acid therapy (Bezurso). J Hepatol 2017;66(1, Suppl):S89.
41. Ghonem NS, Assis DN, Boyer JL. Fibrates and cholestasis. Hepatology 2015; 62(2):635–43.
42. Hirschfield GM, Mason A, Luketic V, et al. Efficacy of obeticholic acid in patients with primary biliary cirrhosis and inadequate response to ursodeoxycholic acid. Gastroenterology 2015;148(4):751–61.
43. Nevens F, Andreone P, Mazzella G, et al. A placebo-controlled trial of obeticholic acid in primary biliary cholangitis. N Engl J Med 2016;375(7):631–43.
44. Levy C. Evolving role of obeticholic acid in primary biliary cholangitis. Hepatology 2017. https://doi.org/10.1002/hep.29726.
45. Kew MC, Varma RR, Dos Santos HA, et al. Portal hypertension in primary biliary cirrhosis. Gut 1971;12(10):830–4.
46. Gores GJ, Wiesner RH, Dickson ER, et al. Prospective evaluation of esophageal varices in primary biliary cirrhosis: development, natural history, and influence on survival. Gastroenterology 1989;96(6):1552–9.
47. Colina F, Pinedo F, Solís JA, et al. Nodular regenerative hyperplasia of the liver in early histological stages of primary biliary cirrhosis. Gastroenterology 1992;102(4 Pt 1):1319–24.
48. Ali AH, Sinakos E, Silveira MG, et al. Varices in early histological stage primary biliary cirrhosis. J Clin Gastroenterol 2011;45(7). e66–71.
49. Levy C, Zein CO, Gomez J, et al. Prevalence and predictors of esophageal varices in patients with primary biliary cirrhosis. Clin Gastroenterol Hepatol 2007;5(7): 803–8.
50. Bressler B, Pinto R, El-Ashry D, et al. Which patients with primary biliary cirrhosis or primary sclerosing cholangitis should undergo endoscopic screening for oesophageal varices detection? Gut 2005;54(3):407–10.
51. de Franchis R, Baveno VI Faculty. Expanding consensus in portal hypertension: report of the Baveno VI consensus workshop: stratifying risk and individualizing care for portal hypertension. J Hepatol 2015;63(3):743–52.

52. Jones DE, Metcalf JV, Collier JD, et al. Hepatocellular carcinoma in primary biliary cirrhosis and its impact on outcomes. Hepatology 1997;26(5):1138–42.
53. Trivedi PJ, Lammers WJ, van Buuren HR, et al. Stratification of hepatocellular carcinoma risk in primary biliary cirrhosis: a multicentre international study. Gut 2016;65(2):321–9.
54. Heimbach JK, Kulik LM, Finn RS, et al. AASLD guidelines for the treatment of hepatocellular carcinoma. Hepatology 2018;67(1):358–80.

Individualizing Care
Management Beyond Medical Therapy

Laura Cristoferi, MD[a], Alessandra Nardi, PhD[b], Pietro Invernizzi, MD, PhD[a], George Mells, MRCP, PhD[c], Marco Carbone, MD, PhD[a,d],*

KEYWORDS

- Primary biliary cholangitis • Precision medicine • Risk-stratification
- Autoimmune liver disease • Individualized care • Novel therapies • Omics

KEY POINTS

- The forthcoming availability of several novel drugs in primary biliary cholangitis (PBC) coupled with the rise of high-throughput omics technologies prompt changing the paradigm of the management of the disease.
- Precision medicine (PM), through the application of omics-based approaches, should enable identifying disease variants, stratifying patients according to disease trajectory, risk of disease progression, and likelihood of response to different therapeutic options in PBC.
- The development of PM needs specific interventions, such as sequencing more genomes, creating bigger biobanks, and linking biological information to health data in electronic medical record.
- The authors envisage that a diagnostic work-up of PBC patients will include information on genetic variants and molecular signature that may define a particular subtype of disease and provide an estimate of treatment response and survival.

Primary biliary cholangitis (PBC) is a chronic, autoimmune liver disease characterized by nonsuppurative granulomatous cholangitis, causing progressive duct destruction and portal fibrosis that progresses slowly to biliary cirrhosis. A substantial proportion of cases eventually develops cirrhosis with attendant complications, such as portal hypertension, chronic liver failure, or hepatocellular cancer (HCC). PBC, therefore, remains a leading indication for liver transplantation (LT).

Advances over the past several years have improved the ability to individualize care in PBC. This is prescient: individualizing care is the aim of precision medicine (PM),

The authors have nothing to disclose.
[a] Division of Gastroenterology and Hepatology, Department of Medicine and Surgery, University of Milan Bicocca, Piazza dell'Ateneo Nuovo, 1, 20126 Milan, Italy; [b] Department of Mathematics, Tor Vergata University of Rome, Via della Ricerca Scientifica 1, Rome, Italy; [c] Academic Department of Medical Genetics, University of Cambridge, Hills Road 1, Cambridge, UK; [d] Academic Department of Medical Genetics, University of Cambridge, Cambridge, UK
* Corresponding author. Division of Gastroenterology and Hepatology, Department of Medicine and Surgery, University of Milan Bicocca, Piazza dell'Ateneo Nuovo, 1, 20126 Milan, Italy.
E-mail address: marco.carbone@unimib.it

Clin Liver Dis 22 (2018) 545–561
https://doi.org/10.1016/j.cld.2018.03.006
1089-3261/18/© 2018 Elsevier Inc. All rights reserved.

described as "an emerging approach for disease treatment and prevention that takes into account individual variability in genes, environment, and lifestyle for each person."[1] The aim of PM is to enable health care workers and biomedical researchers to more accurately predict which treatment and prevention strategies for a particular disease will work in which groups of patients. It contrasts with a 1-size-fits-all approach, in which disease treatment and prevention strategies are developed for the average patient, with less consideration for interindividual variation.[1]

PM relies on biomarkers (or panels of biomarkers) that accurately predict key outcomes, such as treatment response or disease progression (**Fig. 1**). Biomarkers may be measurements in blood, urine, saliva, or other biofluids—but the concept also encompasses features on imaging and histology. Omics-based approaches, coupled with computational and bioinformatics methods, provide an unprecedented opportunity to accelerate biomarker discovery. Such approaches include genetic analysis (genome-wide genotyping of common to rare variants, exome sequencing, and whole-genome sequencing) and a plethora of approaches for profiling the epigenome, transcriptome, proteome, and metabolome (**Fig. 2**). PM is applicable to PBC, as it is to other chronic inflammatory conditions, especially now with the current and forthcoming availability of more efficacious medications.

The clinical features and investigations that already enable individualizing the care of PBC patients are reviewed—and how emerging biomedical technologies might improve the ability to individualize management of PBC patients in the future is speculated on. The premise throughout is that individualized care for PBC, current or future, should achieve the following major objectives:

- Identification of disease variants that may require different management, such as PBC with autoimmune features or the premature ductopenic variant
- Stratification of patients according to different disease trajectories that might require different forms of surveillance, such as portal hypertensive progression; hepatocellular failure-type progression, or progression to HCC

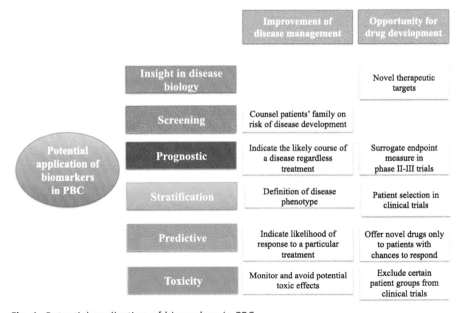

Fig. 1. Potential application of biomarkers in PBC.

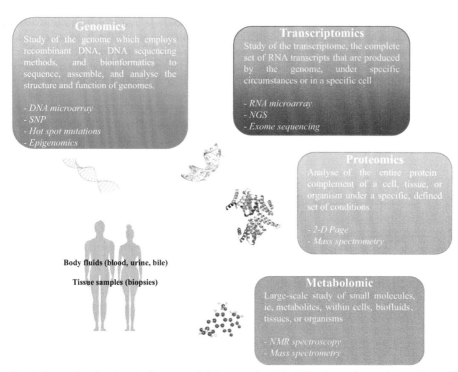

Genomics
Study of the genome which employs recombinant DNA, DNA sequencing methods, and bioinformatics to sequence, assemble, and analyse the structure and function of genomes.

- *DNA microarray*
- *SNP*
- *Hot spot mutations*
- *Epigenomics*

Transcriptomics
Study of the transcriptome, the complete set of RNA transcripts that are produced by the genome, under specific circumstances or in a specific cell

- *RNA microarray*
- *NGS*
- *Exome sequencing*

Proteomics
Analyse of the entire protein complement of a cell, tissue, or organism under a specific, defined set of conditions

- *2-D Page*
- *Mass spectrometry*

Body fluids (blood, urine, bile)

Tissue samples (biopsies)

Metabolomic
Large-scale study of small molecules, ie, metabolites, within cells, biofluids, tissues, or organisms

- *NMR spectroscopy*
- *Mass spectrometry*

Fig. 2. Example of omics platforms available to study PBC. DNA, deoxyribonucleic acid; NGS, next-generation sequencing; NMR, nuclear magnetic resonance; RNA, ribonucleic acid.

- Stratification based on the risk of disease progression
- Stratification based on the likelihood of response to, and side-effects from, different therapeutic options.

In each case, stratification should ideally reflect the underlying mechanism because this informs ongoing development or repurposing of pharmacotherapies. Beyond these major objectives, the authors anticipate that PM initiatives will identify hitherto unknown disease subphenotypes.

STRATIFICATION OF DISEASE VARIANTS

Clinical variants with different disease course have been described. It remains unclear whether these clinical entities are distinct conditions (resulting from unique pathologic processes) or extremes of phenotype (resulting from shared pathologic processes). Either way, it is important to identify patients with variant syndromes because they have different disease trajectories and benefit from different management. PM initiatives should provide insight, if carefully designed.

Primary Biliary Cholangitis with Features of Autoimmune Hepatitis

Also known as PBC/autoimmune hepatitis (AIH) overlap syndrome, primary biliary cholangitis with features of autoimmune hepatitis is a variant of PBC in which there are characteristics of both PBC and AIH. Features of AIH coexist in 8% to 10% of patients with PBC.[2] There is ongoing debate about the nature of PBC with AIH features, whether it is simply the presence of 2 disorders (ie, PBC and AIH) in one individual, a distinct condition with characteristics of PBC and AIH, or one end of the spectrum of hepatic activity in PBC. One reason for ongoing debate is that interface hepatitis, a hallmark of AIH, is also common in PBC, albeit less florid and without other, characteristic histologic features of AIH, such as rosetting and emperipolesis.

It is important to recognize PBC with AIH features because patients with this variant are likely to benefit from combined treatment with ursodeoxycholic acid (UDCA) and classic immunosuppression. Without immunosuppression, it is associated with earlier development of liver fibrosis and cirrhosis.[3] A diagnosis of PBC with AIH features should be considered in any PBC patient with moderately to highly elevated transaminases, with or without raised IgG. The diagnosis should also be considered in PBC patients with inadequate response to treatment with UDCA treatment after 6 months to 12 months showing elevated transaminases[2] (other than elevated alkaline phosphatase [ALP]). The diagnosis is currently made according to Paris criteria[4] endorsed by the European Association for the Study of the Liver (EASL)[2] (**Box 1**). It follows that a liver biopsy is mandatory to make a diagnosis. For those who satisfy the Paris criteria, international guidelines on PBC[2] recommend treatment with immunosuppression (combined or sequential treatment with corticosteroids and azathioprine) in the short term and medium term. A potential problem with the Paris criteria, however, is that they were developed without tests of specificity or sensitivity. This is not a criticism: there is no gold standard against which the Paris criteria may be tested. They might, however, be specific at the cost of sensitivity, meaning they may fail to identify all patients who could benefit from immunosuppression in addition to UDCA. The most recent EASL guidelines on AIH[5] recommend immunosuppressive treatment of AIH patients at lower cutoffs for transaminase or IgG levels and a modified histologic activity index as low as 4 of 18 points. A trial of glucocorticosteroids may, therefore, be warranted in PBC patients with prominent interface hepatitis demonstrated on liver biopsy, even if they do not fulfill the Paris criteria for diagnosis of overlap.

The authors' practical approach is to focus the treatment on the disease that seems to be the predominant entity. The authors suggest treating with immunosuppression if histology shows moderate to severe interface hepatitis, regardless of biochemical (transaminases) activity. Also, the authors suggest not overdiagnosing overlap

---

Box 1
Diagnostic criteria of primary biliary cholangitis–autoimmune hepatitis overlap syndrome

PBC criteria

ALP >2 × ULN or GGT >5 × ULN

AMA >1:40

Liver biopsy specimen showing florid bile duct lesions

AIH criteria

ALT >5 × ULN or a positive test for anti–smooth muscle antibodies

IgG >2 × ULN

Liver biopsy showing moderate or severe periportal or periseptal lymphocytic piecemeal necrosis

Diagnostic criteria of PBC-AIH overlap syndrome of which at least 2 of 3 accepted criteria for PBC and AIH, respectively, should be present. Histologic evidence of moderate to severe lymphocytic piecemeal necrosis (interface hepatitis) is mandatory for the diagnosis.
Data from Chazouillères O, Wendum D, Serfaty L, et al. Primary biliary cirrhosis-autoimmune hepatitis overlap syndrome: clinical features and response to therapy. Hepatology 1998;28(2):296–301.

presentations, given the common presence of mildly to moderately raised transaminases associated with cholestasis (likely a surrogate marker of the interface hepatitis that the authors observe associated with the florid duct lesions of PBC) and that generally responds well to choleretic agents.

Better characterization of PBC with features of AIH is a priority for PM initiatives. The aim is to identify PBC patients who would benefit from immunosuppression, ideally at diagnosis and ideally without recourse to a liver biopsy. Transcriptomic analysis of liver tissue might identify transcriptional biomarkers that can then be sought in circulation. RNA sequencing is not well suited for diagnostic use due to its complexity, computational intensity, limited throughput, and need for expert technicians. In addition, it is challenging to perform RNA sequencing analyses with small amounts of tissue, especially formalin-fixed paraffin-embedded (FFPE) biopsies, which is a limiting factor in large-scale studies. Transcriptomic analysis can be performed on FFPE biopsies using the NanoString (South Lake Union, Seattle, WA, USA) nCounter platform analyzing total mRNA level of hundreds of genes. This might highlight the expression of regulatory genes encoding essential inflammatory chemokines, interleukin, complement that might offer a signature of treatment response to immunosuppressive therapy.[6] Tissue markers should then be correlated with circulating markers. An approach that might yield suitably accurate circulating biomarkers includes immunoassays based on Luminex (Austin, Texas) xMAP (multianalyte profiling) technology that enable simultaneous detection and quantitation of multiple secreted proteins (cytokines, chemokines, growth factors, and so forth).[7] This high-throughput technology produces results comparable to ELISA but with greater efficiency, speed, and dynamic range, allowing a correlation of the composition of the portal tract infiltrate and transcriptomics readout with peripheral immune-phenotype before and after immunosuppression therapy.

The relevant studies will not, however, be easy. PBC with AIH features is a rare variant of a rare disease; therefore, recruiting an adequately powered sample will be difficult. Potential biomarkers must be tested against the current standard, which, as discussed previously, might be flawed. The study would require liver biopsy of PBC patients without AIH features; this is unlikely to be popular among support groups. Potential biomarkers must be tested against biochemical and histologic response to immunosuppression.

Premature Ductopenic Variant

The premature ductopenic variant is a poorly described variant of PBC, with only 4 cases reported in the literature.[8] It is defined histologically by extreme ductopenia disproportionate to the extent of liver fibrosis. Although the extent of fibrosis may be limited initially, progression to cirrhosis might be inevitable in the long term. Laboratory tests show a marked elevation of cholestatic markers (ALP and gamma glutamyl transferase [GGT]). The bilirubin may be elevated without features cirrhosis or portal hypertension. Owing to markedly decreased quality of life, LT is generally required within a few years of presentation.

Whether this is a disease variant or an extreme form of PBC is unknown. When this variant is suspected, a liver biopsy is required to confirm the diagnosis. This may be useful to inform prognosis and guide management. Patients with this variant typically develop jaundice early in the disease course. As a result, they may satisfy listing criteria for LT before they have cirrhosis and liver failure. Provided the symptoms of cholestasis are adequately controlled, however, LT may be safely deferred. Conversely, pruritus is severe and notoriously difficult to control in this variant. For PBC patients known to have premature ductopenia, it may be appropriate to progress rapidly through the stepwise treatment of cholestatic pruritus and consider LT for quality of life sooner rather than later.

There is no specific therapy for the premature ductopenic variant. Anecdotally, response to UDCA is often poor. The efficacy of obeticholic acid and off-label medications, such as fibrates and budesonide, is untested. Clinicians may be hesitant to offer obeticholic acid, which may exacerbate pruritus, to a patient with severe itch. This has to be weighed, however, against the potential benefit of bile duct regeneration and future symptoms improvement. However this approach has not been proved yet.

PM might have a major role to define this severe variant and highlight pathways of treatment.

In the hypothesis that these patients have different bile acid (BA) pools that are increased in their hydrophobicity beyond the capacity of UDCA to moderate or atypical patterns of handling of UDCA itself, a first approach might be to study the phenotype and quantity of circulating BA and liver tissue BA using mass spectrometry–based targeted metabolomics approach. A major challenge, however, is to select patients with this rare condition for study; this implies a major collaborative national or international effort to identify patients with severe itch and jaundice who should then undergo liver biopsy for confirmation diagnosis.

STRATIFICATION OF PATIENTS BY DIFFERENT DISEASE TRAJECTORIES

Preliminary data suggest there may be different patterns of disease progression in PBC. The Japanese Society of Hepatology describes 3 clinical types (**Fig. 3**). A majority of patients progress gradually and remain in the asymptomatic stage for longer than a decade (gradual progressive type). Some patients who progress to portal hypertension presenting without jaundice (portal hypertension type) and others progress rapidly to jaundice and ultimately hepatic failure (jaundice/hepatic failure type). The jaundice/hepatic failure type tends to affect relatively younger patients compared

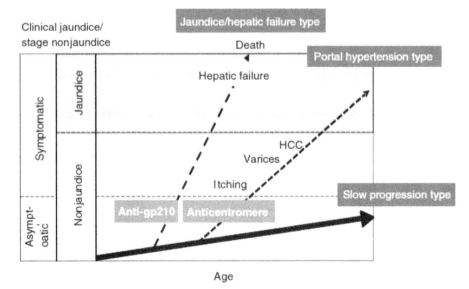

Fig. 3. Potential trajectories based on the autoantibody profile in PBC. (*From* Working Subgroup (English version) for Clinical Practice Guidelines for Primary Biliary Cirrhosis. Guidelines for the management of primary biliary cirrhosis: the Intractable Hepatobiliary Disease Study Group supported by the Ministry of Health, Labour and Welfare of Japan. Hepatol Res 2014;44 Suppl S1:71–90; with permission.)

with the other 2 types. Patients with the jaundice/hepatic failure–type PBC are often positive for anti-gp210 antibody, whereas those with the portal hypertension–type PBC have anticentromere antibodies. The latter antibodies are characteristic of systemic sclerosis (SSc) but are also found in PBC patients without coexistent SSc.[9–11] The only two, old, studies describing this clinical entity looking at the underlying pathologic damage suggest that portal hypertension is initially of presinusoidal type and then as the disease progresses is joined by a sinusoidal component.[12,13] Alternatively, given the strong association with anticentromere antibodies, the mechanism might be that of noncirrhotic portal hypertension occurring in SSc and other connective tissue diseases. As a form of noncirrhotic portal hypertension, this type of progression of PBC is generally recognized by (1) the presence of unequivocal signs of portal hypertension; (2) the absence of cirrhosis, advanced fibrosis, or other causes of chronic liver diseases; and (3) the absence of thrombosis of the hepatic veins or of the portal vein at imaging. In these patients, the liver function is usually preserved; the treatment is based on the monitoring and prevention of complications of portal hypertension, with only few patients requiring LT for unmanageable portal hypertension or liver failure. A target proteomic approach looking at markers on inflammation and/or fibrosis and their dynamic over time might be appropriate to better define different disease trajectories.

STRATIFICATION OF PATIENTS BY RISK OF DISEASE PROGRESSION
Stage of Disease

Measures of liver fibrosis, that is, the stage of disease, are relevant in prognostication because in PBC; as in other liver diseases, they predict treatment response and liver failure.[14,15] Liver biopsy is the gold standard to assess liver fibrosis. Its invasiveness with significant potential complications and the poor patient acceptance, however, coupled with its inherent shortcomings related to sampling error have led to an exponential interest in the identification and use of noninvasive markers of liver fibrosis. To be included in clinical practice, noninvasive markers should predict treatment response, survival, and the risk of cancer and portal hypertension.

Pathologic features

Liver biopsy for staging of PBC lost favor after the publication of a study by Garrido and Hubscher[16]: in this study, the investigators evaluated fibrosis using Menghini needle from simulated needle biopsy in fields approximately the size of conventional needle biopsy and from whole-section scanning in areas with little and extensive fibrosis. They showed considerable variation in the stage of fibrosis across each of 50 explanted PBC livers, evaluated using the staging system of Ludwig and colleagues.[17] There have been no subsequent studies to verify or challenge this observation. There is less variability in staging using the new system of Nakanuma.[18] In this system, the stage of disease is based on the degree of fibrosis, bile duct loss, and cholestasis assessed by deposition of orcein-positive granules, whereas the grade of necroinflammatory activity is based on cholangitis, interface hepatitis, and lobular hepatitis. The accumulation of orcein-positive granules occurs evenly across the PBC liver, which means that staging using the Nakanuma system is more reliable.[19,20] Even so, the widespread availability of noninvasive measures of fibrosis means that liver biopsy for staging of PBC is somewhat obsolete. Liver biopsy does, however, remain useful in certain settings. Nowadays, the main indications are to confirm the diagnosis of PBC when PBC-specific antibodies are absent and confirm a diagnosis of PBC with AIH features. Liver biopsy is also useful to confirm ductopenia and assess the relative contribution of each liver injury when a comorbid liver disease is present, such as nonalcoholic steatohepatitis. In patients with inadequate response to UDCA, liver biopsy may provide the explanation. For example, it may identify a previously unsuspected variant syndrome, steatohepatitis, or interface hepatitis of moderate or greater severity.

Liver biopsy could undoubtedly inform risk stratification in PBC. For example, the Nakanuma[18] stage and grade have been shown to correlate with clinicolaboratory features. Recent data have shown an association between interface hepatitis, bridging fibrosis, and cirrhosis and long-term outcomes in PBC independently from UDCA treatment, confirming historical data.[14,15] Furthermore, the presence of ductopenia/bile duct loss has been reported to be a predictor of PBC progression.[21] These data suggest that liver biopsy could be as important for treatment stratification in PBC as it is in AIH and other liver conditions—but the balance of risk versus benefit and patient acceptability need to be considered. This is exactly the area of unmet need that PM should address.

Ideally, analysis of circulating byproducts (eg, epigenetic factors, such as microRNAs, cell-free DNA, glucose, and fatty acid and amino acid metabolites from high-throughput omics profiling, among others), namely liquid biopsy, could provide access to molecular information related to the severity of portal inflammation, biliary damage, cholestasis, and fibrosis and thus improve patients' stratification and allow evaluation of disease biology dynamically over time. To develop such noninvasive surrogate test of liver pathology, a major effort would be required to select a cohort of PBC patients who undergo deep phenotyping of liver tissue samples and biofluids (such as serum, plasma, peripheral blood mononuclear cells, and urine) at different time points. Building up a well-sized cohort in such a rare condition and performing follow-up liver biopsies are challenging. Nonetheless, this is a promising horizon toward which further research efforts should be directed.

Non-invasive markers of fibrosis

Liver stiffness measure (LSM) by transient elastography, aspartate aminotransferase (AST)-to-platelet ratio index (APRI), and enhanced liver fibrosis (ELF) represent alternative and potentially complementary approaches to assessing liver fibrosis and are associated with minimal discomfort and hazard to the patient when compared with biopsy.

LSM has been regarded as a good marker to exclude or confirm severe fibrosis or cirrhosis in PBC. The largest study (N = 103) demonstrated high specificity and sensitivity (>90%) of transient elastography in distinguishing severe fibrosis from cirrhosis in PBC patients.[22] A threshold of LSM greater than 9.6 kPa (F4) at diagnosis was associated with a 5-fold increase in the risk of future liver decompensation or LT. The results were not as strong when it came to intermediate fibrosis (F2: sensitivity 0.67, specificity 1.0). This may be due to the presence of inflammation and cholestasis that could overestimate the measurement.[22]

Investigators also show a predictive role of longitudinal assessment of LSM: a progression of greater than or equal to 2.1 kPa/y in the overall cohort was associated with 8-fold increased risk of liver decompensation, LT, or death.[22] Before proposing regular assessments of LSM as standard practice, however, for example, on an annual basis, these data would require external validation in a large cohort, in longitudinal fashion. Also, whether the risk estimate is independent of the achievement of treatment response has to be clarified.

There is convincing evidence for the use of APRI in prognostication of PBC. In a recent study of 386 PBC patients, the APRI measured at baseline or after 1 year of therapy with UDCA independently predicted LT-free survival. Measured at baseline,

APRI greater than 0.54 best discriminated good versus poor prognosis. Measured after 1 year of treatment, APRI greater than 0.54 identified a subgroup of patients at risk of disease progression despite meeting the Paris I, Paris II, Barcelona, and Toronto definitions of UDCA response.[23]

The ELF score, calculated from serum measurements of hyaluronic acid, tissue inhibitor of metalloproteinase 1, and procollagen type III N-terminal propeptide, is another noninvasive marker proposed in PBC. There is only 1 multicenter study (N = 161) looking at the ELF score in PBC. ELF showed a good ability to stratify patients into groups of differing prognoses. Prediction of decompensations was good, with an area under a receiver operating characteristic curve (AUC) ranging between 0.68 and 0.78 based on how many years before the first event the serum was collected; however, no calibration, that is, agreement between predicted versus observed events, was provided.[24]

The development of the ELF score is paradigmatic of the potentiality to transfer biomarkers (proteomic markers, in this case) from discovery to clinical practice; it also highlights the pitfalls and limitations of this. Despite encouraging results, ELF score has not been adopted with enthusiasm in clinical practice in PBC, and overall in hepatology, and its use is currently limited to clinical trials where fibrosis is an endpoint (eg, https://clinicaltrials.gov/ct2/show/NCT01672853). The main limitation for its use include the high cost of the equipment and the need for regular recalibration and trained operators to ensure accuracy and reproducibility of the results. There are also concerns regarding its biological meaning and interpretation: for instance, it is unclear whether ELF is a marker of disease severity or disease stage; fluctuations over time have not been studied and this prevents its application as dynamic biomarker; also, stratified analysis for influence factors, such as gender, age and ethnicity, are lacking.[25] More data on ELF score application in patients with PBC are needed to make firm recommendations on its use in this condition A head-to-head comparison with the most robust, currently available prognostic tests, such as the continuous scoring systems (UK-PBC and GLOBE scores) and the transient elastography, would be of interest.

Treatment Response Profile

First-line treatment of PBC is UDCA.[26] Although a majority of patients have an improvement of the liver biochemistry after this therapy, 20% to 40% of patients have insufficient or no response to UDCA. Since 2016, obeticholic acid has been approved by the Food and Drug Administration and European Medicines Agency as a second-line treatment in association with UDCA in nonresponders to first-line therapy or in those intolerant to UDCA monotherapy. Moreover, several molecules targeting pathways involved in cholestasis or immune-related mechanisms might soon be available. It follows the importance of risk-stratification of patients' management based on the treatment response profile to allocate the best treatment to the right patient and improve the overall management.

Age and gender

Age and gender were shown to influence response to treatment with UDCA in PBC in the UK-PBC national cohort.[27] Gender was not confirmed, however, to be a predictor of treatment response in the international cohort of the Global PBC Study Group.[28]

Younger age at diagnosis was strongly and independently associated with response to UDCA, with an approximately linear relationship between age and the probability of response; rates ranged from 90% for patients greater than 70 years to 50% for those younger than age 30. The authors suggest that the relationship between age at diagnosis and likelihood of UDCA response was explicable by the effect of hormones, such that high estrogen levels increase resistance to effective treatment.[27] Furthermore, age and gender seemed to correlate with symptoms. Young girls were more likely to have fatigue and pruritus than older and male patients. The Newcastle group showed that fatigue is associated with a reduced survival.[29] Whether this translates in a worse outcome for young women is not clear.

Liver biochemistry

It is well established that the liver function tests (LFTs) on treatment with UDCA strongly predict LT-free survival in PBC.[30] This observation has prompted the development of several prognostic models based on the UDCA response that may be used to stratify patients according to their risk of developing chronic liver failure.

UDCA biochemical response can be assessed using either a qualitative definition based on binary variables or quantitative scoring systems computed from continuous parameters.[2] All these definitions and scores have been developed to be used only after 1 year of UDCA therapy to stratify according to treatment response.

Qualitative definitions Qualitative definitions use thresholds of the LFTs, such as bilirubin, transaminases, and ALP, after 6 months to 24 months of treatment with UDCA on a stable, optimized dose (13–15 mg/kg/d) to dichotomize patients into responders or nonresponders. The best-known of these binary definitions are reported in **Box 2**. Their accuracy in predicting death or LT has been validated externally[27] and they have all been proposed in the recent Clinical Practice Guidelines of EASL 2017.[2] Where binary definitions are used for risk stratification, it is advised to use a definition with higher sensitivity but lower specificity. Possibly for this reason, the POISE trial definition of UDCA nonresponse (total bilirubin >1 × upper limit of normal [ULN] or ALP ≥1.67 × ULN) seems to have become the commercial standard, included in the eligibility criteria or endpoints of the phase I/II study of FFP104 by Fast Forward Pharmaceuticals (Utrecht, Netherlands); phase II study of LJN452 by Novartis (Basel, Switzerland),

---

Box 2
Biochemical response criteria for risk stratification in ursodeoxycholic acid–treated primary biliary cholangitis patients and characteristics of the cohorts where they were developed

Response Definitions and Prognostic Models	Definition and Parameters Evaluated	Type of Prediction	Number of Patients	Centers
Paris I, 2008	ALP <3 × ULN, AST <2 × ULN and bilirubin ≤1 mg/dL after 1 y	Dichotomous	292	Single center
Barcelona, 2006	>40% decrease of ALP or normalization after 1 y	Dichotomous	192	Single center
Toronto, 2010	ALP ≤1.67 × ULN after 2 y	Dichotomous	69	Single center
Paris II, 2011	ALP ≤1.5 × ULN, AST ≤1.5 × ULN and bilirubin ≤l mg/dL after 1 y	Dichotomous	165	Single center
Rotterdam, 2009	Normalization of abnormal bilirubin and/or albumin after 1 y	Dichotomous	375	Single center
GLOBE score, 2015	Age, bilirubin, albumin, ALP, platelets	Continuous	2488	15 tertiary centers
UK-PBC score, 2016	Bilirubin, alanine aminotransferase (ALT)/AST ALP, platelets, albumin	Continuous	1916	155 secondary and tertiary centers

and phase II study of MBX-8025 by CymaBay (Newark, California, USA) Therapeutics (for details, see https://clinicaltrials.gov/). EASL advocates ALP less than 1.5 × ULN as the threshold at which long-term risk becomes clinically meaningful compared with a control healthy population.[2]

The main advantage of dichotomous definition is that they are easy to use. Such definitons do, however, have limitations because they could potentially lead to loss of important predictive information. Most importantly, they imply there are only 2 levels of risk, which is inaccurate. There is a continuous relationship between the individual LFT and the risk of liver death or LT.[31] Thus, dichotomous definitions fail to quantify intermediate levels of risk. Furthermore, they ignore the relationship between risk and time. They do not indicate whether the high-risk patient will need an LT tomorrow or 15 years in the future.

Quantitative scoring systems Proposed by the UK-PBC Research Group and the Global PBC Study Group,[28,31] quantitative scoring systems enable hepatologists to overcome the limitations of the binary risk stratification. In particular, these models quantify an individual's risk in relation to time. In comparison with the binary definition of response that only evaluate parameters of disease activity, they include surrogate markers of disease stage. Both UK-PBC and GLOBE outperform the Paris I definition.[32]

Each risk score includes the LFTs after treatment with UDCA as well as surrogate measurements of disease stage (see **Box 2**). In addition, the GLOBE score includes the age at diagnosis. In both risk scores, all the predictive variables are continuous—and treated as such. The UK-PBC risk score estimates the risk of LT or liver-related death occurring within 5 years, 10 years, or 15 years. The GLOBE score predicts LT-free survival at 3 years, 5 years, 10 years, and 15 years. Both risk scores were shown to outperform previous models, with C statistics at 15 years in the validation cohorts of 0.90 and 0.82, respectively.

In clinical practice, the UK-PBC and GLOBE scores should be most useful to identify patients who would obtain greatest benefit from further risk-reduction using second-line therapy. This is timely with several potential disease-modifying agents for PBC in phase II or III clinical trials. The UK-PBC and GLOBE scores may also be used to identify low-risk patients, for whom follow-up in primary care may be appropriate. There are no clear-cut thresholds that should prompt addition of second-line therapies or de-escalation of follow-up back to primary care. These thresholds vary from one patient to the next, influenced by the patient profile (age, fibrosis stage, and severity of itch, among others), side effects, and cost-effectiveness of a specific agent.

To date, metabolomics analysis of various classes of blood metabolites has been proposed only to define distinct profiles in patients with PBC. It would also allow, however, classifying patient responsiveness to therapies. The circulating metabolome capturing different metabolites classes (eg, BAs, aminoacids, acylcarnitines, Krebs cycle intermediates, lipids species, among the others), some of which in key biochemical pathways are known to be involved in PBC responsiveness, might be able to be defined by open (untargeted) and close (targeted) approaches. These might be integrated in the predicting model of treatment response to UDCA the authors recently proposed to develop enhanced predictive approaches for identification of high-risk patients earlier in the disease and facilitating application of enhanced therapy in a more timely fashion.[33]

Primary Biliary Cholangitis–Specific Autoantibody Profile

The anti-gp210 targets glycoprotein 210 of the nuclear pore complex. It is reportedly associated with more aggressive disease. In 3 studies from Italy and Japan, the presence of anti-gp210 antibodies was associated with more advanced disease, suggesting that anti-gp210 antibodies might be related to hepatocellular failure-type progression.[32] More recently, antibodies against hexokinase (HK1) and a nuclear protein involved in the metabolism of collagen (KL-p) have been shown sensitive and specific for detection of PBC and could be useful in diagnosis in Anti-mitochondrial M2 antibody (AMA-M2) negative, gp210 antibody negative, and sp100 antibody-negative patients. Furthermore, investigators found a correlation between the presence of antibodies anti-HK1 and disease progression, with lower transplant-free survival.[34] The PBC-specific antinuclear antibodies (ANAs) are still of limited validity in clinical practice because studies showing their prognostic role are limited and only retrospective. Longitudinal, large-scale studies using time-to-event data are needed to confirm their role as reliable markers of prognosis.

PERSPECTIVES OF PRECISION MEDICINE IN PRIMARY BILIARY CHOLANGITIS

To facilitate the identification of high-risk individuals for cost-effective disease monitoring and second-line therapies, mounting efforts have been put forth to develop risk prediction models, including biochemical variables with good accuracy and calibration regarding survival. The next step is the identification and incorporation of novel biomarkers, including genetic and molecular biomarkers, to allow identification of disease variants and trajectory, and to estimate the risk of disease progression and the likelihood of treatment response, paving the way for PM in PBC.

The PM initiative ongoing in PBC, as in many other fields of medicine, promises a new era of health care with targeted disease treatment and management. This features a longitudinal study of national and international cohorts of 1000 or more people with large quantity of data and biospecimens necessary to conduct a wide range of studies, with the aim of customizing interventions based on a person's profile.

Conducting a large study cohort study is challenging from several aspects: identification of financial resources needed for implementing such a large-scale project; time required to obtain meaningful results—this is a major problem in PBC due to its indolent nature, where prospective studies of outcomes would span decades to allow for a robust number of endpoints to occur; obtaining permission for data sharing and the need for researchers to recontact/consent participants; concerns about privacy, security, and access to individual data and health records; and coordination, transparency, and governance.

PM is expected to benefit from combining genetic and molecular studies with high-throughput methods, that is, genomics, transcriptomics, proteomics, and metabolomics, among others. These methods permit the determination of thousands of molecules within a tissue or biological fluid that can configure the signature of a disease. The use of these methods is demanding in terms of the design of the study, acquisition, storage, analysis, and interpretation of the data.

When carried out within the adequate medical context, genetic screens are powerful tools for identifying new genes and variations within genes that are involved in specific physiopathologic processes. An example in hepatology is the variant of patatin-like phospholipase domain-containing protein 3 gene (PNPLA3) that has been associated with the susceptibility and histologic severity of nonalcoholic fatty liver disease (NALFD).[35] PNPLA3 has been proposed as a novel biomarker for (gene-based) classification of NALFD and should be considered in the diagnostic work-up of this disease.

Genetic information will likely help advance the field of pharmacogenomics. Many single-nucleotide polymorphisms (SNPs) have been used to predict outcomes of specific pharmacologic agents. Some SNPs are used to predict whether an individual is susceptible to side effects from a certain class of drugs. Several groups, including the authors', are trying to create simpler tools that combine genetic and molecular data along with clinical and demographic parameters to predict treatment response to UDCA. In theory, this could be used at the outset to decide whether to escalate treatment of high-risk patients, offering second-line treatment at the outset.

An example of how genomics can be brought to real practice is the 100,000 Genomes Project, which was launched in 2012 in the United Kingdom. This project is performing whole-genome sequencing of 100,000 genomes from 70,000 individuals with rare diseases, their families, and patients with cancer. The main aim of this program is to set up a genomic medicine service for National Health Service patients with potential benefits in disease prevention, management, and treatment. It will also stimulate the development of diagnostics, devices, medicines, and treatments based on a new understanding of the genetic and molecular basis of disease. Finally, it will build partnerships between National Health Service, academia, and industry.

Genomic technologies have made feasible investigating the expression of thousands of genes, that is, transcriptomics, at a time using large sets of samples. The clinical application of transcriptomics profiling to reveal novel gene expression signatures is challenging in a complex disease like PBC for the following reasons. PBC might result from a large number of different genes and biological pathways and several phenotypes; therefore, large cohorts of well-characterized patients are necessary to obtain genomic signatures of clinical relevance. Also, pathogenic (that may be immune-related) and prognostic genes signatures (that may be related to fibrosis progression rather than severity of biliary inflammation) might contain a large number of genes and the prediction algorithms may be complex and not easy to transfer to routine clinical practice. Finally, there is the problem of false-positive tests inherent to all high-throughput techniques where large data sets are analyzed. That said, when used correctly, transcriptomics technologies may be translated into scoring systems that can reproducibly predict clinical outcomes. An example in hepatology is the development of a simple risk score classifier based on the expression of a small number of genes that can predict in a reproducible manner overall survival of patients after surgical resection for HCC.[36]

Another branch of omics-based technology is the high-throughput identification and quantification of small-sized molecules, that is, metabolomics. There is increased interest in understanding which metabolic differences between normal and diseased tissues can lead to the development of more selective and effective treatments. The main aim of metabolomics research is the discovery of specific metabolic profiles in serum, urine, feces, tissues, and other biological materials that are associated with disease features, response to specific treatments, or survival. Blood is the most commonly collected (as serum or plasma) and stored biological fluid in epidemiologic studies and has been the most often used sample in metabolomics analyses to date. Because blood components are under tight homeostatic regulation, the extent of variation in blood metabolite concentration is limited. Urine samples represent a good alternative to blood and have greater capture of exogenous compounds, such as microbiota, drugs, and diet, and urine composition can vary a lot, especially in disease states. A 24-hour collection is preferred over spot urine collection because it provides a complete picture of cumulative metabolite excretion over a 24-hour period. However, 24-hour samples are difficult to collect for epidemiologic studies.

The development of metabolomics-based diagnostic and prognostic tests has the same problems inherent to all high-throughput techniques, that is, the detection of true relationships between a group of metabolites and disease, minimizing the risk of false-positive associations. An additional complication in metabolomics, compared with other omics-based methods, is the preparation and storage of the samples, due to large differences in solubility and stability among metabolites. This is particularly important in relation to epidemiologic studies because samples regularly undergo freeze-thaw cycles that may unpredictably affect the analytical results. Metabolic profiling can run in either targeted or untargeted mode. Targeted profiling separates a limited number of specific metabolites of known identity and is a more hypothesis-driven approach. In PBC, such an approach might be focused on markers of BA physiology, inflammation, and fibrosis. Untargeted approaches are applied to capture metabolic classes that escape target analysis (eg, Krebs cycle intermediates, short-chain fatty acids, nucleotides). Untargeted analysis does not require an a priori hypothesis and can be used to discover novel metabolic associations and disease pathways. Data density is high, however, and because analysis is not optimized for specific metabolites, metabolite identification and quantification may be difficult. Several targeted attempts to identify a metabolomics signature are ongoing in PBC; these highlighted altered metabolic pathways associated with glucose, fatty acid, and amino acid metabolites.[37,38] Effort is required to associate the metabolomics profile with clinical features, such as disease subphenotypes, symptoms, disease course, treatment response, and survival.

Before initiating such studies, it is of primary importance to have a robust hypothesis, which dictates the entire omics workflow and greatly influences the study outcomes. The hypothesis dictates which technologies to choose from (eg, genomic and transcriptomic approaches to study the immunologic signature of the disease; metabolomics approaches on plasma and urine to study the cholestatic component; and proteomic approach to identify markers of the different patterns of fibrosis progression in PBC), the sample to study (eg, circulating cells vs infiltrating cells and whole blood cells vs peripheral blood mononuclear cells), and which approaches to use (eg, targeted vs untargeted metabolomics study) to carry on the study. As a next step, integration of omics data (transomics) is useful, complementary, and more informative than if single omics stood alone, despite being challenging.

Omics-based research to develop PM, however, requires more than just accumulating data. First of all, it is necessary to develop standard protocols that yield consistent results in different laboratories so that data can be built into a single repository. Another problem is the integration of all the data generated by omics-based screens (such as RNAs, proteins, metabolites, protein-protein interactions, protein-lipid interactions, protein-nucleic acid interactions, and so on). Finally, practical application will necessitate the creation of tools by which omics information can be filtered and made readily accessible to clinicians who will incorporate it into medical decision making at the point of care. A key component to advance PM from the academic setting to the point of care in the community is the incorporation of genetic and molecular databases directly into a universal electronic medical record (EMR) system. An effective EMR system prompts practitioners to follow certain diagnostic or treatment algorithms based on an individual's information and reference genomic/molecular datasets stored in the EMR.

PM, when fully realized, has great potential to change the way patients are managed with PBC today. Knowing the genetic and/or molecular variations linked to specific disease phenotype might influence the way disease is screened for drugs are selected and disease progression is surveyed. Ideally, all patients who enter a health care system in the future will have their DNA/molecular profile routinely sequenced and analyzed at admission and entered into a database to enhance patient care. The cost of obtaining, analyzing, storing, and integrating this information will have to be balanced with the potential overall savings to the health care system.

SUMMARY

In view of forthcoming availability of novel drugs that might have a positive impact on morbidity and mortality of patients with PBC and thanks to the rise of high-throughput omics technologies, the PBC field is now moving more quickly toward clinical translation to support PM. PM development has a great potential to change the standard of care in diagnostics, therapeutics, and clinical trials in this disease. In the future, a diagnostic work-up of PBC patients may include information on genetic variants and molecular signature that may define a particular subtype of disease and provide an estimate of treatment response and survival. To reach this point, specific interventions are needed, such as sequencing more genomes, creating bigger biobanks, and linking biological information to health data in EMR. This hopefully will help to shed light on the pathogenic mechanisms of this condition and translate knowledge into new therapies and care pathways.

REFERENCES

1. Collins FS, Varmus H. A new initiative on precision medicine. N Engl J Med 2015; 372(9):793–5.
2. Hirschfield GM, Beuers U, Corpechot C, et al. EASL clinical practice guidelines: the diagnosis and management of patients with primary biliary cholangitis. J Hepatol 2017;67(1):145–72.
3. Poupon R, Chazouilleres O, Corpechot C, et al. Development of autoimmune hepatitis in patients with typical primary biliary cirrhosis. Hepatology 2006;44(1):85–90.
4. Chazouillères O, Wendum D, Serfaty L, et al. Primary biliary cirrhosis-autoimmune hepatitis overlap syndrome: clinical features and response to therapy. Hepatology 1998;28(2):296–301.
5. European Association for the Study of the Liver. EASL clinical practice guidelines: autoimmune hepatitis. J Hepatol 2015;63(4):971–1004.
6. Millar B, Wong LL, Green K, et al. Autoimmune hepatitis patients with poor treatment response have a distinct liver transcriptome: implications for personalised therapy. J Hepatol 2017;66(1):S364.
7. Ercole A, Magnoni S, Vegliante G, et al. Current and emerging technologies for probing molecular signatures of traumatic brain injury. Front Neurol 2017;8:450.
8. Vleggaar FP, van Buuren HR, Zondervan PE, et al, Dutch Multicentre PBC Study Group the DMP Study. Jaundice in non-cirrhotic primary biliary cirrhosis: the premature ductopenic variant. Gut 2001;49(2):276–81.
9. Liberal R, Grant CR, Sakkas L, et al. Diagnostic and clinical significance of anti-centromere antibodies in primary biliary cirrhosis. Clin Res Hepatol Gastroenterol 2013;37(6):572–85.
10. Nakamura M, Kondo H, Tanaka A, et al. Autoantibody status and histological variables influence biochemical response to treatment and long-term outcomes in Japanese patients with primary biliary cirrhosis. Hepatol Res 2015;45(8):846–55.
11. Nakamura M, Kondo H, Mori T, et al. Anti-gp210 and anti-centromere antibodies are different risk factors for the progression of primary biliary cirrhosis. Hepatology 2007;45(1):118–27.
12. Navasa M, Parés A, Bruguera M, et al. Portal hypertension in primary biliary cirrhosis. J Hepatol 1987;5(3):292–8.
13. Kew MC, Varma RR, Dos Santos HA, et al. Portal hypertension in primary biliary cirrhosis. Gut 1971;12(10):830–4.
14. Corpechot C, Abenavoli L, Rabahi N, et al. Biochemical response to ursodeoxycholic acid and long-term prognosis in primary biliary cirrhosis. Hepatology 2008; 48(3):871–7.
15. Carbone M, Sharp SJ, Heneghan MA, et al. P1198: histological stage is relevant for risk-stratification in primary biliary cirrhosis. J Hepatol 2015;62:S805.

16. Garrido MC, Hubscher SG. Accuracy of staging in primary biliary cirrhosis. J Clin Pathol 1996;49(7):556–9. Available at: http://www.ncbi.nlm.nih.gov/pubmed/8813953. Accessed January 15, 2018.

17. Ludwig J, Dickson ER, McDonald GS. Staging of chronic nonsuppurative destructive cholangitis (syndrome of primary biliary cirrhosis). Virchows Arch A Pathol Anat Histol 1978;379(2):103–12. Available at: http://www.ncbi.nlm.nih.gov/pubmed/150690. Accessed January 15, 2018.

18. Nakanuma Y, Zen Y, Harada K, et al. Application of a new histological staging and grading system for primary biliary cirrhosis to liver biopsy specimens: interobserver agreement. Pathol Int 2010;60(3):167–74.

19. Desmet VJ. Histopathology of cholestasis. Verh Dtsch Ges Pathol 1995;79:233–40. Available at: http://www.ncbi.nlm.nih.gov/pubmed/8600686. Accessed January 15, 2018.

20. Goldfischer S, Popper H, Sternlieb I. The significance of variations in the distribution of copper in liver disease. Am J Pathol 1980;99(3):715–30. Available at: http://www.ncbi.nlm.nih.gov/pubmed/7386600. Accessed January 15, 2018.

21. Kumagi T, Guindi M, Fischer SE, et al. Baseline ductopenia and treatment response predict long-term histological progression in primary biliary cirrhosis. Am J Gastroenterol 2010;105(10):2186–94.

22. Corpechot C, Carrat F, Poujol-Robert A, et al. Noninvasive elastography-based assessment of liver fibrosis progression and prognosis in primary biliary cirrhosis. Hepatology 2012;56(1):198–208.

23. Trivedi PJ, Bruns T, Cheung A, et al. Optimising risk stratification in primary biliary cirrhosis: AST/platelet ratio index predicts outcome independent of ursodeoxycholic acid response. J Hepatol 2014;60(6):1249–58.

24. Mayo MJ, Parkes J, Adams-Huet B, et al. Prediction of clinical outcomes in primary biliary cirrhosis by serum enhanced liver fibrosis assay. Hepatology 2008;48(5):1549–57.

25. Lichtinghagen R, Pietsch D, Bantel H, et al. The Enhanced Liver Fibrosis (ELF) score: normal values, influence factors and proposed cut-off values. J Hepatol 2013;59(2):236–42.

26. Poupon R, Poupon R, Calmus Y, et al. Is ursodeoxycholic acid an effective treatment for primary biliary cirrhosis? Lancet 1987;329(8537):834–6.

27. Carbone M, Mells GF, Pells G, et al. Sex and age are determinants of the clinical phenotype of primary biliary cirrhosis and response to ursodeoxycholic acid. Gastroenterology 2013;144(3):560–9.e7.

28. Lammers WJ, Hirschfield GM, Corpechot C, et al. Development and validation of a scoring system to predict outcomes of patients with primary biliary cirrhosis receiving ursodeoxycholic acid therapy. Gastroenterology 2015;149(7):1804–12.e4.

29. Jones DE, Al-Rifai A, Frith J, et al. The independent effects of fatigue and UDCA therapy on mortality in primary biliary cirrhosis: results of a 9year follow-up. J Hepatol 2010;53(5):911–7.

30. Leuschner U, Fischer H, Kurtz W, et al. Ursodeoxycholic acid in primary biliary cirrhosis: results of a controlled double-blind trial. Gastroenterology 1989;97(5):1268–74. Available at: http://www.ncbi.nlm.nih.gov/pubmed/2551765. Accessed January 16, 2018.

31. Carbone M, Sharp SJ, Flack S, et al. The UK-PBC risk scores: derivation and validation of a scoring system for long-term prediction of end-stage liver disease in primary biliary cholangitis. Hepatology 2016;63(3):930–50.

32. Yang F, Yang Y, Wang Q, et al. The risk predictive values of UK-PBC and GLOBE scoring system in Chinese patients with primary biliary cholangitis: the additional effect of anti-gp210. Aliment Pharmacol Ther 2017;45(5):733–43.

33. Carbone M, Nardi A, Carpino G, et al. Pre-treatment risk stratification in primary biliary cholangitis: A predictive model to guide first-line combination therapy. 50(1):21–2.

34. Reig A, Garcia M, Shums Z, et al. The novel hexokinase 1 antibodies are useful for the diagnosis and associated with bad prognosis in primary biliary cholangitis. J Hepatol 2017;66(1):S355–6.

35. Sookoian S, Pirola CJ. Meta-analysis of the influence of I148M variant of patatin-like phospholipase domain containing 3 gene (PNPLA3) on the susceptibility and histological severity of nonalcoholic fatty liver disease. Hepatology 2011;53(6): 1883–94.

36. Nault J-C, De Reyniès A, Villanueva A, et al. A hepatocellular carcinoma 5-gene score associated with survival of patients after liver resection. Gastroenterology 2013;145(1):176–87.

37. Hao J, Yang T, Zhou Y, et al. Serum metabolomics analysis reveals a distinct metabolic profile of patients with primary biliary cholangitis. Sci Rep 2017;7(1):784.

38. Bell LN, Wulff J, Comerford M, et al. Serum metabolic signatures of primary biliary cirrhosis and primary sclerosing cholangitis. Liver Int 2015;35(1):263–74.

Natural History of Primary Biliary Cholangitis in the Ursodeoxycholic Acid Era

Role of Scoring Systems

Aparna Goel, MD, Woong Ray Kim, MD*

KEYWORDS

• PBC • Ursodeoxycholic acid • Prognosis • Scoring systems • Predictive models

KEY POINTS

- Although the natural history of primary biliary cholangitis (PBC) is variable, mathematical models may be used to predict patient outcomes, incorporating variables such as age, bilirubin, albumin, coagulopathy, and stages of fibrosis.
- Although ursodeoxycholic acid (UDCA) has significantly altered the natural history of PBC by improving transplant-free survival, a significant proportion of patients do not respond to UDCA.
- Prognostic models for UDCA-treated patients have been developed to reflect patients' baseline liver function and biochemical response to treatment.
- As new biomarkers and therapeutic agents are discovered, future models may enhance the accuracy and reliability of the prediction, providing better tools for clinicians and researchers.

INTRODUCTION

Primary biliary cholangitis (PBC), previously referred to as primary biliary cirrhosis, is a progressive cholestatic liver disease characterized by the destruction of small intrahepatic bile ducts.[1] The gradual and sustained loss of bile ducts leads to periportal inflammation, fibrosis, and cirrhosis with its ensuing complications. It is a rare disease with an estimated prevalence of 19 to 402 per million persons and approximately 120,000 people are affected in the United States.[2] The disease primarily afflicts middle-aged women and is characterized by fatigue and pruritus, which can be debilitating.[3] The autoimmune features are a hallmark of PBC, with more than 95% of

Disclosure Statement: The authors have nothing to disclose.
Division of Gastroenterology and ·Hepatology, Stanford University, Alway Building, Room M211, 300 Pasteur Drive, Stanford, CA 94305, USA
* Corresponding author.
E-mail address: wrkim@stanford.edu

patients having a detectable antimitochondrial antibody (AMA). The presence of AMA along with an elevated alkaline phosphatase level is sufficient to diagnose PBC and liver biopsy is only required in atypical cases.

Ursodeoxycholic acid (UDCA) was the only treatment of PBC until the approval of obeticholic acid (OCA) in 2016. UDCA delays progression of disease, especially when started early in the disease course and hence improves transplant-free survival. However, nearly 40% of patients do not respond to UDCA. For those with an incomplete response or intolerability to UDCA, OCA has a significant biochemical response, although the long-term survival benefits of OCA are yet to be determined. Additional therapies for PBC are currently under investigation and show promising results.

For the last 3 decades, prediction models have been used in PBC to help clinicians stratify patients at highest risk of death or liver transplantation. The first of these models was created before the widespread use of UDCA. With longer term data and larger cohorts, older models continue to be modified and newer models created. This article describes the natural history of PBC in the pre-UDCA and UDCA eras, and the various prognostic scores that have been studied in PBC over time.

OUTCOMES AND PROGNOSIS OF PRIMARY BILIARY CHOLANGITIS WITHOUT THERAPY
Natural History of Primary Biliary Cholangitis in the Pre–Ursodeoxycholic Acid Era

PBC is a chronic disease that progresses over a span of decades to cause end-stage liver disease. Before the availability of UDCA, PBC was usually diagnosed at advanced, symptomatic stages of liver disease. The median survival at the time of diagnosis was substantially lower than the general population, ranging from 6 to 10 years.[4,5] With the widespread use of screening liver chemistries and laboratory tests to detect AMA, patients have been diagnosed at earlier, asymptomatic stages. The proportion of asymptomatic patients who ultimately develop symptomatic liver disease varies in studies and ranges from 36% to 89% in a period of 5 to 17 years.[6] The median survival in asymptomatic patients tends to be longer compared with symptomatic patients, although it still averages 6 to 10 years after the development of symptoms.[6]

Histologic severity predicts survival in patients with PBC. In a study of 225 subjects with PBC who were not on any effective therapy, most developed histologic progression of disease within 2 years. Fifty percent of subjects with stage II fibrosis developed cirrhosis by 4 years and only 20% of subjects showed histologic stability. Overall, the rate of histologic progression without treatment is estimated at 1 stage every 1.5 years.[5] The development of hepatic decompensation, manifesting as ascites, bleeding, hepatic encephalopathy, or hyperbilirubinemia, was estimated at 15% to 25% over the course of 5 years.

Prognostic Models in the Pre–ursodeoxycholic Acid Era

Patients with PBC have variable disease courses, hence prognosis varies greatly. Factors that are independently associated with worse outcomes include older age, elevated serum bilirubin, lower albumin, coagulopathy, presence of edema, and advanced degrees of fibrosis. The mathematical ability to estimate prognosis is beneficial for patient counseling and clinical decision-making, such as determining the need and urgency of liver transplantation. Several natural history models estimating transplant-free survival with biochemical, clinical, and histologic features have been developed (**Table 1**). The first 2 models required a liver biopsy, a factor that significantly limited their widespread adoption. The Mayo model overcame this shortcoming by using readily available noninvasive variables and was widely accepted in clinical practice after demonstrating validity in several independent cohorts.

Table 1
Prediction models developed in the pre–ursodeoxycholic acid era for estimating transplant-free survival in primary biliary cholangitis patients

Model	Derivation Cohort	Prognostic Score			
Roll 1983[28]	280 subjects with asymptomatic and symptomatic disease	R = 1.037 (age [y]) + 2.1 (hepatomegaly = 1) + 0.26 (portal fibrosis = 1) + (2.26 [if bilirubin>5] or 0.48 [if bilirubin<1.5])			
European I (Christensen) 1985[29]	248 subjects in azathioprine placebo-controlled trial Time-fixed model	R = 2.51 ($\log_{10}$ bilirubin) + $0.0069^{(age[y]-20/10)}$ - 0.05 (albumin) + 0.88 (cirrhosis = 1) + 0.68 (central cholestasis = 1) + 0.52 (azathioprine = 0)			
Bonsel (AZG) 1990[30]	131 subjects with PBC and nonalcoholic cirrhosis who did not receive liver transplant Time-fixed model	R = 0.0065 (bilirubin) + 0.0605 (age[y]) - 0.0517 (albumin) + 1.1827 (HBsAg = 1) + 2.0849 (neurologic complications = 1) + 1.2804 (varices = 1) + 0.1866 (quick-time prolongation) + 0.9183 (ascites = 1) + 0.7468 (clinical icterus = 1)			
Mayo I 1989[31]	312 subjects enrolled in D-penicillamine trials at Mayo Clinic & 106 for data validation Time-fixed model	R = 0.871 ($\log_e$ bilirubin) + 0.039 (age [y]) + 2.53 ($\log_e$ albumin) + 2.38 (prothrombin time) + 0.859 (edema severity = 0,0.5,1)			
European II 1993[32]	248 subjects in azathioprine placebo-controlled trial Time-dependent model	R = 2.53 ([$\log_{10}$ bilirubin]-1.53) + 1.39 (ascites = 1) − 0.085 (albumin-34.3) + 0.040 (age [y]-55) + 0.65 (gastrointestinal bleeding = 1)			
Mayo II 1994[33]	312 subjects enrolled in D-penicillamine trials at Mayo Clinic and 106 for data validation with follow-up through 1988 Time-dependent model	R = 0.051 (age [y]) + 1.209 ($\log_e$ bilirubin) + 2.754 ($\log_e$ prothrombin time) + 0.675 (edema) − 3.304 ($\log_e$ albumin)			
Mayo III 2000[34]	Same as above Mayo risk score (418 subjects total)		**0**	**1**	**2**	**3**
		Age	<38	38–62	≥63	—
		Bilirubin	<1	1–1.7	1.6–6.4	≥6.4
		Albumin	>4.1	2.8–4.1	<2.8	—
		Prothrombin time	—	Normal	Prolonged	—
		Edema	Absent	Present	—	—
Newcastle model 2002[7]	770 subjects from 1987–1994 in Northeast England Time-fixed model	R = 0.0742 (age [y]) + 0.2610 $\log_e$ [ALP/ALP ULN] −2.53 (albumin/LLN) + 0.195 × $\log_e$ (bilirubin/ULN)			

Abbreviations: HBsAg, hepatitis b surface antigen; $\log_{10}$, logarithm; $\log_e$, natural logarithm; R, Risk score.

The initial Mayo and European models were derived from data collected at a single timepoint. These models were subsequently modified using interval data from follow-up visits to refine survival predictions over the short term. In 2000, the Mayo risk score was further simplified to facilitate use in clinical practice and provide minimal listing criteria for liver transplant candidates. A score of 6 in the abbreviated model corresponded to a 1-year survival rate of 90.6%, matching the minimal listing criteria for liver transplantation. The Newcastle score, developed in 2002, used a geographically diverse group of patients spanning the pre-UDCA era and the UDCA era.[7]

Although it is not certain how well these models have been used practically, the Mayo model has perhaps been the most frequently referenced for research and patient care. **Fig. 1** illustrates how the Mayo model may be used to predict survival of

A

	Patient		
	A	B	C
Age (years)	53	58	50
Total Bilirubin (mg/dL)	1.2	2.8	5.3
Albumin (g/dL)	3.9	3.2	2.9
Prothrombin time (seconds)	10.1	14.5	16.2
Edema score[a]	0	0	1
Mayo Risk Score (R)	4.24	6.58	8.20

B

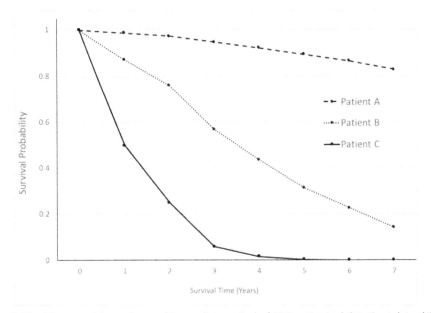

Fig. 1. The Mayo model may be used to predict survival of PBC patients. (*A*) Patient data. (*B*) Survival probability and time. [a] Edema score: 0 if no edema without diuretics, 0.5 if no edema with diuretic therapy, 1 if edema despite diuretic therapy.

a PBC patient. In **Fig. 1**A, 3 patients with progressively advanced PBC are presented. Patient A has no signs of hepatic decompensation with only mildly abnormal serum bilirubin, whereas patient B has more abnormal biochemical dysfunction without clinical decompensation (namely, peripheral edema). Patient C, although the youngest of the 3, has clearly advanced PBC. Mayo risk scores are calculated according to the equation shown in **Table 1** (Mayo I). Based on the scores, survival probabilities up to 7 years may be calculated by the survival function shown in **Fig. 1**B. As expected, predicted survival of patients A through C is according to the risk score. The advantage of using this model is that it provides numerical survival estimates, providing more tangible information than clinical intuition even by an experienced hepatologist. The mathematical calculation necessary to implement the Mayo model can be undertaken by online calculators. **Fig. 2** is a screenshot of the example of patient C presented in **Fig. 1**.

OUTCOMES OF PATIENTS IN THE URSODEOXYCHOLIC ACID ERA
Impact of Ursodeoxycholic Acid on Outcomes of Primary Biliary Cholangitis

The introduction of UDCA in the early 1990s markedly reshaped the history of PBC and led to a substantial improvement in patient outcomes. UDCA is thought to have a

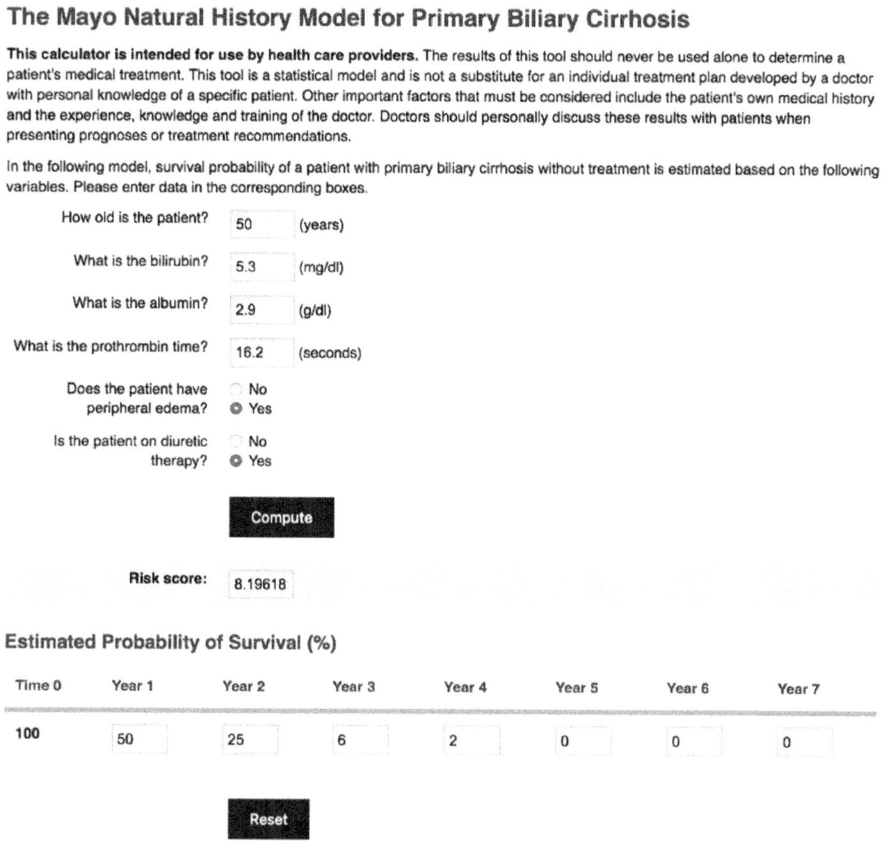

The Mayo Natural History Model for Primary Biliary Cirrhosis

This calculator is intended for use by health care providers. The results of this tool should never be used alone to determine a patient's medical treatment. This tool is a statistical model and is not a substitute for an individual treatment plan developed by a doctor with personal knowledge of a specific patient. Other important factors that must be considered include the patient's own medical history and the experience, knowledge and training of the doctor. Doctors should personally discuss these results with patients when presenting prognoses or treatment recommendations.

In the following model, survival probability of a patient with primary biliary cirrhosis without treatment is estimated based on the following variables. Please enter data in the corresponding boxes.

How old is the patient?	50	(years)
What is the bilirubin?	5.3	(mg/dl)
What is the albumin?	2.9	(g/dl)
What is the prothrombin time?	16.2	(seconds)
Does the patient have peripheral edema?	○ No ◉ Yes	
Is the patient on diuretic therapy?	○ No ◉ Yes	

Compute

Risk score: 8.19618

Estimated Probability of Survival (%)

Time 0	Year 1	Year 2	Year 3	Year 4	Year 5	Year 6	Year 7
100	50	25	6	2	0	0	0

Reset

Fig. 2. Online calculator of Mayo model (using former term primary biliary cirrhosis). Based on patient C from **Fig. 1**. (*From* Dickson ER1, Grambsch PM, Fleming TR, et al. Prognosis in primary biliary cirrhosis: model for decision making. Hepatology 1989;10(1):4; with permission.)

beneficial effect in the treatment of PBC by increasing the hydrophilicity of the circulating bile acid pool; stimulating hepatocellular and bile duct secretions, which provides cytoprotection against bile acid and cytokine-induced injury; and offering immunomodulation.[8] Initial studies from the late 1980s showed a significant improvement in liver biochemistries of patients with PBC treated with UDCA, leading to an exhaustive number of randomized controlled trials, observational studies, and combined analyses.[9] Overall, these studies have shown that UDCA improves biochemical indices, delays histologic progression of disease, delays development of esophageal varices, and reduces the need for liver transplantation. A selection of relevant studies of UDCA in PBC with brief conclusions is shown in **Table 2**.

The long-term observational studies previously noted have unequivocally shown a survival benefit in patients treated with UDCA, especially in those with early stages of disease that demonstrate a biochemical response. Although several meta-analyses failed to show a beneficial effect of UDCA, these analyses notably included studies of less than 2 years treatment duration, inadequate treatment doses of UDCA, and underpowered samples.[10–12] A meta-analysis that included studies of longer than 2 years duration or more than 100 patients corroborated individual study findings of the beneficial effect of UDCA.[13]

Unfortunately, approximately 40% of patients with PBC will have an inadequate biochemical response to UDCA.[14,15] These patients have more rapid progression of disease and 5 times higher risk of death or liver transplantation.[15] Several criteria of biochemical response to UDCA have been defined to estimate the long-term outcomes of patients with PBC (**Table 3**). Nearly all criteria agree that normalization or near-normalization of alkaline phosphatase predicts a favorable outcome. Most criteria assess response after 1 year of treatment, although more recent data suggest that assessment at 6 months may be equally predictive.[16]

Predicting Survival in the Ursodeoxycholic Acid Era

The applicability of the Mayo risk score described in **Table 1** was questioned after the introduction of UDCA. Because UDCA can have a significant effect on bilirubin level, it was unclear if the Mayo risk score would capture that improvement in survival. The maximal effect of UDCA on serum bilirubin is expected within several months of the start of therapy. A study of 222 subjects originally included in a 2-year Canadian multicenter trial of UDCA demonstrated that repeating the Mayo risk score 6 months after treatment adequately discriminated subjects at low, medium, and high risk of death.[17] Another study of 180 subjects included in an UDCA trial showed that the Mayo risk score calculated at the time of study entry overestimated the risk of death but recalculating the Mayo risk score after 6 months of therapy accurately predicted survival.[18] Other studies suggest that the Mayo risk score overestimates the risk of death when applied before the start of treatment, particularly in patients with early stages of disease.[19–21] Nonetheless the Mayo risk score has limitations. Because the model was derived from patients at a tertiary referral center, it may not be representative of the global PBC population. Additionally, the clinical assessment of edema in the score is subjective.

The Child-Pugh score and the Model for End-Stage Liver Disease (MELD) are used to predict survival and organ allocation in patients with end-stage liver disease. Although both of the scores have been widely accepted as reliable indicators of survival across various types of chronic liver disease, how well PBC patients with end-stage liver disease are served in the current MELD system has been questioned. When MELD was first developed, PBC patients were thought to be advantaged because multivariable analysis suggested that their short-term mortality was expected

Table 2

Studies evaluating ursodeoxycholic acid for the treatment of primary biliary cholangitis with various endpoints and brief conclusions

Study	Study Design	Study Duration	Study Outcome	Conclusion
Leuschner,[35] 1989	RCT	9 mo	Biochemical, histology	UDCA-treated subjects had decline in biochemical parameters by 48%–79% within 24 wk, 60% improved histologic score vs 13% in placebo
Poupon,[36] 1991	RCT	2 y	Biochemical, histology	Significant decrease in biochemical tests in UDCA-treated group. No change in fibrosis between groups but improvement in histologic score
Battezzati,[37] 1993	RCT	6 mo	Symptoms, biochemistry	Improvement in pruritus and biochemistries (bilirubin, alkaline phosphatase, GGT, AST, IgG, and IgM) in UDCA-treated ($P<.01$)
Poupon,[38] 1994	RCT	2–4 y	DC, LT, death	RR 0.28 for disease progression in UDCA group vs placebo ($P<.002$). RR 0.32 for transplantation or death in UDCA group vs placebo ($P = .005$)
Turner,[39] 1994	RCT	2 y	Biochemistry	Improved bilirubin, alkaline phosphatase, AST in UDCA-treated subjects
Lindor,[40] 1994	RCT	2 y	Histology, DC, LT, death	Treatment failure delayed in UDCA-treated subjects ($P = .0003$)
Combes,[41] 1995	RCT	2 y	Biochemistry, histology	Improvements in biochemistries in stage I or II disease. Improved histology in UDCA (10–12 mg/kg) group vs placebo
Lindor,[42] 1996	RCT	3 y	Death or LT	RR 2.6 ($P = .04$) in placebo group vs UDCA
Batts,[43] 1996	RCT	2 y	Biochemistry, histology	No significant changes in the degree of inflammation or histologic stage in UDCA-treated group
Poupon,[44] 1997	3 RCT data combined	2–4 y	LT	RR 1.9 for transplant-free survival in UDCA group vs placebo ($P<.001$), especially in histologic stage IV group
Eriksson,[45] 1997	RCT	2–4 y	Biochemistry, histology, survival	Improved serum enzymes but not histology and survival at UDCA dose of 7.7 mg/kg
Lindor,[46] 1997	Observational	4 y	Esophageal varices	16% UDCA-treated vs 58% placebo developed varices ($P<.001$)
Angulo,[47] 1999	RCT	5–9 y	Histology	13% vs 49% progressed to cirrhosis with UDCA vs placebo

(continued on next page)

Table 2
(continued)

Study	Study Design	Study Duration	Study Outcome	Conclusion
Poupon et al,[20] 1999	Observational cohort	10 y	LT, survival	78% 10-y transplant-free survival in UDCA-treated patients significantly higher than Mayo model prediction (P<.04)
Goulis et al,[12] 1999	Meta-analysis of 17 studies	6 mo	Biochemistry, LT, death	No difference in liver transplantation or death rate between UDCA-treated subjects and placebo
Corpechot,[48] 2000	RCT	2 y	Histology	7% vs 34% progressed with UDCA vs placebo (P<.002)
Gluud & Christensen,[10] 2001	Meta-analysis 16 RCTs	3 mo–5 y	Biochemistry, LT, death	Improved biochemistries with UDCA but no improvement in mortality or liver transplantation
Papatheodoridis et al,[11] 2002	RCT	7.3 y	DC, LT, death	No significant difference in liver decompensation, liver death, or transplantation
Poupon,[49] 2003	4 RCT data combined	3 y	Histology	UDCA delays histologic progression in early stages (I or II) of the disease
Corphecot,[50] 2005	Observational cohort	8 y	Histology, LT, death	• Transplant-free survival was 84% and 66% at 10 and 20 y, respectively, which was lower than general population but higher than Mayo model prediction (P<.01) • Survival rate in subjects with stage I or II disease similar to general population
Shi et al,[13] 2006	Meta-analysis of 7 studies	2–7.3 y	Biochemistry, LT, death	• UDCA might result in 28% reduction in the risk of dying or undergoing liver transplantation • Sensitivity analysis of long-term studies, >100 subjects and placebo-controlled, indicate UDCA improves transplant-free survival
Parés et al,[15] 2006	Observational series	6.8 y	Death, LT or DC	97% transplant-free survival in UDCA responders vs 83% in nonresponders (P = .001)
Lammers et al,[14] 2014	Meta-analysis	7.3 y	LT, death	Transplant-free survival in UDCA-treated group 90% at 5 y, 78% at 10 y and 66% at 15 y compared with 79%, 59%, and 32%, respectively, in placebo

Abbreviations: DC, hepatic decompensation; LT, liver transplantation; RCT, randomized controlled trial; RR, relative risk.

Table 3
Criteria defining biochemical response to ursodeoxycholic acid treatment in primary biliary cholangitis

Criteria	Definition	Timeframe to Assess Response
Mayo[18,51]	Decrease in alkaline phosphatase <2 × ULN	6 mo
Barcelona[15]	Decrease in alkaline phosphatase 40% from baseline or to normal value	1 y
Paris I[52]	Decrease in alkaline phosphatase to ≤3 × ULN, decease in AST to ≤2 × ULN and normal bilirubin	1 y
Rotterdam[53]	Normalization of bilirubin or albumin, when 1 or both were abnormal before treatment	1 y
Toronto[54]	Alkaline phosphatase ≤1.67 × ULN	2 y
Ehime[55]	Decrease in GGT >70% of the baseline level or a normal level	6 mo
Lammers[14]	Alkaline phosphatase level <2 × ULN and/or bilirubin <1 × ULN	1 y
Paris II[56]	Decrease in alkaline phosphatase to <1.5 × ULN or AST <1.5 × ULN and normal bilirubin	1 y

Abbreviations: AST, aspartate aminotransferase; GGT, gamma glutamyltransferase; ULN, upper limit of normal.

to be lower compared with patients with parenchymal liver disease with the same MELD score.[22] Subsequently, however, several studies have shown that patients with PBC may face a higher rate of death on the liver transplant waitlist compared with patients with other causes of liver disease, such as hepatitis C virus. This may be due to older age, lower albumin, dyslipidemia, and cardiovascular disease in patients with PBC.[23] Based on these data, some investigators have suggested considering MELD exception points for PBC.[23]

Additional predictive models have been proposed in recent years (**Table 4**). Trivedi and colleagues[24] reported that the aspartate aminotransferase to platelet ratio index (APRI) at baseline or 1 year after treatment (APRI-r1) of greater than 0.54 predicts liver transplantation or death despite response to UDCA. The APRI score was initially developed as a surrogate marker of fibrosis in chronic viral hepatitis patients and in essence, detects preclinical fibrosis in patients with PBC. Although a useful adjunct to biochemical response criteria, APRI and APRI-r1 have limited ability to accurately predict survival rates.

The albumin-bilirubin (ALBI) score was derived using a cohort of 61 Chinese subjects with PBC who were followed for 18.3 years.[25] It was initially developed to assess liver synthetic function in patients with hepatocellular carcinoma. The ALBI score stratified subjects into 3 different survival groups. Group 1 patients (score ≤−2.6) had the best 2-year, 5-year, and 10-year event-free survival rates of 100% throughout. Group 2 patients (score −2.6 to −1.39) and group 3 patients (score >−1.39) had 2-year, 5-year, and 10-year event-free survival rates of 100% and 88.5%, 81.7% and 57.1%, and 14.3% and 0.0%, respectively. Although the score is relatively simple to calculate, it is derived retrospectively from a limited sample size that had few events and has not been validated.

The GLOBE score was developed using prospectively collected data from 2488 subjects at 15 liver centers in 8 North American and European countries with a median follow-up of 7.3 years. This international, multicenter collaboration aimed to create a

Table 4
Prognostic scores in primary biliary cholangitis in the ursodeoxycholic acid–treatment era

Model	Derivation Cohort	Prognostic Score
APRI or APRI-r1[24]	386 subjects and validation cohort of 629 subjects	([AST/AST ULN] × 100)/platelets (10^9/L)
Albumin-bilirubin (ALBI) score[25]	61 Chinese subjects followed for 18.3 y	-0.085 × (albumin) + 0.66 × $\log_{10}$ (bilirubin)
GLOBE score[26]	2488 subjects and validated in 1631 subjects in Europe and North America	0.044378 (age at start of UDCA therapy) + 0.93982 × $\log_e$ (bilirubin12/ bilirubin ULN) + 0.335648 + $\log_e$ (ALP12/ ALP ULN) − 2.266708 (albumin at 12 months/albumin LLN) − 0.002581 (platelet 10^9/L at 12 mo) + 1.216865.
UK-PBC score[28]	1916 patients from UK research cohort and validated in 1249 patients	Baseline survivor function‾EXP (0.0288* [ALP12 × ULN] −1.722) − 0.0423* ([ALT12 × ULN/10‾-1] − 8.676) + 1.4199 * (LN [bilirubin12 × ULN/10]+2.710)−1.960* (albumin × LLN −1.177)−0.4162* (platelets × LLN −1.874) Baseline survivor function = 0.982 (at 5 y), 0.941 (at 10 y), 0.893 (at 15 y)

Abbreviations: *, multiplication; ALP, alkaline phosphatase; ALP12, alkaline phosphatase after 12 months of UDCA; ALT, alanine aminotransferase; APRI, AST to platelet ratio index; bilirubin12, bilirubin after 12 months of UDCA; LLN, lower limit of normal; UK, United Kingdom; ULN, upper limit of normal.

unifying predictive score that minimizes geographic variance in patients who were treated with UDCA for 1 year.[26] The score incorporates 5 objective variables, including age at the start of UDCA therapy and levels of bilirubin, albumin, alkaline phosphatase, and platelet count 1 year after UDCA therapy. Subjects with a GLOBE score greater than 0.30 had more than 5 times higher risk of death or transplantation compared with a matched general population (hazard ratio 5.51, 95% CI 4.52–6.72, $P<.0001$) with 5-year, 10-year, and 15-year transplant-free survival rates of 79.7%, 57.4%, and 42.5%, respectively. In contrast, subjects with a GLOBE score less than or equal to 0.30 were considered UDCA-responders and had a life-expectancy comparable with a matched general population. The 5-year, 10-year, and 15-year transplant-free survival rates were 98.0%, 92.0%, and 82.3%, respectively ($P<.0001$). The overall predictive ability of the GLOBE score, assessed by the C-statistic, was 0.81 in the derivation cohort and 0.80 in the validation cohort. This was in comparison with the C-statistics of the several other biochemical response criteria (Barcelona, Paris-I, Rotterdam, Toronto, Paris-II) evaluated in the cohort, which ranged from 0.57 to 0.70. Although the calculation of the GLOBE score is relatively complex, it incorporates readily available clinical data and the cutoff risk threshold of 0.30 simplifies decision-making. The GLOBE score has not been externally validated yet but has been applied to other cohorts showing similarly accurate predictive capability.[27]

Most recently, Carbone and colleagues[28] developed and validated the United Kingdom (UK)-PBC score. This score is unique in that it combines variables that define UDCA treatment response in addition to measures of hepatic fibrosis and function at baseline to determine risk of end-stage liver disease at 5, 10, and 15 years. The UK-PBC score yielded a C-statistic of 0.92 in the derivation cohort. When used in the validation cohort, the area under receiver operating characteristic curve (AUC) was 0.96,

0.95, and 0.94 for 5-year, 10-year, and 15-year risk scores. This was better than the AUC calculated using the Barcelona, Paris I, Toronto, and Paris II criteria, which ranged from 0.56 to 0.81. The large sample size of 3165 subjects used to derive this model, in addition to risk estimates at definite time points in the future, are significant advantages of the UK-PBC score. Although a specific risk threshold is not presented with this score, the investigators suggest that the risk estimates should inform individualized clinical decision-making depending on patient age and comorbidities. As the score stands at this point, albumin and platelet count are only included at baseline and it is unclear if changes in these values after years of treatment would alter risk estimates.

When evaluating a patient with PBC in clinical practice, these scoring systems can be used to obtain helpful prognostic information. For example, after starting a patient on UDCA, 1 of the biochemical response criteria can be used to determine if a patient has had an adequate treatment response on UDCA. For those who have not achieved an appropriate response, further management may involve OCA or enrollment in a clinical trial. Prognostic information using the Mayo, GLOBE, or UK-PBC scores can also be calculated from the patient's clinical and laboratory data. These scores provide a basis for clinical decision-making and counseling. For patients deemed at low risk of death or transplantation, follow-up intervals can be extended or referral to a liver transplant center can be delayed. The opposite would be true for those at high risk of death or transplantation.

Fig. 3 demonstrates an exercise in which the Mayo model and the UK-PBC model may be compared in a patient who has received 1 year of UDCA. Data obtained at baseline and updated after 1 year of therapy are applied as appropriate. Because serum bilirubin concentrations carry the most weight in both models, survival probability at 5 years was compared with all other variables being held as normal. For this illustration, the authors set the age for the Mayo model for the median of the UK-PBC data, for example, 55 years. It is helpful to see that the estimates are roughly comparable to each other. The UK-PBC model tended to be more optimistic than the Mayo model for patients with lower bilirubin concentrations ($\leq$5 mg/dL), whereas for patients with bilirubin of 10 mg/dL, the reverse is true. Although these estimates are 5% to 10% points off from each other, the difference does not seem material to clinical decision-making in most circumstances.

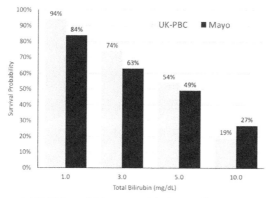

Fig. 3. Comparison of UK-PBC and Mayo models in an illustrative patient after 1 year of UDCA therapy. Data applied to the models include age (55 years), total bilirubin (1.0 mg/dL, upper limit of normal), albumin (3.2 g/dL, lower limit of normal), prothrombin time (10 seconds), no edema, alkaline phosphatase 120 U/L (upper limit of normal), ALT 45 U/L (upper limit of normal), and platelets (150,000 mm^3, lower limit of normal).

SUMMARY

More than a dozen predictive scoring systems have been developed in PBC patients with or without UDCA therapy in various study populations with different endpoints. These indicate the need to risk stratify patients with PBC to help guide their management and provide reliable prognoses. It remains to be determined whether a single scoring system is sufficient and applicable in all clinical scenarios or if several systems need to be used for specific circumstances. The exercise shown in **Fig. 3** comparing the Mayo risk score (derived from untreated patients) and the UK-PBC model (developed and validated specifically among UDCA-treated patients) seems to suggest that a representative model might be useful for multiple purposes.

The landscape of therapeutics for patients with chronic liver disease as of 2018 is brighter than ever. With the approval of OCA, the unmet need of PBC patients incompletely responding to UDCA has been at least partially addressed. With further gain in the insight of the molecular mechanisms of liver disease, several other compounds are being developed. However, until PBC can be cured in a manner similar to hepatitis C virus, the authors anticipate that there will always be a need to risk stratify patients. In the clinical setting, scoring systems may be used to guide optimal management and provide appropriate counseling for patients. Those at higher risk of death or liver transplantation should be referred to a liver transplant center, considered for additional therapy, and monitored more closely. Those at lower risk of adverse outcomes can be reassured and monitored less frequently, possibly by local gastroenterologists or primary care.

Scoring systems have proven useful for research as well. As several promising new therapeutic agents enter clinical trials for PBC, it will be important to identify the population of patients at high risk of death and liver transplantation who should be enrolled in these studies. There also needs to be standardization of determining biochemical effectiveness of these newer therapies. For example, in the placebo-controlled trial with OCA, subjects who did not meet a modified Toronto criteria (alkaline phosphatase >1.67 × ULN or abnormal bilirubin but less than 2 × ULN) were selected for study entry. Subjects were stratified based on the Paris-I criteria and the primary composite endpoint was a combination of Toronto and Paris criteria (alkaline phosphatase <1.67 × ULN, with a reduction of at least 15% from baseline, and a total bilirubin level at or below ULN) at 12 months.

The authors believe that prognostic models will continue to be developed and modified over time in part as the natural history of PBC evolves with subsequent treatment. Ideally, prognostic models in PBC should incorporate variables that drive the pathophysiological progression of disease and treatment response in patients. As more genetic, molecular, and immunologic mechanisms in PBC are elucidated, we anticipate biomarkers that correlate closely with the underlying pathophysiological processes will be identified and incorporated in future prognostic systems. Furthermore, methodological innovation, such as machine learning and neural networks, may further add to the precision and accuracy of the models. Ultimately, highly optimized prediction models may guide research and clinical management for the benefit of PBC patients in the future.

REFERENCES

1. Lindor KD, Gershwin ME, Poupon R, et al. Primary biliary cirrhosis. Hepatology 2009;50(1):291–308.
2. Boonstra K, Beuers U, Ponsioen CY. Epidemiology of primary sclerosing cholangitis and primary biliary cirrhosis: a systematic review. J Hepatol 2012;56(5): 1181–8.

3. Selmi C, Bowlus CL, Gershwin ME, et al. Primary biliary cirrhosis. Lancet 2011; 377(9777):1600–9.

4. Christensen E, Crowe J, Doniach D, et al. Clinical pattern and course of disease in primary biliary cirrhosis based on an analysis of 236 patients. Gastroenterology 1980;78(2):236–46. Available at: http://www.ncbi.nlm.nih.gov/pubmed/7350046. Accessed January 10, 2018.

5. Locke GR, Therneau TM, Ludwig J, et al. Time course of histological progression in primary biliary cirrhosis. Hepatology 1996;23(1):52–6.

6. Springer J, Cauch-Dudek K, O'Rourke K, et al. Asymptomatic primary biliary cirrhosis: a study of its natural history and prognosis. Am J Gastroenterol 1999; 94(1):47–53.

7. Prince M, Chetwynd A, Newman W, et al. Survival and symptom progression in a geographically based cohort of patients with primary biliary cirrhosis: follow-up for up to 28 years. Gastroenterology 2002;123(4):1044–51. Available at: http://www.ncbi.nlm.nih.gov/pubmed/12360466. Accessed January 18, 2018.

8. Poupon R. Ursodeoxycholic acid and bile-acid mimetics as therapeutic agents for cholestatic liver diseases: an overview of their mechanisms of action. Clin Res Hepatol Gastroenterol 2012;36(Suppl 1):S3–12.

9. Poupon R, Chrétien Y, Poupon RE, et al. Is ursodeoxycholic acid an effective treatment for primary biliary cirrhosis? Lancet 1987;1(8537):834–6. Available at: http://www.ncbi.nlm.nih.gov/pubmed/2882236. Accessed January 11, 2018.

10. Gluud C, Christensen E. Ursodeoxycholic acid for primary biliary cirrhosis. In: Gluud C, editor. Cochrane database of systematic reviews. Chichester (United Kingdom): John Wiley & Sons, Ltd; 2001. CD000551. https://doi.org/10.1002/14651858.CD000551.

11. Papatheodoridis GV, Hadziyannis ES, Deutsch M, et al. Ursodeoxycholic acid for primary biliary cirrhosis: final results of a 12-year, prospective, randomized, controlled trial. Am J Gastroenterol 2002;97(8):2063–70.

12. Goulis J, Leandro G, Burroughs AK. Randomised controlled trials of ursodeoxycholic-acid therapy for primary biliary cirrhosis: a meta-analysis. Lancet 1999;354(9184):1053–60.

13. Shi J, Wu C, Lin Y, et al. Long-term effects of mid-dose ursodeoxycholic acid in primary biliary cirrhosis: a meta-analysis of randomized controlled trials. Am J Gastroenterol 2006;101(7):1529–38.

14. Lammers WJ, van Buuren HR, Hirschfield GM, et al. Levels of alkaline phosphatase and bilirubin are surrogate end points of outcomes of patients with primary biliary cirrhosis: an international follow-up study. Gastroenterology 2014;147(6): 1338–49.e5 [quiz: e15].

15. Parés A, Caballería L, Rodés J. Excellent long-term survival in patients with primary biliary cirrhosis and biochemical response to ursodeoxycholic acid. Gastroenterology 2006;130(3):715–20.

16. Zhang L-N, Shi T-Y, Shi X-H, et al. Early biochemical response to ursodeoxycholic acid and long-term prognosis of primary biliary cirrhosis: results of a 14-year cohort study. Hepatology 2013;58(1):264–72.

17. Kilmurry MR, Heathcote EJ, Cauch-Dudek K, et al. Is the Mayo model for predicting survival useful after the introduction of ursodeoxycholic acid treatment for primary biliary cirrhosis? Hepatology 1996;23(5):1148–53.

18. Angulo P, Lindor KD, Therneau TM, et al. Utilization of the Mayo risk score in patients with primary biliary cirrhosis receiving ursodeoxycholic acid. Liver 1999; 19(2):115–21. Available at: http://www.ncbi.nlm.nih.gov/pubmed/10220741. Accessed January 14, 2018.

19. ter Borg PC, Schalm SW, Hansen BE, et al. Prognosis of ursodeoxycholic acid-treated patients with primary biliary cirrhosis. Results of a 10-yr cohort study involving 297 patients. Am J Gastroenterol 2006;101(9):2044–50.

20. Poupon RE, Bonnand AM, Chrétien Y, et al. Ten-year survival in ursodeoxycholic acid-treated patients with primary biliary cirrhosis. The UDCA-PBC study group. Hepatology 1999;29(6):1668–71.

21. Koulentaki M, Moscandrea J, Dimoulios P, et al. Survival of anti-mitochondrial antibody-positive and -negative primary biliary cirrhosis patients on ursodeoxycholic acid treatment. Dig Dis Sci 2004;49(7–8):1190–5. Available at: http://www.ncbi.nlm.nih.gov/pubmed/15387345. Accessed January 18, 2018.

22. Malinchoc M, Kamath PS, Gordon FD, et al. A model to predict poor survival in patients undergoing transjugular intrahepatic portosystemic shunts. Hepatology 2000;31(4):864–71.

23. Singal AK, Fang X, Kaif M, et al. Primary biliary cirrhosis has high wait-list mortality among patients listed for liver transplantation. Transpl Int 2017;30(5):454–62.

24. Trivedi PJ, Bruns T, Cheung A, et al. Optimising risk stratification in primary biliary cirrhosis: AST/platelet ratio index predicts outcome independent of ursodeoxycholic acid response. J Hepatol 2014;60(6):1249–58.

25. Chan AWH, Chan RCK, Wong GLH, et al. New simple prognostic score for primary biliary cirrhosis: albumin-bilirubin score. J Gastroenterol Hepatol 2015; 30(9):1391–6.

26. Lammers WJ, Hirschfield GM, Corpechot C, et al. Development and validation of a scoring system to predict outcomes of patients with primary biliary cirrhosis receiving ursodeoxycholic acid therapy. Gastroenterology 2015;149(7): 1804–12.e4.

27. Yang F, Yang Y, Wang Q, et al. The risk predictive values of UK-PBC and GLOBE scoring system in Chinese patients with primary biliary cholangitis: the additional effect of anti-gp210. Aliment Pharmacol Ther 2017;45(5):733–43.

28. Carbone M, Sharp SJ, Flack S, et al. The UK-PBC risk scores: derivation and validation of a scoring system for long-term prediction of end-stage liver disease in primary biliary cholangitis. Hepatology 2016;63(3):930–50.

29. Christensen E, Neuberger J, Crowe J, et al. Beneficial effect of azathioprine and prediction of prognosis in primary biliary cirrhosis. Final results of an international trial. Gastroenterology 1985;89(5):1084–91.

30. Bonsel G, van 't Veer F, Habbema JD, et al. Use of prognostic models for assessment of value of liver transplantation in primary biliary cirrhosis. Lancet 1990; 335(8688):493–7.

31. Dickson ER, Grambsch PM, Fleming TR, et al. Prognosis in primary biliary cirrhosis: model for decision making. Hepatology 1989;10(1):1–7.

32. Christensen E, Altman DG, Neuberger J, et al. Updating prognosis in primary biliary cirrhosis using a time-dependent Cox regression model. PBC1 and PBC2 trial groups. Gastroenterology 1993;105(6):1865–76.

33. Murtaugh PA, Dickson ER, Van Dam GM, et al. Primary biliary cirrhosis: prediction of short-term survival based on repeated patient visits. Hepatology 1994;20(1 Pt 1): 126–34.

34. Kim WR, Wiesner RH, Poterucha JJ, et al. Adaptation of the Mayo primary biliary cirrhosis natural history model for application in liver transplant candidates. Liver Transpl 2000;6(4):489–94.

35. Leuschner U, Fischer H, Kurtz W, et al. Ursodeoxycholic acid in primary biliary cirrhosis: results of a controlled double-blind trial. Gastroenterology 1989;97(5): 1268–74.

36. Poupon RE, Balkau B, Eschwège E, et al. A Multicenter, Controlled Trial of Urso-diol for the Treatment of Primary Biliary Cirrhosis. N Engl J Med 1991;324(22): 1548–54.
37. Battezzati PM, Podda M, Bianchi FB, et al. Ursodeoxycholic acid for symptomatic primary biliary cirrhosis. Preliminary analysis of a double-blind multicenter trial. Italian Multicenter Group for the Study of UDCA in PBC. J Hepatol 1993;17(3): 332–8.
38. Poupon RE, Poupon R, Balkau B. Ursodiol for the long-term treatment of primary biliary cirrhosis. The UDCA-PBC Study Group. N Engl J Med 1994;330(19): 1342–7.
39. Turner IB, Myszor M, Mitchison HC, et al. A two year controlled trial examining the effectiveness of ursodeoxycholic acid in primary biliary cirrhosis. J Gastroenterol Hepatol 1994;9(2):162–8.
40. Lindor KD, Dickson ER, Baldus WP, et al. Ursodeoxycholic acid in the treatment of primary biliary cirrhosis. Gastroenterology 1994;106(5):1284–90.
41. Combes B, Carithers RL, Maddrey WC, et al. A randomized, double-blind, pla-cebo-controlled trial of ursodeoxycholic acid in primary biliary cirrhosis. Hepatol-ogy 1995;22(3):759–66.
42. Lindor K, Therneau T, Jorgensen R, et al. Effects of ursodeoxycholic acid on sur-vival in patients with primary biliary cirrhosis. Gastroenterology 1996;110(5): 1515–8.
43. Batts KP, Jorgensen RA, Dickson ER, et al. Effects of ursodeoxycholic acid on he-patic inflammation and histological stage in patients with primary biliary cirrhosis. Am J Gastroenterol 1996;91(11):2314–7.
44. Poupon RE, Lindor KD, Cauch-Dudek K, et al. Combined analysis of randomized controlled trials of ursodeoxycholic acid in primary biliary cirrhosis. Gastroenter-ology 1997;113(3):884–90.
45. Eriksson LS, Olsson R, Glauman H, et al. Ursodeoxycholic acid treatment in pa-tients with primary biliary cirrhosis. A Swedish multicentre, double-blind, random-ized controlled study. Scand J Gastroenterol 1997;32(2):179–86.
46. Lindor KD, Jorgensen RA, Therneau TM, et al. Ursodeoxycholic acid delays the onset of esophageal varices in primary biliary cirrhosis. Mayo Clin Proc. 1997; 72(12):1137–40.
47. Angulo P, Batts KP, Therneau TM, et al. Long-term ursodeoxycholic acid delays histological progression in primary biliary cirrhosis. Hepatology 1999;29(3): 644–7.
48. Corpechot C, Carrat F, Bonnand A, et al. The effect of ursodeoxycholic acid ther-apy on liver fibrosis progression in primary biliary cirrhosis. Hepatology 2000; 32(6):1196–9.
49. Poupon RE, Lindor KD, Parés A, et al. Combined analysis of the effect of treat-ment with ursodeoxycholic acid on histologic progression in primary biliary cirrhosis. J Hepatol 2003;39(1):12–6.
50. Corpechot C, Carrat F, Bahr A, et al. The effect of ursodeoxycholic acid therapy on the natural course of primary biliary cirrhosis. Gastroenterology 2005;128(2): 297–303.
51. Momah N, Silveira MG, Jorgensen R, et al. Optimizing biochemical markers as endpoints for clinical trials in primary biliary cirrhosis. Liver Int 2012;32(5):790–5.
52. Corpechot C, Abenavoli L, Rabahi N, et al. Biochemical response to ursodeoxy-cholic acid and long-term prognosis in primary biliary cirrhosis. Hepatology 2008; 48(3):871–7.

53. Kuiper EMM, Hansen BE, de Vries RA, et al. Improved prognosis of patients with primary biliary cirrhosis that have a biochemical response to ursodeoxycholic acid. Gastroenterology 2009;136(4):1281–7.

54. Kumagi T, Guindi M, Fischer SE, et al. Baseline ductopenia and treatment response predict long-term histological progression in primary biliary cirrhosis. Am J Gastroenterol 2010;105(10):2186–94.

55. Azemoto N, Abe M, Murata Y, et al. Early biochemical response to ursodeoxycholic acid predicts symptom development in patients with asymptomatic primary biliary cirrhosis. J Gastroenterol 2009;44(6):630–4.

56. Corpechot C, Chazouillères O, Poupon R. Early primary biliary cirrhosis: Biochemical response to treatment and prediction of long-term outcome. J Hepatol 2011;55(6):1361–7.

Liver Biopsy in Primary Biliary Cholangitis

Indications and Interpretation

Daisong Tan, MD, Zachary D. Goodman, MD, PhD*

KEYWORDS

- Liver biopsy • Histopathology • Primary biliary cholangitis
- Antimitochondrial antibody

KEY POINTS

- Primary biliary cholangitis is a disease characterized by immune-mediated bile duct destruction, followed by inflammation, scarring, and the development of chronic cholestasis and a slow progression to cirrhosis over the course of years.
- Liver biopsy is used in conjunction with clinical evaluation and serologic autoantibody testing to establish the diagnosis, but it is not required in typical cases.
- Liver biopsy is required to establish the diagnosis of PBC or alternative diagnoses in AMA-negative patients with unexplained chronic cholestasis.
- Liver biopsy is useful in assessing stage of disease and degree of progression, and it is the gold standard by which noninvasive tests are evaluated.

INTRODUCTION

Liver biopsy has traditionally been the gold standard in diagnosis of many diffuse or localized liver diseases and in the assessment of their severity.[1] Despite advances in laboratory tests, molecular diagnosis, and imaging, examination of liver biopsy specimens remains a source of otherwise unobtainable qualitative information about the structural integrity of the liver and changes that occur in liver diseases. Although a needle liver biopsy remains a primary tool for the diagnosis of liver diseases and for the staging of liver fibrosis, in the case of primary biliary cholangitis (PBC), liver biopsy is no longer recommended for diagnosis. Instead, careful clinical evaluation to exclude other causes of chronic cholestasis, followed by serologic screening for antimitochondrial antibody (AMA) and PBC-specific antinuclear antibodies, ultrasound, and magnetic resonance cholangiopancreatography imaging are recommended before

The authors have nothing to disclose.
Division of Liver Pathology Research, Center for Liver Diseases, Inova Fairfax Hospital, 3300 Gallows Road, Falls Church, VA 22042, USA
* Corresponding author.
E-mail address: zachary.goodman@inova.org

considering a liver biopsy for diagnosis, whereas response to initial therapy and evaluation of liver stiffness are often sufficient for assessment of short-term prognosis.[2] Liver biopsy is most often indicated when atypical clinical or laboratory features are present or when there is doubt about the diagnosis or stage of disease.

PATHOLOGY AND PATHOGENESIS OF PRIMARY BILIARY CHOLANGITIS

Although early descriptions of patients with this disease date to the mid-nineteenth century, the first series with detailed description and the name "primary biliary cirrhosis," popularly called PBC, was published by Ahrens and colleagues[3] in 1950. Because the initial patients were at the end-stage of the disease, it was named a form of cirrhosis, but subsequent reports of earlier stage disease and elucidation of its natural history made the term a misnomer. Nevertheless, attempts to rename the disease were unsuccessful until the recent change to PBC with retention of the acronym PBC.[4]

Early Stage Primary Biliary Cholangitis

Rubin and coworkers[5] provided the first description of the key early lesion, chronic nonsuppurative destructive cholangitis, also frequently called the florid duct lesion (**Figs. 1–3**).[6] With careful observation, they and subsequent authors deduced the sequence of events and corresponding histologic lesions leading to end-stage cirrhosis.[5–8] The early stage is characterized by immune-mediated destruction of small interlobular bile ducts caused by aberrant expression of the E2 subunit of pyruvate dehydrogenase complex, the same antigen that is the target of AMA. Bile duct epithelial cell damage is mediated primarily by $CD8^+$ cytotoxic T cells along with a variable number of other inflammatory cells. B cells with occasional lymphoid follicles may be present, whereas eosinophils and plasma cells are sometimes numerous. Damaged ducts show epithelial cell irregularity, swelling, or apoptosis, usually with infiltration by lymphocytes and often with disruption of the basement membrane (see **Figs. 1–3**). The ducts may rupture, and there may be neutrophils or granulomatous inflammation in response to bile leaking from the damaged ducts. Affected bile

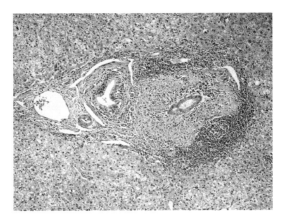

Fig. 1. Early stage PBC. A medium-size portal area with chronic lymphoplasmacytic inflammation and two damaged bile ducts. The duct on the left shows epithelial cell damage with irregular nuclear pseudostratification and infiltration by inflammatory cells, predominant lymphocytes. The duct on the right is more severely damaged with cytoplasmic eosinophilia surrounding granulomatous inflammation (hematoxylin-eosin ×40).

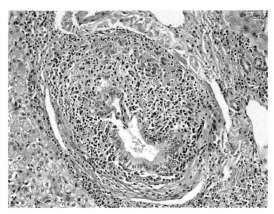

Fig. 2. Early stage PBC. A florid duct lesion with severe epithelial damage and disruption of the duct and its basement membrane. The ductal epithelium is infiltrated by lymphocytes, and the surrounding inflammation contains plasma cells and macrophages, producing a poorly formed granuloma (hematoxylin-eosin ×100).

ducts and portal areas are haphazardly distributed in the liver, so a small needle biopsy may miss diagnostic lesions, especially in the early stage. Sampling error is always a consideration when PBC is considered clinically, but this is minimized by the use of large biopsies and multiple passes. The result of the destructive cholangitis is disappearance of the duct (**Figs. 4** and **5**), frequently leaving a lymphoid aggregate and sometimes periodic acid Schiff–positive amorphous basement membrane material as markers of the lost duct. Because the bile ducts typically run parallel to hepatic artery branches, the finding of an unaccompanied artery is presumptive evidence of a vanishing bile duct disease.

Midstage Primary Biliary Cholangitis and Disease Progression

The portal inflammation that accompanies bile duct destruction frequently extends into the adjacent hepatic parenchyma with damage to the surrounding hepatocytes,

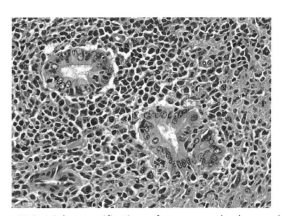

Fig. 3. Early stage PBC. High magnification of two severely damaged bile ducts with numerous surrounding plasma cells and some macrophages indicating granulomatous inflammation on the right side of the field (hematoxylin-eosin ×200).

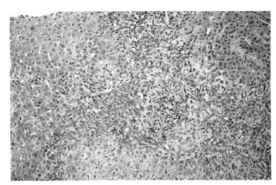

Fig. 4. Midstage PBC. This portal tract has lost its acinar bile duct and there is marked proliferation of periportal ductules (Scheuer stage 2) (hematoxylin-eosin ×100).

producing a lymphoplasmacytic interface hepatitis similar in appearance to that of chronic autoimmune or viral hepatitis (see **Figs. 4** and **5**; **Figs. 6–9**). As the ducts are destroyed, features of chronic cholestasis develop and contribute to the periportal injury through retention of toxic bile acids or "cholate stasis," which produces a xanthomatous appearance in periportal hepatocytes (see **Fig. 7**). Copper and copper binding protein are demonstrated with appropriate stains (see **Fig. 8**), and ductular proliferation may also be present, and periportal hepatocytes undergo ductular metaplasia with production of biliary keratins types 7 and 19 (see **Fig. 9**). Collagen is produced in response to the injury, and portal-portal septa are formed. Midstage PBC typically has bile duct loss with chronic cholestasis and bridging fibrosis, but lesions of early stage disease may still be present.

Cirrhosis in Late-Stage Primary Biliary Cholangitis

With continued fibrosis progression, the liver develops cirrhosis with eventual loss of all small bile ducts and increasing chronic cholestasis (**Fig. 10**). The biliary pattern of cirrhosis differs from cirrhosis of other causes, such as viral hepatitis and alcoholic

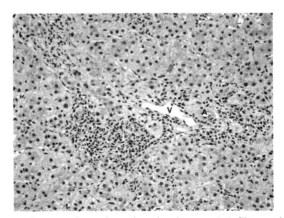

Fig. 5. Midstage PBC. This portal tract has a lymphoplasmacytic infiltrate along with a portal vein branch (V) and a branch of the hepatic artery (A), but it has lost its acinar bile duct. There is considerable periportal interface hepatitis and spotty lobular inflammation, similar to that seen in autoimmune hepatitis (hematoxylin-eosin ×200).

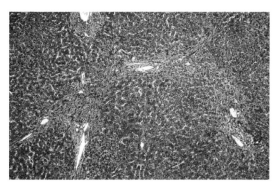

Fig. 6. Midstage PBC. There is loss of many bile ducts resulting in fibrous portal expansion and portal-portal bridging fibrosis (Masson trichrome ×40).

liver disease or nonalcoholic steatohepatitis, in that regeneration is much less prominent, and cirrhotic nodules tend to maintain lobular landmarks with central veins in the middle of the nodule (see **Fig. 10**). There is characteristically a "jigsaw" pattern of fibrosis with nodules that have variable shapes and septa corresponding to the pre-existing biliary tracts.

INDICATIONS FOR LIVER BIOPSY

PBC typically causes a chronic cholestatic disease with insidious onset with a long asymptomatic phase and slow progression over the course of years. A patient presenting with the acute onset of jaundice is unlikely to have PBC. Careful clinical evaluation to exclude hepatocellular diseases and acute biliary obstruction usually uncovers the cause of most instances of acute cholestasis.

Liver biopsy is no longer required for the diagnosis of most cases, but PBC should always be suspected when patients develop chronic persistent cholestasis, and a liver biopsy should be performed when initial diagnostic steps have not revealed the cause of this cholestasis. The diagnosis is initially based on the presence of AMAs and if available the classes of antinuclear antibodies (anti-sp100/anti-gp210) specific for

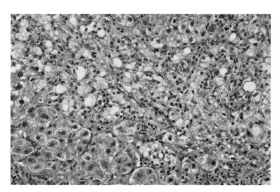

Fig. 7. Midstage PBC. After loss of the bile duct, periportal hepatocytes accumulate bile lipids and bile salts that cannot be excreted, causing the cells to have a foamy appearance that has been called "cholate stasis," as shown in the photomicrograph (hematoxylin-eosin ×200).

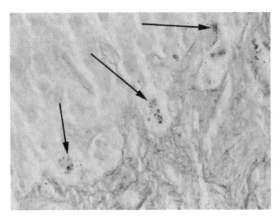

Fig. 8. Midstage PBC. Copper, which is normally excreted into the bile, is retained in periportal hepatocytes after loss of the bile duct. The copper accumulates in lysosomes bound to metallothianein, also called "copper binding protein," which is visualized as brown cytoplasmic granules with the orcein stain (*arrows*) (orcein ×40). The Nakanuma staging system (see **Table 1**) uses this as a measure of the severity of chronic cholestasis.

PBC. If not already performed, imaging (ultrasound, magnetic resonance cholangiopancreatography, endoscopic retrograde cholangiopancreatography and/or endoscopic ultrasound) to evaluate possible large-duct biliary obstruction is useful before proceeding to liver biopsy. Biopsy is most clearly indicated in the situations discussed next.

Negative Antimitochondrial Antibody

Up to 10% of patients fall into the category of negative AMA in a subject with unexplained chronic cholestasis, so biopsy may be necessary to establish the diagnosis

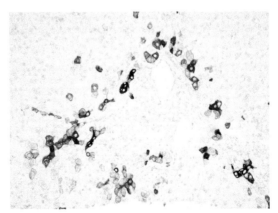

Fig. 9. Midstage PBC. After loss of the bile duct, periportal hepatocytes produce biliary-type keratin proteins (types 7 and 19) as a protection against the toxic bile components that accumulate preferentially in this part of the tissue. This immunostain for keratin 7 shows loss of the bile duct that should be present and positively stained in the center of the portal tract. Instead, the portal tract has a few dark brown–stained ductules and many light brown–stained hepatocytes in the periportal area that should normally have none (keratin 7 ×200).

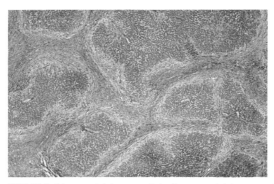

Fig. 10. Late-stage PBC. This Masson trichrome stain (masson trichrome ×20) demonstrated a typical "jigsaw" pattern of advanced biliary cirrhosis. The bile ducts are entirely gone from the portal tracts that are incorporated into the fibrous septa, but residual central veins are present in the centers of the nodules.

or reveal features that lead to an alternative diagnosis. Diseases that are likely to mimic the slowly progressive chronic cholestatic syndrome of PBC include primary sclerosing cholangitis (especially the small duct variant) and hepatic sarcoidosis. Vascular diseases, such as congestive hepatopathy and amyloidosis, may also present with chronic cholestatic liver tests before the underlying cause is clinically apparent. Drug-induced cholestatic liver injury can cause a destructive cholangitis that leads to ductopenia, mimicking the mid to late stage of PBC, but the onset is typically acute with jaundice and cholestasis that does not resolve, rather than the insidious onset and slow progression of PBC. There are also cases of unknown cause that present with end-stage biliary cirrhosis and ductopenia, but they have negative AMA and no florid duct lesions, precluding a diagnosis of PBC, and they have normal cholangiograms and no evidence of inflammatory bowel disease, precluding primary sclerosing cholangitis. These have been called idiopathic adulthood ductopenia.[9]

Suspected Overlap Syndromes

Suspected overlap syndromes or identification of individuals who may benefit from immunosuppressive therapy is a controversial topic because of the variable definitions, lack of standardized criteria for diagnosis, and lack of consensus on clinical management.[10–12] The term overlap syndrome has been used for patients with cholestatic forms of autoimmune hepatitis and hepatitic forms of PBC based on serum enzymes, histology, autoantibodies, or some combination of these. However, the International Autoimmune Hepatitis Group recommends that patients with autoimmune liver disease should be categorized according to the predominant features as autoimmune hepatitis, PBC, or primary sclerosing cholangitis and that those with overlapping features are not considered to have a distinct disease. Anecdotal evidence has suggested a beneficial effect of immunosuppression when features of autoimmune hepatitis are present, but evidence from controlled trials is not available. Nevertheless, the European Association for the Study of the Liver Clinical Practice Guideline[2] recommends consideration of this when supported by biopsy findings that suggest an element of autoimmune hepatitis.

Primary Biliary Cholangitis with Suspicion of Another Diagnosis

Patients with a diagnosis of PBC remain at risk for other forms of liver disease. Because PBC is most prevalent in middle-aged women, other diseases common in this demographic group should always be considered. In particular, nonalcoholic steatohepatitis has become prevalent in the same population at risk for PBC, even though there is no evidence to link the two diseases. A biopsy is required to establish this diagnosis.

GRADING AND STAGING OF LIVER BIOPSIES

Grading and staging have come to have similar meanings in all inflammatory liver diseases. Stage of any disease is how far it has progressed to the end stage, which is usually a stage of advanced cirrhosis and its clinical complications. Intermediate stages have lesser degrees of fibrosis. Grade of a disease relates to the severity of the underlying lesions that produce the type of injury characteristic of that disease. Thus, in chronic viral or autoimmune hepatitis, it is the hepatocellular injury and interface hepatitis that are the principal components of the grade. Chronic biliary tract disease is much more complex and includes the primary injury to the bile ducts followed by bile duct and hepatocellular destruction and inflammation, features of chronic cholestasis, and perpetuation of the injury leading to fibrosis and eventually cirrhosis. It is possible to categorize the degree of injury and scarring into early, midstage, and late-stage disease, and for most purposes a simple classification such as this is adequate for diagnosis and prognosis. More complex systems have been proposed with the potential to convey more detailed information when necessary (**Table 1**).

Scheuer[6,7] proposed a simple four-stage classification based on the progression of lesions affecting individual portal tracts with stage 1 (florid duct lesions) progressing to stage 2 (ductular proliferation), stage 3 (portal fibrosis and bile duct loss), and eventually to stage 4 (cirrhosis). Although widely cited, its use has always been limited by the patchy distribution of lesions within an individual patient's liver. In any individual case, all four stages may be found in the same biopsy. Ludwig's system[13] is similar to that used for chronic hepatitis with stage 1 (portal inflammation) progressing to stage 2 (periportal inflammation and fibrosis), stage 3 (fibrous septa), and finally to stage 4 (cirrhosis). Although simple to apply, key lesions, such as bile duct injury and loss, and chronic cholestatic features are not included, so its usefulness has been limited.

In 2010, Nakanuma and colleagues[14] proposed a PBC staging and grading system that takes into account necroinflammatory activity and histologic heterogeneity of the disease. Three pathologic features used for staging include fibrosis, bile duct loss, and

Table 1
Histologic staging of PBC: comparison of three systems

	Scheuer[6,7]	Ludwig[13]	Nakanuma[14]
Stage 1	Florid duct lesions Bile duct damage Portal inflammation	Portal inflammation	No or minimal progression (fibrosis, bile duct loss, copper binding protein = 0)
Stage 2	Ductular proliferation Portal expansion Interface hepatitis	Periportal inflammation Interface hepatitis	Mild progression (fibrosis, bile duct loss, copper binding protein = 1–3)
Stage 3	Scarring Loss of bile ducts	Fibrous septa	Moderate progression (fibrosis, bile duct loss, copper binding protein = 4–6)
Stage 4	Cirrhosis	Cirrhosis	Advanced progression (fibrosis, bile duct loss, copper binding protein = 7–9)

hepatocellular orcein-positive granules that represent copper binding protein typical of chronic cholestasis. Each of these is scored on a scale of 0 to 3, and the sum of the scores is used to assess degree of histologic progression (see **Table 1**) as mild, moderate, or advanced. Necroinflammatory activity is graded separately for cholangitis based on the extent of active bile duct inflammation and hepatitis based on the extent of interface hepatitis and lobular inflammation. The result is a histologic summary that is much more complete than the previous simple staging systems. Although unlikely to be used in diagnosis, a system such as this may be useful in the setting of a clinical trial.

Regarding the merits of the various staging systems, none has proven valuable enough to resurrect the indication for liver biopsy in PBC. It is nearly always sufficient to characterize the disease as early, midstage (bridging fibrosis), or late stage (cirrhosis) without using any particular system, and in a multivariate analysis, Roll and colleagues[15] showed this to be the only histologic predictor of prognosis. The Scheuer and Ludwig staging systems do not add further prognostic information. The Nakanuma system, which includes consideration of histologic chronic cholestasis and ductopenia, correlates better with laboratory features of the disease and Child-Pugh score, so there may be added prognostic information, particularly in late-stage disease.[16,17] If there should be consideration of a histologic endpoint for a new clinical trial, this would clearly be the best system to use. However, because approval of new agents has been achieved using improvement in serum alkaline phosphatase rather than in the histologic features of the disease,[18] it is unlikely that liver biopsy will be a part of any future trials in this disease.

SUMMARY

Although liver biopsies are not routinely performed for diagnosis of PBC, they remain essential for diagnosis in subjects with negative AMA, and they are a highly accurate way of determining progression of the disease and prognosis, and occasionally revealing additional unsuspected diagnoses.

REFERENCES

1. Rockey DC, Caldwell SH, Goodman ZD, et al. Liver biopsy. Hepatology 2009;49: 1017–44.
2. European Association for the Study of the Liver. EASL clinical practice guidelines: the diagnosis and management of patients with primary biliary cholangitis. J Hepatol 2017;67:145–72.
3. Ahrens EH, Payne MA, Kunkel HG, et al. Primary biliary cirrhosis. Medicine (Baltimore) 1950;29:299–364.
4. Beuers U, Gershwin ME, Gish RG, et al. Changing nomenclature for PBC: from 'cirrhosis' to 'cholangitis'. Hepatology 2015;62:1620–2.
5. Rubin E, Schaffner F, Popper H. Primary biliary cirrhosis: chronic nonsuppurative destructive cholantitis. Am J Pathol 1965;46:387–407.
6. Scheuer PJ. Primary biliary cirrhosis. Proc R Soc Med 1967;60:1257–60.
7. Sherlock S, Scheuer PJ. The presentation and diagnosis of 100 patients with primary biliary cirrhosis. N Engl J Med 1973;289:674–8.
8. Leung PS, Rossaro L, Davis PA, et al. Antimitochondrial antibodies in acute liver failure: implications for primary biliary cirrhosis. Hepatology 2007;46:1436–42.
9. Ludwig J. Idiopathic adulthood ductopenia: an update. Mayo Clin Proc 1998;73: 285–91.

10. Boberg KM, Chapman RW, Hirschfield GM, et al. Overlap syndromes: the International Autoimmune Hepatitis Group (IAIHG) position statement on a controversial issue. J Hepatol 2011;54:374–85.

11. Trivedi PJ, Hirschfield GM. Review article: overlap syndromes and autoimmune liver disease. Aliment Pharmacol Ther 2012;36:517–33.

12. Czaja AJ. Cholestatic phenotypes of autoimmune hepatitis. Clin Gastroenterol Hepatol 2014;12:1430–8.

13. Ludwig J, Dickson ER, McDonald GS. Staging of chronic nonsuppurative destructive cholangitis (syndrome of primary biliary cirrhosis). Virchows Arch A Pathol Anat Histol 1978;379:103–12.

14. Nakanuma Y, Zen Y, Harada K, et al. Application of a new histological staging and grading system for primary biliary cirrhosis to liver biopsy specimens: interobserver agreement. Pathol Int 2010;60:167–74.

15. Roll J, Boyer JL, Barry D, et al. The prognostic importance of clinical and histologic features in asymptomatic and symptomatic primary biliary cirrhosis. N Engl J Med 1983;308:1–7.

16. Kakuda Y, Harada K, Sawada-Kitamura S, et al. Evaluation of a new histologic staging and grading system for primary biliary cirrhosis in comparison with classical systems. Hum Pathol 2013;44:1107–17.

17. Chan AWH, Chan RCK, Wong GLH, et al. Evaluation of histological staging systems for primary biliary cirrhosis: correlation with clinical and biochemical factors and significance of pathological parameters in prognostication. Histopathology 2014;65:174–86.

18. Nevens F, Andreone P, Mazzella G, et al. A placebo-controlled trial of obeticholic acid in primary biliary cholangitis. N Engl J Med 2016;375:631–43.

Antimitochondrial Antibody–Negative Primary Biliary Cholangitis

Is It Really the Same Disease?

David M. Chascsa, MD[a], Keith D. Lindor, MD[a,b],*

KEYWORDS

- Antimitochondrial antibody (AMA) • Primary biliary cholangitis (PBC)
- Antinuclear antibody (ANA) • Ursodeoxycholic acid (UDCA)

KEY POINTS

- Terminology to define patients with histologic and clinical features of primary biliary cholangitis (PBC) without antimitochondrial antibody (AMA)-positivity is confusing, including autoimmune cholangitis, overlap syndromes, and the preferred term AMA-negative PBC.
- AMA-negativity as confirmed with tests of adequate sensitivity and specificity is essential to definitively diagnosis AMA-negative PBC.
- The clinical course of AMA-negative PBC is similar to AMA-positive PBC and current data are insufficient to separate these into 2 distinct disease processes.
- Given their high prevalence, antinuclear antibody and antismooth muscle antibody should be checked in patients suspected of AMA-negative PBC.
- AMA-negative PBC may be treated with ursodeoxycholic acid (UDCA) or a combination of UDCA and immunosuppression as directed by liver histology.

INTRODUCTION

Primary biliary cholangitis (PBC) is a chronic progressive cholestatic liver disease characterized by an elevated alkaline phosphatase (ALP) level and destruction of the small intrahepatic bile ducts, with granuloma formation seen on liver histology and, in almost all cases, a positive antimitochondrial antibody (AMA).[1,2] Diagnostic

Declaration of Interest: There was no financial support provided for the creation of this article. Dr K.D. Lindor was an unpaid advisor for Intercept Pharmaceuticals and Shire Pharmaceuticals. Dr D.M. Chascsa has nothing to declare.
[a] Division of Gastroenterology and Hepatology, Mayo Clinic, 5777 East Mayo Boulevard, Phoenix, AZ 85054, USA; [b] Office of the Provost, Arizona State University, 550 North 3rd Street, Phoenix, AZ 85004, USA
* Corresponding author. 550 North 3rd Street, Phoenix, AZ 85004.
E-mail address: keith.lindor@asu.edu

Clin Liver Dis 22 (2018) 589–601
https://doi.org/10.1016/j.cld.2018.03.009
1089-3261/18/© 2018 Elsevier Inc. All rights reserved.

liver.theclinics.com

criteria as set forth by the American Association for the Study of Liver Disease (AASLD) require the presence of at least 2 of the following: a persistent elevation in ALP greater than 1.5 times the upper limit of normal, the presence of a positive AMA, or diagnostic liver biopsy with characteristic findings.[3] AMA is highly specific for PBC and found in 90% to 95% of cases, though it has been reported in patients with autoimmune-related liver disease and those without clinically apparent liver disease.[4–6] However, a small number of patients with characteristic biopsy findings and clinical manifestations may present with clinical and histologic features indistinguishable from AMA-positive PBC but without the hallmark AMA. It is unclear whether these patients have a unique clinical entity or whether they are on a spectrum of autoimmune-related liver disease with autoimmune hepatitis (AIH) at 1 end, AMA-negative disease in the middle, and PBC with AMA positivity framing the other end.[7,8] PBC may have features of inflammatory hepatitis, thus muddying the water. This confusion has manifested with changing terminology from autoimmune cholangitis to AMA-negative PBC.[9] Additionally, the entity of overlap AIH-PBC has been entertained because there are patients with definite and coexistent histologic features of both AIH and PBC.[10] This article reviews the published work on AMA-negative PBC, its classical presentation, serologic and pathologic findings, response to treatment (medical and transplant), and thus compares these with AMA-positive disease.

TERMINOLOGY

The diagnosis of AMA-negative PBC is challenging due to the heterogeneous histologic findings in each of the 4 stages of PBC and the frequent lack of the classic findings such as the florid duct lesion.[11] The literature has been difficult to interpret because many terms are used to define the same disease entity, including AMA-negative PBC, autoimmune cholangitis, primary autoimmune cholangitis, autoimmune cholangiopathy, immunocholangitis, or (even more broadly) the nonspecific term autoimmune liver disease.[12–16] Conversely, many diseases with nonspecific autoimmunity may be lumped together, creating a heterogeneous group that may include overlap syndromes (**Fig. 1**). Alric and colleagues[17] noted that overlap syndromes represented up to 20% of autoimmune liver diseases. Although they did find some differences between those with overlap that were AMA-positive versus AMA-negative, a morphologic difference between PBC and AMA-negative overlap syndrome could not be elucidated. This confusion also hinders adequate assessment of the natural history of AMA-negative PBC. For the purposes of this article, AMA-negative PBC is defined as a disease process consisting of destructive cholangitis with histologic features of PBC in the absence of a detectable AMA but otherwise fulfilling AASLD diagnostic criteria for PBC. Previously published work referenced in this article may use terms interchangeably.

EPIDEMIOLOGY

PBC is a rare disease with a prevalence of 40 per 100,000 overall and 65 per 100,000 in women in North America.[18] AMA-negative PBC is much less frequent, accounting for only 5% to 10% of cases of PBC, though in certain populations the prevalence may approach 13% to 18%.[19–21] Disease prevalence varies by population. For instance, Southeast Alaskan Natives have been shown to have an overall higher incidence of PBC (combined AMA-negative and AMA-positive) at 71.5 per 100,000, with 21 in 100,000 cases of AMA-negative PBC.[22] Notably, in this particular study, subjects were diagnosed as having autoimmune cholangitis.

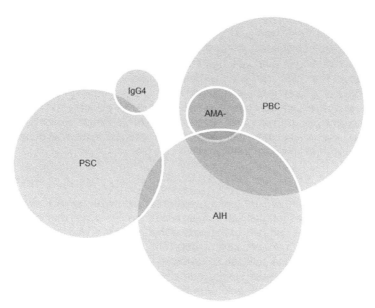

Fig. 1. The complexity and overlap of the multiple autoimmune liver diseases that affect the liver parenchyma and biliary tree. AMA-negative PBC shares similar histologic and clinical findings of AMA-positive PBC. Thus AMA-negative is contained entirely within the sphere of PBC. It may have features that overlap with AIH, including serologic markers (antinuclear antibody [ANA] and antismooth muscle antibody [ASMA]), and histologic findings. Primary sclerosing cholangitis (PSC) and IgG4-related cholangiopathy are additional autoimmune-related liver diseases that affect the biliary tree.

It is generally accepted that PBC affects women 10 times more than men. AMA-negative disease follows a similar pattern and seems to affect women much more frequently.[23] Many of the reported studies have no male subjects, though in a small single-center study aimed at the utility of using CD1a immunostaining in the diagnosis of PBC, and including 12 AMA-negative PBC subjects, the gender ratio was reported as high as 1:3 for affected men to women.[24]

Multiple risk factors and exposures have been implicated as increasing the risk of PBC, from nail polish to cigarette smoking.[25] Probably the strongest risk factor is a family history, specifically an affected first-degree relative. Given the small number of studies of subjects with AMA-negative disease, it is not possible to directly prove this association in the AMA-negative population; however, it stands to reason that the case would be similar. A study from British Columbia noted a common ancestry of subjects with AMA-negative PBC, suggesting a genetic predisposition.[19] Although familial clustering has been reported, to date there is no known causative gene. However, 1 candidate is the CTLA4 gene located on chromosome 2q33. There are multiple known polymorphisms, and a 49 A/G polymorphism is thought to increase susceptibility to AMA-positive PBC as shown in a Chinese cohort; specifically the G allele.[26] The odds ratio for this allele was 1.23 for AMA-positive disease compared with those with AMA-negative PBC. Similar findings were found by Juran and colleagues[27] in a white population. Single nucleotide polymorphisms (SNPs), specifically rs231735, around the 3′ region of the CTLA4 gene have also been implicated. These findings were noted in 17% of AMA-positive, 4% of AMA-negative, and 9% of unaffected controls, respectively.[28]

In summary, it does not seem that AMA-negative disease displays significant epidemiologic variation from AMA-positive disease. There is female predominance. The geographic areas of incidence are similar, though one must be careful of publication bias. Most interesting is that, although it is known that risk of PBC is increased if a close relative has PBC, there have been reports of the coexistence of AMA-negative PBC–autoimmune cholangitis and typical PBC occurring within families, suggesting a possible genetic connection between AMA-positive and AMA-negative disease.[29] However, in their study including 26 AMA-negative subjects, Stone and colleagues[30] showed that there were haplotype differences in the HLA genes between those with AMA-positive and AMA-negative disease.

PATHOGENESIS

PBC is an autoimmune destructive process that targets the small intrahepatic bile ducts. Targets of mitochondrial antibodies include the 2-oxo acid dehydrogenase enzymes, specifically the subunits of pyruvate dehydrogenase, which are thought to be the stimulus for T-cell–mediated inflammation and bile duct destruction. Interestingly, a study by Tsuneyama and colleagues[31] showed that, in 7 of 9 AMA-negative subjects of both genders and all disease stages, confirmed by both immunofixation and immunoblot, staining patterns of monoclonal antibodies were identical, suggesting that the targets of AMA-positive and AMA-negative autoantibodies were the same. Of the 2 subjects who were AMA-negative and did not react, 1 had scleroderma and 1 had Sjögren. The investigators concluded they may have had an overlap syndrome and not specifically PBC. Despite these similarities, it has been noted that the intensity of inflammation is more robust in AMA-negative disease, which may be due to elevated vitronectin (a regulator of proteolysis) levels.[32]

CLINICAL FEATURES

AMA-negative PBC is in some sense a diagnosis of exclusion after evaluation for cholestatic liver disease, such as drug-induced liver disease; large or small duct primary sclerosing cholangitis (PSC); other biliary pathologic conditions; and AMA-positive PBC (**Fig. 2**).

AMA-negative PBC has been proposed to exist on a spectrum with AMA-positive disease, and even the nomenclature that includes PBC suggests that the clinical syndrome must parallel that of AMA-positive disease irrespective of the underlying mechanism of hepatic injury. Multiple studies have looked to compare the presentations and natural history of AMA-positive PBC with AMA-negative PBC. They are a heterogeneous group of small studies from many countries, thus drawing direct comparisons is not possible. However, in aggregate they provide insight into the clinical manifestations of AMA-negative PBC.

The manifestations of AMA-negative PBC are that of a cholestatic liver profile with an elevated ALP, greater than 1.5 times the upper limit of normal, in keeping with a diagnosis of PBC. The presence of coexistent symptoms is variable. The typical patient is a middle-aged woman with a median age of 55 years; a demographic shared by AMA-positive PBC.[33,34] The female-to-male ratio varies from as low as 3:1 to as high as 29:1, with many studies including no male subjects.[24,34,35] ALP levels do not seem to significantly differ between AMA-positive and AMA-negative cohorts.[35] Careful history must be performed to exclude the presence of drug-induced liver injury, overt large bile duct, or biliary pathologic conditions (eg, PSC, choledocholithiasis), and to definitively exclude the presence of an AMA. Older studies are limited in this regard because newer assays have become available that have identified AMA

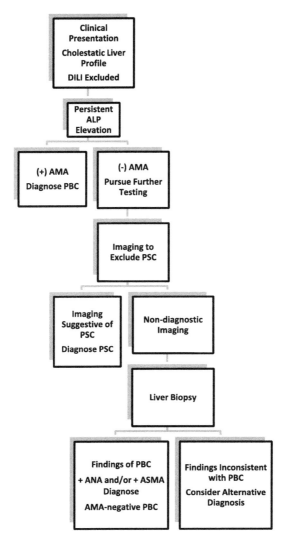

Fig. 2. Diagnostic algorithm. In the patient with the appropriate clinical presentation, with cholestatic liver enzyme profile and persistently elevated ALP, and in whom drug-induced liver injury (DILI) has been excluded, biliary pathologic conditions should be suspected. AMA negativity excludes AMA-positive PBC. In those who are AMA-negative, imaging can be used to exclude large-duct PSC. Liver biopsy will confirm the diagnosis of AMA-negative PBC. ANA and ASMA may be positive. If liver biopsy is not suggestive, alternate causes should be considered.

in subjects who were previously negative. Although it is known that the tests are now more sensitive, seroconversion also occurs. Interestingly, AMA status may alternate over time, resulting in reclassification of disease from AMA-positive to AMA-negative and vice versa.[8]

Clinical features of AMA-negative PBC are thought to parallel those of patients with AMA-positive disease without significant variance, as reported by several studies spanning the globe from Asia, North America, and Europe (**Box 1**).[7,20,36,37] Fatigue

---

Box 1
Unique features of antimitochondrial antibody–negative primary biliary cholangitis compared with antimitochondrial antibody–positive disease

- Negative AMA
- High prevalence of positive antinuclear antibody (ANA) and antismooth muscle antibody (ASMA)
- Lower or normal IgM levels
- More significant inflammation on biopsy
- Possibly more severe clinical course
- Coexistence of other autoimmune conditions

---

and pruritus are the most common symptoms affecting nearly a third to a half of patients.[15,34] However, others have found that pruritus, although the most common symptom, was present in fewer AMA-negative patients.[23] It should be noted that a significant number of patients may be completely asymptomatic.[35] Tsou and Yeh[38] showed a significantly higher prevalence of asymptomatic AMA-negative individuals. Michieletti and colleagues[15] described 20 Canadian subjects who were AMA-negative and thus were declined enrollment in a trial for ursodeoxycholic acid (UDCA) but who were otherwise matched demographically and biochemically with AMA-positive subjects. Three subjects became AMA-positive with repeated testing. The groups were similar with respect to the presence of jaundice, fatigue, pruritus, xanthelasma, hypothyroidism, polyarthralgias, Sicca syndrome, calcinosis, raynaud phenomenon, esophageal dysmotility, sclerodactyly, and telangiectasia (CREST), Raynaud phenomenon, and diabetes.

Whether AMA-negative patients have a more severe clinical course compared with AMA-positive patients is debatable. Several studies have suggested that there is no difference in clinical outcomes, progression to decompensated liver disease, development of hepatocellular carcinoma, or transplant-free or overall survival.[13,30,33] Progression of liver disease, defined as worsening biochemical markers, including bilirubin, international normalized ratio or albumin, or need for liver transplant, occurs in 15% of AMA-negative patients compared with 45% of AMA-positive patients.[30] Survival free of liver failure is similar between AMA-negative and AMA-positive patients: 85% at 4 years and 70% at 7 years, respectively.[13] These findings contrast with those of Juliusson and colleagues[34] who found differences in complication-free survival between AMA-positive and AMA-negative subjects, with AMA-negative subjects having statistically significantly shorter complication-free survival. This included an increase in the prevalence of cirrhosis in AMA-negative subjects and that varices were present in 10% of AMA-negative subjects, with 10% also suffering a variceal bleeding. In this study, the prevalence of varices in AMA-positive subjects was not reported, though only 1% suffered a variceal bleed. This suggests a more severe disease course. However, this is in contrast to a larger study that reported a prevalence of varices of greater than 30% in AMA-positive subjects, with 15% of that cohort suffering a variceal bleed.[39]

The presence of coexistent autoimmunity is well-described in AMA-positive PBC, and these associations exist in AMA-negative disease as well. Despite absence of AMA, antinuclear antibody (ANA) has been reported with extremely high prevalence in AMA-negative PBC as compared with AMA-positive subjects. In a study of 71 subjects with AMA-negative PBC, two-thirds of subjects had at least 1 coexistent autoimmune-related disease; 25% had more than 1.[34] Sjögren is the most commonly concurrent syndrome, though rheumatoid arthritis, scleroderma, and CREST syndrome have all been reported with higher prevalence in the AMA-negative population.[23] Although the prevalence of most autoimmune conditions is not significantly different from AMA-positive disease, Raynaud has been encountered more often.[13] Further confusing the picture of whether AMA-negative PBC is a variant of PBC is the presence of antismooth muscle antibody (ASMA) in some patients. Although ANA and ASMA are more prevalent in AMA-negative patients, their presence does not affect disease course.[40] However, it should be mentioned that patients with detectable ANA or ASMA have been diagnosed with PBC and later with an overlap of AIH in some cases.[10]

SEROLOGIC TESTING

The serologic profiles of those with AMA-positive and AMA-negative PBC show striking similarities with the following few notable exceptions. The AMA is absent at diagnosis, however may change over time. Additionally, mild serum transaminase elevations may be seen in AMA-negative PBC in conjunction with the elevated ALP.[15,41] Higher prevalence of ANA, ASMA, and lower or normal serum IgM levels have been seen in AMA-negative PBC, though clinical significance is unclear.

Antimitochondrial Antibody

AMA is the serologic fingerprint of PBC, present in greater than 90% of cases. Thus, absence of the AMA is considered essential for diagnosing AMA-negative disease. However, the inability to reliably detect AMA can result in an incorrect diagnosis. There are 3 major methods for detecting AMAs: immunofluorescence (IF), enzyme-linked immunosorbent assay (ELISA), and immunoblot. IF detects components of both AMA and ANA and is a good screening test but is operator-dependent.[41] Immunoblot is the most sensitive test at 85%; ELISA is 78% to 81% sensitive.[20] Whether IF, ELISA, or immunoblot are used, rediagnosis from AMA-negative to AMA-positive disease occurs in 3% to 22% of patients with fluctuations in AMA titers and the ability to detect the antibody.[8,34,42] Low-level AMA titers less than 1:40 may result in false-negative testing.[41,43] Treatment of the disease may also influence AMA detectability, though these fluctuations do not seem to influence disease outcome.[44] Repeated AMA testing, which is not routinely recommended clinically, has shown to increase the prevalence of AMA over time.[45] However, a study by Mytilinaiou and colleagues[46] showed that, after 5 years of follow-up, 31 of 33 initially AMA-negative subjects remained so. As such, it cannot be concluded that there is natural progression from AMA-negative disease to AMA-positive, especially given that AMA may predate the development of symptoms in a significant number of subjects. Nakanuma and colleagues[35] showed that even in subjects who were AMA-negative, many were positive for antibodies against r-mitochondrial polypeptides PDC-E2, BCOADC-E2, and PDC-E1, again suggesting that currently available tests to detect AMA may still lack adequate sensitivity. In this particular study, 20% of AMA-negative subjects still had no detectable antibody.

Antinuclear Antibody

ANAs are directed at a host of nuclear targets. The difference in prevalence of ANA positivity between AMA-positive and AMA-negative subjects may be perhaps the most striking difference between the 2 groups. Although up to 50% of AMA-positive individuals may have a detectable ANA, 60% to 100% of AMA-negative subjects do, though ANA titers do not differ.[13,15,34] There are several distinct ANA profiles found in PBC. One is a nonspecific pattern. The others are quite specific, such as the rim-like nuclear membrane and multiple nuclear dot patterns on IF, corresponding to gp210 and sp100 antigens in ELISA. These more specific ANA patterns are found in 30% to 50% of AMA-negative subjects with a sensitivity of 30% and specificity of 99%.[41,47,48] Screening for these targets along with pMIT3 provides a test with 83.8% sensitivity and 94% specificity for diagnosing AMA-negative PBC, and may identify an additional 45% of patients who previously tested AMA-negative but have PBC.[48,49] Anti-kelch–like 12 and antihexokinase 1 are additional ANAs, with greater than 95% specificity for PBC patients and present in up to 35% of those that are AMA-negative.[50]

Additional Serologies

Additional serologies noted to be different between those who are AMA-negative compared with AMA-positive, include normal or lower level IgM, and higher C-reactive protein.[37,47,51] ASMA has been found in up to 20% to 40% of AMA-negative patients compared with 10% of those who were AMA-positive. Nearly 80% of AMA-negative patients will test positive for either ANA or ASMA.[13,34] Anti–*Saccharomyces cerevisiae* (ASCA) antibodies have also been detected in nearly half of patients with AMA-negative disease.[52] The presence of ASCA was associated with more severe liver injury; however, the total number of subjects was small. *Novosphingobium aromaticivorans* antibody was noted to react with a high proportion of AMA-positive subjects and up to 12% of AMA-negative subjects, suggesting that there may be possible molecular mimicry.[43] Antibodies targeting carbonic anhydrase II have also been found in 50% of AMA-negative PBC patients; however, this positivity is believed to be a marker of general autoimmunity as opposed to a specific biomarker of the disease because they are found with significant frequency in other autoimmune liver diseases.[53]

HISTOLOGIC FINDINGS

Classic histologic features of AMA-positive PBC include nonsuppurative cholangitis and small bile duct injury. The florid duct lesion is pathognomonic for the disease but is not commonly encountered. Additional findings compatible with a diagnosis of PBC include portal inflammation, ductular proliferation, cholestasis, and interface hepatitis. The latter can cause diagnostic confusion with AIH.[41] Given the lack of serologic biomarkers, the diagnosis of AMA-negative PBC relies on histology similar to that found in AMA-positive PBC. Similarity between AMA-positive and AMA-negative disease has been shown by lack of difference in disease stage at diagnosis, granuloma formation, portal inflammation, or piecemeal necrosis between positive and negative patients.[35] However, Michieletti and colleagues[15] showed that AMA-negative specimens lacked piecemeal and periportal inflammation, arguing against an AIH, or even overlap with AIH and PBC. Additional stains such as copper and CK7 may aid in diagnosis.[41]

T-cell–mediated inflammation is thought to be the driver of hepatic injury in PBC. AMA-positive biopsies showed a significantly more robust lymphocytic infiltrate compared with negative counterparts, defined as autoimmune cholangitis with AMA-negativity but positive ANA.[37] However, there was no significant difference in the amount or presence of plasma cells, eosinophils, or neutrophils. A study by Graham and colleagues[24] showed no difference in the density of Langerhans antigen–presenting cells per bile duct. More severe bile duct injury has been shown in AMA-negative biopsies in the setting of identical clinical and histologic features.[32,54]

B-cell infiltration has also been assessed and there was no difference in the overall level of CD20-positive cells between positive and negative biopsies.[54]

TREATMENT RESPONSE

Assessment of treatment response for AMA-negative PBC has been difficult to catalog owing to a large number of very small and heterogeneous studies. Lack of understanding of the exact pathologic mechanism of the disease process and inability to consistently classify the disease has hindered adequate assessment. If AMA-negative PBC represents a variant of PBC, then one would expect a response to UDCA. However, given the abundance of autoimmune biomarkers, immunosuppressive medications could also reasonably be expected to provide benefit. The results of liver transplantation seem to be equivalent between AMA-positive and AMA-negative patients.[14] Reported outcomes with living donor liver transplantation in AMA-negative PBC are very limited.[55]

In AMA-positive PBC, adequate biochemical response to UDCA is between 60% and 80%.[11,56] Treatment with UDCA at standard treatment dosages (13–15 mg/kg/d in divided doses) was shown to have equivalent efficacy in AMA-positive and AMA-negative patients.[7,57,58] In their review of 52 subjects from 13 studies, Gisbert and colleagues[59] noted in those with autoimmune cholangitis or AMA-negative PBC that UDCA improved biochemical markers in 83% of subjects. However, there were no specific factors that predicted a response to UDCA. No studies have assessed the efficacy of obeticholic acid in AMA-negative PBC.

A retrospective study evaluated treatment response in 22 subjects: 12 with AIH-PBC overlap and 10 AIH-AMA-negative PBC overlap. Treatment consisted of UDCA alone in only 3 subjects with AIH-PBC, and a combination of UDCA and immunosuppressants in the remaining AIH-PBC subjects and all AIH-AMA-negative patient subjects.[36] Complete remission was noted in 90% of the AMA-negative group compared with 50% in the AIH-PBC cohort. However, other studies have shown that nearly 88% to 100% of patients with AMA-negative disease will be unable to achieve adequate disease control with UDCA, steroids, or a combination.[60] A review of several cases of AMA-negative PBC showed that immunosuppression may help approximately half of patients with AMA-negative PBC.[59]

SUMMARY

AMA is present in 9 out of 10 patients with PBC. However, AASLD diagnostic criteria require at least 2 of 3 features to be present, including a persistent elevation in ALP greater than 1.5 times the upper limit of normal, positive AMA, or consistent biopsy features to make a diagnosis of PBC. Patients are diagnosed with AMA-negative PBC when they have a clinical picture consistent with PBC but lack an AMA. Thus they meet criteria for the diagnosis of PBC. Additionally, associated symptoms, comorbid medical conditions, and response to medical and surgical therapy seem to be relatively in line with the clinical course of those with AMA-positive disease. The progression to liver cirrhosis and decompensation suggest that AMA-negative patients may have a more severe course. Because it is not entirely clear what the underlying pathologic mechanism is for the injury related to either AMA-positive or AMA-negative disease, the authors agree with Vierling,[61] who stated there was insufficient evidence to suggest they are 2 different diseases. The term AMA-negative PBC certainly helps to highlight that these patients have a disease process that parallels AMA-positive PBC. However, it is important to note that there is not clear progression from AMA-negative to AMA-positive disease. In summary, as currently understood, it cannot be concluded that there is a significant difference between AMA-negative and AMA-positive PBC.

REFERENCES

1. Kaplan MM. Primary biliary cirrhosis. N Engl J Med 1996;335(21):1570–80.
2. Beuers U, Gershwin ME, Gish RG, et al. Changing nomenclature for PBC: from 'cirrhosis' to 'cholangitis'. Clin Res Hepatol Gastroenterol 2015;39(5):e57–9.
3. Lindor KD, Gershwin ME, Poupon R, et al. Primary biliary cirrhosis. Hepatology 2009;50(1):291–308.
4. Doniach D, Walker G. Mitochondrial antibodies (AMA). Gut 1974;15(8):664–8.
5. Nezu S, Tanaka A, Yasui H, et al. Presence of antimitochondrial autoantibodies in patients with autoimmune hepatitis. J Gastroenterol Hepatol 2006;21(9):1448–54.
6. Li CH, Xu PS, Wang CY, et al. The presence of anti-mitochondrial antibodies in Chinese patients with liver involvement in systemic lupus erythematosus. Rheumatol Int 2006;26(8):697–703.
7. Liu B, Shi XH, Zhang FC, et al. Antimitochondrial antibody-negative primary biliary cirrhosis: a subset of primary biliary cirrhosis. Liver Int 2008;28(2):233–9.
8. Kadokawa Y, Omagari K, Ohba K, et al. Does the diagnosis of primary biliary cirrhosis of autoimmune cholangitis depend on the 'phase' of the disease? Liver Int 2005;25(2):317–24.
9. SanchezPobre P, Castellano G, Colina F, et al. Antimitochondrial antibody-negative chronic nonsuppurative destructive cholangitis - atypical primary biliary cirrhosis or autoimmune cholangitis? J Clin Gastroenterol 1996;23(3):191–8.
10. Jesic R, Boricic I, Krstic MN, et al. Autoimmune cholangitis - AMA-negative syndrome. Arch Gastroenterohepatol 2002;21(1–2):31–5.
11. Kaplan MM, Gershwin ME. Primary biliary cirrhosis. N Engl J Med 2005;353(12): 1261–73.
12. Gordon SC, Quattrociocchi-Longe TM, Khan BA, et al. Antibodies to carbonic anhydrase in patients with immune cholangiopathies. Gastroenterology 1995; 108(6):1802–9.
13. Invernizzi P, Crosignani A, Battezzati PM, et al. Comparison of the clinical features and clinical course of antimitochondrial antibody-positive and -negative primary biliary cirrhosis. Hepatology 1997;25(5):1090–5.
14. Lacerda MA, Ludwig J, Dickson ER, et al. Antimitochondrial antibody-negative primary biliary cirrhosis. Am J Gastroenterol 1995;90(2):247–9.
15. Michieletti P, Wanless IR, Katz A, et al. Antimitochondrial antibody negative primary biliary-cirrhosis - a distinct syndrome of autoimmune cholangitis. Gut 1994;35(2):260–5.
16. Taylor SL, Dean PJ, Riely CA. Primary autoimmune cholangitis. An alternative to antimitochondrial antibody-negative primary biliary cirrhosis. Am J Surg Pathol 1994;18(1):91–9.
17. Alric L, Thebault S, Selves J, et al. Characterization of overlap syndrome between primary biliary cirrhosis and autoimmune hepatitis according to antimitochondrial antibodies status. Gastroenterol Clin Biol 2007;31(1):11–6.
18. Kim WR, Lindor KD, Locke GR 3rd, et al. Epidemiology and natural history of primary biliary cirrhosis in a US community. Gastroenterology 2000;119(6):1631–6.
19. Arbour L, Rupps R, Field L, et al. Characteristics of primary biliary cirrhosis in British Columbia's first nations population. Can J Gastroenterol 2005;19(5): 305–10.
20. Muratori P, Muratori L, Gershwin ME, et al. 'True' antimitochondrial antibody-negative primary biliary cirrhosis, low sensitivity of the routine assays, or both? Clin Exp Immunol 2004;135(1):154–8.

21. Sfakianaki O, Koulentaki M, Tzardi M, et al. Peri-nuclear antibodies correlate with survival in Greek primary biliary cirrhosis patients. World J Gastroenterol 2010; 16(39):4938–43.

22. Hurlburt KJ, McMahon BJ, Deubner H, et al. Prevalence of autoimmune liver disease in Alaska natives. Am J Gastroenterol 2002;97(9):2402–7.

23. Sakauchi F, Mori M, Zeniya M, et al. Antimitochondrial antibody negative primary biliary cirrhosis in Japan: utilization of clinical data when patients applied to receive public financial aid. J Epidemiol 2005;16(1):30–4.

24. Graham RPD, Smyrk TC, Zhang LZ. Evaluation of Langerhans cell infiltrate by CD1a immunostain in liver biopsy for the diagnosis of primary biliary cirrhosis. Am J Surg Pathol 2012;36(5):732–6.

25. Gershwin ME, Selmi C, Worman HJ, et al. Risk factors and comorbidities in primary biliary cirrhosis: a controlled interview-based study of 1032 patients. Hepatology 2005;42(5):1194–202.

26. Chen RR, Han ZY, Li JG, et al. Cytotoxic T-lymphocyte antigen 4 gene+49A/G polymorphism significantly associated with susceptibility to primary biliary cirrhosis: a meta-analysis. J Dig Dis 2011;12(6):428–35.

27. Juran BD, Atkinson EJ, Larson JJ, et al. Carriage of a tumor necrosis factor polymorphism amplifies the cytotoxic T-lymphocyte antigen 4 attributed risk of primary biliary cirrhosis: evidence for a gene-gene interaction. Hepatology 2010; 52(1):223–9.

28. Juran BD, Lazaridis KN. Update on the genetics and genomics of PBC. J Autoimmun 2010;35(3):181–7.

29. Agarwal K, Jones DEJ, Watt FE, et al. Familial primary biliary cirrhosis and autoimmune cholangitis. Dig Liver Dis 2002;34(1):50–2.

30. Stone J, Wade JA, Cauch-Dudek K, et al. Human leukocyte antigen class II associations in serum antimitochondrial antibodies (AMA)-positive and AMA-negative primary biliary cirrhosis. J Hepatol 2002;36(1):8–13.

31. Tsuneyama K, Van De Water J, Van Thiel D, et al. Abnormal expression of PDC-E$_2$ on the apical surface of biliary epithelial cells in patients with antimitochondrial antibody-negative primary biliary cirrhosis. Hepatology 1995;22(5):1440–6.

32. Deng C, Chaojun H, Wang L, et al. Serological comparative proteomics analysis of mitochondrial autoantibody-negative and -positive primary biliary cirrhosis. Electrophoresis 2015;36(14):1588–95.

33. Simionov I, Gheorghe L, Becheanu G. Antimitochondrial antibodies - negative primary biliary cirrhosis - a variant of primary biliary cirrhosis. AFH 2009; 14(1–2):9–13.

34. Juliusson G, Imam M, Björnsson ES, et al. Long-term outcomes in antimitochondrial antibody negative primary biliary cirrhosis. Scand J Gastroenterol 2016; 51(6):745–52.

35. Nakanuma Y, Harada K, Kaji K, et al. Clinicopathological study of primary biliary cirrhosis negative for antimitochondrial antibodies. Liver 1997;17(6):281–7.

36. Ozaslan E, Efe C, Akbulut S, et al. Therapy response and outcome of overlap syndromes: autoimmune hepatitis and primary biliary cirrhosis compared to autoimmune hepatitis and autoimmune cholangitis. Hepatogastroenterology 2010; 57(99–100):441–6.

37. Watanabe S, Deguchi A, Uchida N, et al. Histopathologic comparison of antimitochondrial antibody-positive primary biliary cirrhosis and autoimmune cholangiopathy. Hepatol Res 2001;19(1):41–51.

38. Tsou YK, Yeh CT. Primary biliary cirrhosis in antimitochondrial antibody-negative patients: Chang Gung Memorial Hospital experience. Chang Gung Med J 2003; 26(5):323–9.

39. Gores GJ, Wiesner RH, Dickson ER, et al. Prospective evaluation of esophageal varices in primary biliary cirrhosis: development, natural history, and influence on survival. Gastroenterology 1989;96(6):1552–9.

40. Zhang FK, Jia JD, Wang BE. Clinical evaluation of serum antimitochondrial antibody-negative primary biliary cirrhosis. Hepatobiliary Pancreat Dis Int 2004; 3(2):288–91.

41. Ozaslan E, Efe C, Gokbulut Ozaslan N. The diagnosis of antimitochondrial antibody-negative primary biliary cholangitis. Clin Res Hepatol Gastroenterol 2016;40(5):553–61.

42. Liaskos C, Norman GL, Moulas A, et al. Prevalence of gastric parietal cell antibodies and intrinsic factor antibodies in primary biliary cirrhosis. Clin Chim Acta 2010;411(5–6):411–5.

43. Selmi C, Balkwill DL, Invernizzi P, et al. Patients with primary biliary cirrhosis react against a ubiquitous xenobiotic-metabolizing bacterium. Hepatology 2003;38(5): 1250–7.

44. Vleggaar FP, Van Buuren HR. No prognostic significance of antimitochondrial antibody profile testing in primary biliary cirrhosis. Hepatogastroenterology 2004;51(58):937–40.

45. Munoz LE, Thomas HC, Scheuer PJ, et al. Is mitochondrial antibody diagnostic of primary biliary cirrhosis? Gut 1981;22(2):136–40.

46. Mytilinaiou MG, Meyer W, Scheper T, et al. Diagnostic and clinical utility of antibodies against the nuclear body promyelocytic leukaemia and Sp100 antigens in patients with primary biliary cirrhosis. Clin Chim Acta 2012;413(15–16):1211–6.

47. Hu CJ, Deng CW, Song G, et al. Prevalence of autoimmune liver disease related autoantibodies in Chinese patients with primary biliary cirrhosis. Dig Dis Sci 2011; 56(11):3357–63.

48. Bizzaro N, Covini G, Rosina F, et al. Overcoming a "probable" diagnosis in antimitochondrial antibody negative primary biliary cirrhosis: study of 100 sera and review of the literature. Clin Rev Allergy Immunol 2012;42(3):288–97.

49. Liu H, Norman GL, Shums Z, et al. PBC screen: an IgG/IgA dual isotype ELISA detecting multiple mitochondrial and nuclear autoantibodies specific for primary biliary cirrhosis. J Autoimmun 2010;35(4):436–42.

50. Norman GL, Yang CY, Ostendorff HP, et al. Anti-kelch-like 12 and anti-hexokinase 1: novel autoantibodies in primary biliary cirrhosis. Liver Int 2015;35(2):642–51.

51. Fallatah HI, Akbar HO. Autoimmune liver disease - are there spectra that we do not know? Comp Hepatol 2011;10:9.

52. Hu C, Deng C, Zhang S, et al. Clinical significance and prevalence of anti-*Saccharomyces cerevisiae* antibody in Chinese patients with primary biliary cirrhosis. Clin Exp Med 2013;13(4):245–50.

53. Comay D, Cauch-Dudek K, Hemphill D, et al. Are antibodies to carbonic anhydrase II specific for anti-mitochondrial antibody-negative primary biliary cirrhosis? Dig Dis Sci 2000;45(10):2018–21.

54. Jin QL, Moritoki Y, Lleo A, et al. Comparative analysis of portal cell infiltrates in antimitochondrial autoantibody-positive versus antimitochondrial autoantibody-negative primary biliary cirrhosis. Hepatology 2012;55(5):1495–506.

55. Hashimoto E, Taniai M, Yatsuji S, et al. Long-term clinical outcome of living-donor liver transplantation for primary biliary cirrhosis. Hepatol Res 2007;37:S455–61.

56. Carbone M, Mells GF, Pells G, et al. Sex and age are determinants of the clinical phenotype of primary biliary cirrhosis and response to ursodeoxycholic acid. Gastroenterology 2013;144(3):560–569 e7 [quiz: e13–4].
57. Kim WR, Poterucha JJ, Jorgensen RA, et al. Does antimitochondrial antibody status affect response to treatment in patients with primary biliary cirrhosis? Outcomes of ursodeoxycholic acid therapy and liver transplantation. Hepatology 1997;26(1):22–6.
58. Li CP, Hwang SJ, Chan CY, et al. Clinical evaluation of primary biliary cirrhosis in Chinese patients without serum anti-mitochondrial antibody. Zhonghua Yi Xue Za Zhi (Taipei) 1997;59(6):334–40.
59. Gisbert JP, Jones EA, Pajares JM, et al. Is there an optimal therapeutic regimen for antimitochondrial antibody-negative primary biliary cirrhosis (autoimmune cholangitis)? Aliment Pharmacol Ther 2003;17(1):17–27.
60. Czaja AJ, Carpenter HA, Santrach PJ, et al. Autoimmune cholangitis within the spectrum of autoimmune liver disease. Hepatology 2000;31(6):1231–8.
61. Vierling JM. Autoimmune cholangiopathy. Clin Liver Dis 1999;3(3):571–84.

Overlap Syndrome of Autoimmune Hepatitis and Primary Biliary Cholangitis

Uyen To, MD, Marina Silveira, MD*

KEYWORDS

- Overlap syndrome • Autoimmune hepatitis • Primary biliary cholangitis

KEY POINTS

- Multiple criteria have been used to diagnose and characterize patients with overlap syndrome, including the Paris criteria, the International Autoimmune Hepatitis Group (IAIHG) scoring system, the revised IAIHG scoring system, and the simplified IAIHG scoring system.
- Patients with overlap syndrome have significantly higher rates of portal hypertension, esophageal varices, gastrointestinal bleeding, ascites, death, and need of liver transplant.
- Several retrospective studies comparing treatment with ursodeoxycholic acid alone or in combination with immunosuppression (steroids or a thiopurine) suggest combination therapy may result in improved outcomes.

INTRODUCTION

Over the last 2 decades, there has been increasing attention to a rare clinical subgroup of patients who appear to have a combination of autoimmune liver disease, an "overlap" of conditions such as autoimmune hepatitis (AIH), primary biliary cholangitis (PBC), and primary sclerosing cholangitis (PSC), that are classically thought to have independent mechanisms. It remains unclear whether overlap syndrome is a variant of PBC, AIH, or an individual entity unto itself, because PBC and AIH share histologic findings, such as ductal injury, which can be seen in AIH, and interface hepatitis, which can be seen as part of PBC.[1,2] The consecutive occurrence of the 2 disorders supports the notion of coincident autoimmune diseases, consistent with the fact that autoimmune disorders are often associated with one another. A series of investigations have attempted to define the affected populations, determine the clinical significance of such presentation, propose diagnostic criteria, and evaluate treatment strategies in this subset of patients. In this review, the authors focus on the overlap syndrome of AIH and PBC (AIH-PBC overlap), highlighting the latest published studies on this topic.

Disclosure Statement: Dr M. Silveira has done consulting for Conatus. Dr U. To has nothing to disclose.
Department of Digestive Diseases, Yale University, New Haven, CT, USA
* Corresponding author. 333 Cedar Street LMP 1080, PO Box 208019, New Haven, CT 06510.
E-mail address: Marina.silveira@yale.edu

Clin Liver Dis 22 (2018) 603–611
https://doi.org/10.1016/j.cld.2018.03.010
1089-3261/18/© 2018 Elsevier Inc. All rights reserved.

DEFINITION AND DIAGNOSTIC CRITERIA

PBC-AIH overlap is the most commonly described overlap syndrome, but the term can also be used in reference to overlap of PSC and AIH.[3] Although there is no formal definition of what constitutes PBC-AIH overlap syndrome, the term is typically used to describe patients with clinical features of both antimitochondrial antibodies (AMA)-positive PBC and AIH.[4] The spectrum of presentation and clinical characteristics in individual autoimmune liver diseases has complicated the development of a uniform consensus definition for overlap syndrome.[3] As a result, several distinct criteria have been used to diagnose patients with overlap syndrome of AIH and PBC, including the Paris criteria, the International Autoimmune Hepatitis Group (IAIHG) scoring system, the revised IAIHG scoring system, and the simplified IAIHG scoring system.[5–8]

The Paris criteria were designed to standardize the characterization of patients with AIH-PBC overlap syndrome and are defined by the presence of at least 2 of the 3 accepted key criteria of each disease, as summarized in **Box 1**.[5] It is the most commonly used criteria for overlap syndrome and has been endorsed by the European Association for the Study of the Liver (EASL) and the American Association Society of Liver Disease (AASLD) with the caveat that the histologic finding of interface hepatitis is required to establish the diagnosis of overlap syndrome.[4,9,10]

The original[6] and revised[7] IAIHG scoring systems have also been frequently used to assess for the presence of overlap syndrome in patients with known PBC (the revised IAIHG scoring system is summarized in **Table 1**); however, their effectiveness as diagnostic tools has been questioned.[7] Application of these criteria can be clinically burdensome for the diagnosis of AIH-PBC overlap, given the multiple items required in the scoring system.[7] The scoring systems were also created by an expert panel for the purpose of comparing AIH studies from multiple institutions and to distinguish AIH from PBC, not to diagnose AIH in patients with PBC.[8] As such, both the original and the revised IAIHG scoring systems assign a negative score to the findings of positive AMA or biliary changes on liver biopsy.[11] As a result of the frequent utilization of the scoring systems in the diagnosis of overlap syndrome, the position paper by the

---

Box 1
Paris criteria

Autoimmune hepatitis

1. Alanine aminotransferase (ALT) $\geq 5\times$ upper normal limit

2. Immunoglobulin G (IgG) $\geq 2\times$ ULN or presence of antismooth muscle antibodies

3. Liver biopsy with moderate or severe periportal or periseptal lymphocytic piecemeal necrosis

Primary biliary cholangitis

1. Alkaline phosphatase (ALP) $\geq 2\times$ upper normal limit or gamma-glutamyl transferase $\geq 5\times$ upper normal limit

2. Presence of AMA

3. Liver biopsy with florid bile duct lesions

At least 2 of 3 accepted criteria for PBC and AIH, respectively, should be present. Histologic evidence of moderate to severe lymphocytic piecemeal necrosis (interface hepatitis) is mandatory for the diagnosis.

From Chazouilleres O, Wendum D, Serfaty L, et al. Primary biliary cirrhosis-autoimmune hepatitis overlap syndrome: clinical features and response to therapy. Hepatology 1998;28(2):297; with permission.

Table 1
Revised International Autoimmune Hepatitis Group scoring system

	Points
Female gender	2
ALP:AST ratio	
<1.5	2
1.5–3.0	0
>3.0	−2
Serum globulin or IgG above normal	
>2.0	3
1.5–2.0	2
1.0–1.5	1
<1	0
ANA, SMA, LKM1	
>1:80	3
1: 80	2
1: 40	1
<1:40	0
Illicit drug use history	
Positive	−4
Negative	1
Average alcohol intake daily	
<25 g/d	2
>60 g/d	−2
Histologic findings	
Interface hepatitis	3
Lymphoplasmacytic infiltrate	1
Rosette formation	1
None of the above	−5
Biliary changes	−3
Other changes	2
Other autoimmune disease	2
AMA positivity	−4
Hepatitis viral markers	
Positive	−3
Negative	3
Aggregate score without treatment	
Definite AIH	>15
Probable AIH	10–15

Abbreviations: ANA, antinuclear antibody; AST, aspartate aminotransferase; LKM1, liver kidney microsomal antibody; SMA, smooth muscle antibody.

From Alvarez F, Berg PA, Bianchi FB, et al. International Autoimmune Hepatitis Group Report: review of criteria for diagnosis of autoimmune hepatitis. J Hepatol 1999;31(5):934; with permission.

IAIHG suggests that the scoring systems "should not be used to establish subgroups of patients."[7] Because of the cumbersome nature of the original and revised IAIHG scoring criteria, the simplified criteria for diagnosis of AIH have also been applied to patients with PBC for the diagnosis of overlap syndromes. The simplified criteria are composed of specific autoantibodies, level of immunoglobulin G, specific histologic findings on liver biopsy, and the absence of viral hepatitis (**Table 2**).[8] Although it is an easier diagnostic tool to use than the original and revised IAIHG scoring systems, similar limitations to its use in the diagnosis of overlap syndromes apply.

When comparing the criteria used in diagnosing overlap syndrome, wide variability in the sensitivity and specificities has been reported. A recent Chinese study evaluated the diagnostic performance of Paris criteria and the revised and simplified IAIHG scoring systems in 65 patients with PBC in whom a liver biopsy was available.[12] The study identified 2 patients by the Paris criteria, 13 in the IAIHG revised scoring system, and 10 in the simplified scoring system.[12] In this study, overlap syndrome of PBC-AIH was defined as the presence of PBC and AIH simultaneously or sequentially as defined by the Paris criteria or if they met the following criteria: (i) ALT levels higher than the upper limit of normal (ULN); (ii) IgG levels higher than the ULN; (iii) histologically confirmed moderate or severe interface hepatitis; and (iv) patients with a therapeutic response to immunosuppressive treatment. When using this diagnostic criteria for PBC-AIH overlap syndrome, the simplified IAIHG scoring system was the most sensitive and specific for diagnosis of AIH-PBC overlap syndrome, with a sensitivity of 90% and a specificity of 98.2%,[12] followed by the IAIHG revised scoring system. The Paris criteria showed a high specificity of 100% but relatively low sensitivity (20%) in the diagnosis of AIH-PBC overlap syndrome. In contrast, a Dutch study including 134 patients diagnosed with either PBC, AIH, or AIH-PBC overlap syndrome evaluated the diagnostic performance of the Paris criteria, revised IAIHG scoring system, and the simplified IAIHG scoring system in a similar fashion and showed that the sensitivity and specificity of the Paris criteria for the diagnosis of overlap syndrome were 92% and 97%, respectively. The investigators concluded the Paris criteria may be more accurate than the revised or simplified IAIHG scoring systems.[11] When comparing the revised or simplified IAIHG scoring system, a large study from

Table 2 Simplified International Autoimmune Hepatitis Group scoring system	
	Points
ANA or SMA	
≥1:40	1
ANA or SMA ≥1:80 or LKM1 ≥1:40 or SLA-positive	2
Serum IgG	
>Upper limit of normal	1
>1.1 times upper limit of normal	2
Histologic findings	
Compatible with AIH	1
Typical of AIH	2
Hepatitis viral markers	
Negative	2
Aggregate score without treatment	
Definite AIH	≥7
Probable AIH	≥6

Abbreviation: SLA, soluble liver antigen antibody.

From Hennes EM, Zeniya M, Czaja AJ, et al. Simplified criteria for the diagnosis of autoimmune hepatitis. Hepatology 2008;48(1):171; with permission.

the Mayo Clinic, including 368 patients with PBC, showed that the simplified IAIHG scoring system was more specific in patients with PBC. In this cohort, approximately 12% of patients with PBC were found to have "probable" AIH-PBC overlap using the revised IAIHG scoring system, but only 6% of patients with PBC met criteria for overlap using the simplified scoring system.[13] Variability in these conflicting conclusions highlights the challenges faced by clinicians and researchers when diagnosing overlap syndrome. The determination of the most adequate set of criteria to use for diagnosis of overlap syndrome is further confounded by both a lack of an established gold standard for comparison and potential variability among different patient populations.

EPIDEMIOLOGY

One result of this lack of consensus in the diagnostic criteria is a wide range in reported prevalence of AIH-PBC overlap. The prevalence of PBC and AIH in one study ranged from 2.1% to 19% using the Paris criteria and IAIHG revised criteria, respectively.[5] The extent to which a second diagnosis is sought in a patient with autoimmune liver disease is also an important factor in estimation of prevalence within this condition and whether patients who develop consecutive overlap features are captured in studies may also influence prevalence estimations.

An important observation regarding AIH-PBC overlap syndrome is that Hispanic patients with PBC had a significantly higher prevalence of overlap syndrome (based on Paris criteria or simplified IAIHG criteria) than non-Hispanic patients (31% vs 13%, respectively).[14] Differences in the frequency of complications, such as ascites, esophageal varices, variceal bleeding, or encephalopathy, occurred more frequently among patients of Hispanic origin, although this did not reach statistical significance. Similarly, a recent study evaluating the clinical patterns of autoimmune liver disease in Cuba revealed the prevalence AIH-PBC overlap was 15% based on the Paris criteria, almost as high as the prevalence of PBC alone (20.7%) among a cohort of 106 patients with autoimmune liver diseases,[15] supporting higher prevalence of AIH-PBC in patients of Hispanic origin. These findings highlight the importance of establishing clear diagnostic criteria, to appropriately identify whether certain ethnicities are more likely to develop overlap syndrome and implement appropriate screening in these groups.

CLINICAL PRESENTATION

Patients may develop overlap syndrome sequentially, presenting with PBC first and then developing AIH, or may present simultaneously with both diseases.[15,16] Overlap syndrome should be suspected in patients with AIH and PBC whose clinical course deviates from the classical course of disease in the absence of a known trigger, such as viral infections or drug-induced liver injury. In patients with PBC who present with high transaminases and hypergammaglobulinemia, overlap syndrome should be suspected. Similarly, in patients with a diagnosis of AIH, the presence of cholestatic features should also raise the possibility of an overlap syndrome. Sudden deterioration of liver function or suboptimal response to treatment of a previously well-controlled autoimmune liver disease should also raise the suspicion of an overlap syndrome.

In a retrospective study of 1065 patients with both PBC and AIH, Efe and colleagues[17] showed that 1.8% of patients developed overlap syndrome (based on Paris criteria) after a mean of 6.5 years of follow-up. No serologic or histologic findings predicted the development of AIH-PBC overlap, although it was noteworthy that the baseline rates of SMA positivity and moderate/severe interface hepatitis were slightly higher in patients with PBC who developed AIH-PBC overlap than those who did not.[17] Specifically, the presence of AMA positivity in patients with a diagnosis of

AIH did not predict the development of AIH-PBC overlap syndrome during follow-up.[17,18] Conversely, in a study by Muratori and colleagues,[19] clinical characteristics, laboratory findings, histologic features, and treatment responses were compared between 15 patients with overlap syndrome to 120 patients of PBC and 120 patients of AIH; concomitant AMA and anti–double-stranded DNA seropositivity were found to be significantly higher in those with overlap syndrome than those with PBC or AIH who did not develop overlap (47% vs 2%).[19] Although it is not clear why some patients with PBC develop AIH or vice versa, the finding that patients with AIH-characteristic HLA antigen type B8, DR3, or DR4 may be more likely to develop a hepatitis in the setting of PBC suggests an underlying genetic susceptibility.[1,15]

Clinically, patients with overlap syndrome have predilection to other autoimmune diseases, oftentimes more than one.[20] In one retrospective study of 71 patients with overlap syndrome, 43.6% patients had other associated autoimmune diseases, including thyroid disease (18.3%), Sjögren syndrome (8.4%), celiac disease (4.2%), psoriasis (4.2%), rheumatoid arthritis (4.2%), vitiligo (2.8%), and systemic lupus erythematosus (2.8%).[20]

NATURAL HISTORY

The natural history of patients with AIH-PBC overlap syndrome can be variable. Patients with overlap syndrome have been described to exhibit significantly higher rates of portal hypertension, esophageal varices, gastrointestinal bleeding, ascites, and death or need for liver transplantation (LT) compared with those with AIH or PBC alone.[21] In a recent study comparing 277 patients with PBC alone to 46 patients with overlap syndrome (based on Paris criteria),[22] those with overlap syndrome had a decreased 5-year adverse event–free survival than patients with PBC alone (58% vs 81%).[22] Laboratory parameters in patients with overlap syndrome associated with a poorer prognosis include a total bilirubin $\geq 2.7 \times$ ULN, similar to what has been shown in patients with PBC, in which bilirubin has been shown to be the best predictor of survival.[22,23] Surprisingly, the study also showed that those patients with AIH-PBC overlap with AST $\geq 4.6 \times$ ULN had a better prognosis compared with those with lower baseline AST. In contrast, in patients with PBC alone, higher AST levels were related to poorer outcomes with a cutoff of $2.9 \times$ ULN, a result that the investigators could not entirely explain.[22] In another study performed in Korea including 158 patients with AIH, PBC, and AIH-PBC overlap syndrome, patients with overlap syndrome (based on revised and simplified IAIHG scoring systems) developed cirrhosis more rapidly than those with AIH alone and had decreased clinical responses to ursodeoxycholic acid (UDCA) and steroid therapy, whereas hepatic decompensations were similar between the 2 groups.[24] However, the differences between the outcomes in patients with AIH-PBC overlap and PBC alone were not as clear.[24] These findings highlight the importance of early diagnosis and intervention in patients with overlap syndromes.

MANAGEMENT AND TREATMENT

The management of patients with overlap syndrome has not been standardized, because there have been no large randomized control trials (RCT), likely as a result of low prevalence of the disease. Several small RCT have compared treatment with UDCA alone or in combination with immunosuppression (steroids or, less frequently, a thiopurine), with variable results. In a recent meta-analysis by Zhang and colleagues,[25] 8 RCT including a total of 214 patients with AIH-PBC overlap were analyzed, comparing the use of UDCA to the combination of corticosteroids and

UDCA for therapy in AIH-PBC overlap syndrome. In this meta-analysis, outcomes evaluated included symptoms of pruritus and jaundice, changes in ALP and ALT, histologic regression, death, or need for LT, and adverse events. Although combination therapy with UDCA and steroids did significantly improve ALP, ALT, and histologic regression without significant difference in adverse events compared with UDCA alone, it did not improve symptoms of pruritus and jaundice, or lead to reduction of death or need for LT.[25] Although there was concern of study bias in the meta-analysis due to the small number and low quality of the studies, the investigators still concluded that combination therapy was superior because of the improvement in biochemical markers. A recent study evaluating factors that would predict corticosteroid response in overlap syndrome revealed that those who responded had more severe interface hepatitis on their histology and serum IgG levels greater than $1.3 \times$ ULN (the latter having 97% specificity and 60% sensitivity for steroid responsiveness),[26] suggesting that perhaps response to corticosteroids can further support the diagnosis of overlap syndrome and should be considered as diagnostic criteria as proposed in previous studies. In fact, the most recent EASL guidelines recommended the addition of steroid therapy to UDCA for those with severe interface hepatitis and consideration of steroid therapy for patients with moderate interface hepatitis.[27] In the AASLD guidelines, UDCA with or without other immunosuppressive agents is recommended for treatment of overlap syndrome, but it highlights the lack of evidence regarding the optimal therapy and timing of the treatment.[4] In previous retrospective studies, lack of response to UDCA and immunosuppressive therapy was observed in patients with advanced fibrosis.[28,29] Thus, those who do not respond to combination therapy with UDCA and steroids can be trialed on alternative immunosuppression, such as azathioprine or mycophenolate mofetil.[30,31] Despite the findings provided by these studies, the management and treatment of patients with overlap syndrome still require ongoing research to evaluate optimal time of treatment, ideal pharmacologic agents, and their dosage and administration and duration of therapy.

SUMMARY

Because of the variable clinical, laboratory, and histologic presentations of patients with overlap syndrome, it can be difficult to establish a definitive diagnosis. Overlap syndrome should be considered if a patient with PBC presents with transaminitis and hypergammaglobulinemia or in a patient with AIH who has cholestasis or if there is a deterioration of liver function in a patient who previously had well-controlled autoimmune liver disease. Although high-quality data are lacking, studies suggest that patients with AIH-PBC overlap may benefit from combination therapy with UDCA and corticosteroids and/or steroid-sparing agents. Timely and accurate diagnosis and early intervention may potentially improve long-term adverse outcomes in patients with overlap syndrome. On the other hand, overdiagnoses can lead to unnecessary overtreatment and adverse medication effects. Thus, standardized, algorithm-based, diagnostic criteria incorporating laboratory and histologic parameters, and perhaps response to therapy, are required. As AIH-PBC overlap syndrome is a rare disease, improved understanding and treatment will certainly require collaboration between multiple institutions to develop standard diagnostic criteria and therapeutic interventions to appropriately guide further trials regarding therapy.

REFERENCES

1. Vierling JM. Autoimmune hepatitis and overlap syndromes: diagnosis and management. Clin Gastroenterol Hepatol 2015;13(12):2088–108.

2. Verdonk RC, Lozano MF, van den Berg AP, et al. Bile ductal injury and ductular reaction are frequent phenomena with different significance in autoimmune hepatitis. Liver Int 2016;36(9):1362–9.
3. Boberg KM, Chapman RW, Hirschfield GM, et al. Overlap syndromes: the International Autoimmune Hepatitis Group (IAIHG) position statement on a controversial issue. J Hepatol 2011;54(2):374–85.
4. Lindor KD, Gershwin ME, Poupon R, et al. Primary biliary cirrhosis. Hepatology 2009;50(1):291–308.
5. Chazouilleres O, Wendum D, Serfaty L, et al. Primary biliary cirrhosis-autoimmune hepatitis overlap syndrome: clinical features and response to therapy. Hepatology 1998;28(2):296–301.
6. Johnson PJ, McFarlane IG. Meeting report: International Autoimmune Hepatitis Group. Hepatology 1993;18(4):998–1005.
7. Alvarez F, Berg PA, Bianchi FB, et al. International Autoimmune Hepatitis Group Report: review of criteria for diagnosis of autoimmune hepatitis. J Hepatol 1999;31(5):929–38.
8. Hennes EM, Zeniya M, Czaja AJ, et al. Simplified criteria for the diagnosis of autoimmune hepatitis. Hepatology 2008;48(1):169–76.
9. European Association for the Study of the Liver. EASL Clinical Practice Guidelines: management of cholestatic liver diseases. J Hepatol 2009; 51(2):237–67.
10. Chazouilleres O, Wendum D, Serfaty L, et al. Long term outcome and response to therapy of primary biliary cirrhosis-autoimmune hepatitis overlap syndrome. J Hepatol 2006;44(2):400–6.
11. Kuiper EM, Zondervan PE, van Buuren HR. Paris criteria are effective in diagnosis of primary biliary cirrhosis and autoimmune hepatitis overlap syndrome. Clin Gastroenterol Hepatol 2010;8(6):530–4.
12. Liu F, Pan ZG, Ye J, et al. Primary biliary cirrhosis-autoimmune hepatitis overlap syndrome: simplified criteria may be effective in the diagnosis in Chinese patients. J Dig Dis 2014;15(12):660–8.
13. Neuhauser M, Bjornsson E, Treeprasertsuk S, et al. Autoimmune hepatitis-PBC overlap syndrome: a simplified scoring system may assist in the diagnosis. Am J Gastroenterol 2010;105(2):345–53.
14. Levy C, Naik J, Giordano C, et al. Hispanics with primary biliary cirrhosis are more likely to have features of autoimmune hepatitis and reduced response to ursodeoxycholic acid than non-Hispanics. Clin Gastroenterol Hepatol 2014;12(8): 1398–405.
15. Lohse AW, zum Buschenfelde KH, Franz B, et al. Characterization of the overlap syndrome of primary biliary cirrhosis (PBC) and autoimmune hepatitis: evidence for it being a hepatitic form of PBC in genetically susceptible individuals. Hepatology 1999;29(4):1078–84.
16. Poupon R, Chazouilleres O, Corpechot C, et al. Development of autoimmune hepatitis in patients with typical primary biliary cirrhosis. Hepatology 2006; 44(1):85–90.
17. Efe C, Ozaslan E, Heurgue-Berlot A, et al. Sequential presentation of primary biliary cirrhosis and autoimmune hepatitis. Eur J Gastroenterol Hepatol 2014; 26(5):532–7.
18. Dinani AM, Fischer SE, Mosko J, et al. Patients with autoimmune hepatitis who have antimitochondrial antibodies need long-term follow-up to detect late development of primary biliary cirrhosis. Clin Gastroenterol Hepatol 2012;10(6):682–4.

19. Muratori P, Granito A, Pappas G, et al. The serological profile of the autoimmune hepatitis/primary biliary cirrhosis overlap syndrome. Am J Gastroenterol 2009; 104(6):1420–5.
20. Efe C, Wahlin S, Ozaslan E, et al. Autoimmune hepatitis/primary biliary cirrhosis overlap syndrome and associated extrahepatic autoimmune diseases. Eur J Gastroenterol Hepatol 2012;24(5):531–4.
21. Silveira MG, Talwalkar JA, Angulo P, et al. Overlap of autoimmune hepatitis and primary biliary cirrhosis: long-term outcomes. Am J Gastroenterol 2007;102(6): 1244–50.
22. Yang F, Wang Q, Wang Z, et al. The Natural history and prognosis of primary biliary cirrhosis with clinical features of autoimmune hepatitis. Clin Rev Allergy Immunol 2016;50(1):114–23.
23. Dickson ER, Grambsch PM, Fleming TR, et al. Prognosis in primary biliary cirrhosis: model for decision making. Hepatology 1989;10(1):1–7.
24. Park Y, Cho Y, Cho EJ, et al. Retrospective analysis of autoimmune hepatitis-primary biliary cirrhosis overlap syndrome in Korea: characteristics, treatments, and outcomes. Clin Mol Hepatol 2015;21(2):150–7.
25. Zhang H, Yang J, Zhu R, et al. Combination therapy of ursodeoxycholic acid and budesonide for PBC-AIH overlap syndrome: a meta-analysis. Drug Des Devel Ther 2015;9:567–74.
26. Wang Q, Selmi C, Zhou X, et al. Epigenetic considerations and the clinical reevaluation of the overlap syndrome between primary biliary cirrhosis and autoimmune hepatitis. J Autoimmun 2013;41:140–5.
27. European Association for the Study of the Liver. Electronic address: easloffice@easloffice.euEuropean Association for the Study of the Liver. EASL Clinical Practice Guidelines: the diagnosis and management of patients with primary biliary cholangitis. J Hepatol 2017;67(1):145–72.
28. Efe C, Ozaslan E, Kav T, et al. Liver fibrosis may reduce the efficacy of budesonide in the treatment of autoimmune hepatitis and overlap syndrome. Autoimmun Rev 2012;11(5):330–4.
29. Ozaslan E, Efe C, Heurgue-Berlot A, et al. Factors associated with response to therapy and outcome of patients with primary biliary cirrhosis with features of autoimmune hepatitis. Clin Gastroenterol Hepatol 2014;12(5):863–9.
30. Baven-Pronk AM, Coenraad MJ, van Buuren HR, et al. The role of mycophenolate mofetil in the management of autoimmune hepatitis and overlap syndromes. Aliment Pharmacol Ther 2011;34(3):335–43.
31. Wolf DC, Bojito L, Facciuto M, et al. Mycophenolate mofetil for autoimmune hepatitis: a single practice experience. Dig Dis Sci 2009;54(11):2519–22.

Current Status of Liver Transplantation for Primary Biliary Cholangitis

Maria T. Aguilar, MD[a], Elizabeth J. Carey, MD[b],*

KEYWORDS

- Primary biliary cholangitis • Liver transplant • Ursodeoxycholic acid
- Obeticholic acid • Recurrent PBC • Mayo Risk Score • GLOBE score • UK-PBC

KEY POINTS

- With the discovery of the antimitochondrial antibody (AMA) the prevalence of primary biliary cholangitis (PBC) has risen. Yet, the proportion of liver transplants (LT) indicated for PBC has decreased by 20%.
- The widespread use of ursodeoxycholic acid (UDCA) has substantially altered the disease course of PBC.
- Several risk scores have been developed to assess transplant-free survival with PBC. Newer scores, such as the GLOBE score and UK PBC, use noninvasive, objective data to evaluate UDCA response.
- Indications for LT in PBC are similar to other etiologies of end-stage liver disease (ESLD). However, additional indications specific to PBC include a Mayo Risk Score of 7.8 and intractable pruritus.
- Recurrent PBC (rPBC) is not an uncommon complication of LT in PBC patients; however, recurrence has not been shown to have an impact on patient or graft survival.

INTRODUCTION

Primary biliary cholangitis (PBC) is an autoimmune liver disease characterized by the progressive destruction of small intralobular bile ducts resulting in hepatocellular injury, fibrosis, and cirrhosis. The serologic hallmark of PBC is the antimitochondrial antibody (AMA), a disease-specific autoantibody found in 90% to 95% of patients and less than 1% of healthy individuals. PBC is serologically diagnosed when alkaline phosphatase (ALP) is persistently elevated in the presence of AMA.[1] Liver biopsy is

The authors have nothing to disclose.
[a] Division of Gastroenterology and Hepatology, Mayo Clinic, 13400 East Shea Boulevard, Scottsdale, AZ 85259, USA; [b] Division of Gastroenterology and Hepatology, Mayo Clinic, 5777 East Mayo Boulevard, Phoenix, AZ 85054, USA
* Corresponding author.
E-mail address: carey.elizabeth@mayo.edu

Clin Liver Dis 22 (2018) 613–624
https://doi.org/10.1016/j.cld.2018.03.011
1089-3261/18/© 2018 Elsevier Inc. All rights reserved.

liver.theclinics.com

required when there is a high suspicion for PBC in the absence of AMA. Histologic diagnosis requires evidence of portal inflammation.

The introduction of ursodeoxycholic acid (UDCA) as first-line therapy has significantly improved the disease course of PBC. However, 40% of patients treated with UDCA have a partial or absent biochemical response to therapy, and 3% to 5% of patients are intolerant and experience adverse events.[2] Before the widespread use of UDCA, liver transplantation (LT) was the only treatment option for PBC, and remains the only means for cure. PBC was the most common indication for LT in the 1980s and although the absolute number of patients registered for LT has increased steadily, the proportion indicated for PBC has decreased by 20%.[3,4] PBC is currently the sixth most common indication for LT. Prognosis in PBC is independent of symptoms, yet overall survival of asymptomatic patients is shorter than the predicted survival of an age- and gender-matched control population.[5]

URSODEOXYCHOLIC ACID

The clinical course of PBC has dramatically changed over the last 20 years with earlier disease recognition and widespread use of UDCA. Before the Food and Drug Administration (FDA) approved obeticholic acid (OCA) in 2016, UDCA was the only drug approved for the treatment of patients with PBC. UDCA improves liver function tests and histology and prolongs transplant-free survival.[6–9] The recommended dose of UDCA is 13 to 15 mg/kg/d. UDCA may normalize overall patient survival when given during early stages of the disease. Yet, up to 40% of patients do not respond to UDCA. Risk factors associated with nonresponse to UDCA include male gender, females younger than 45 years old, and patients with advanced disease at diagnosis.[2] Poor or absent response to UDCA is the strongest predictor of poor outcome in patients with PBC.

Before UDCA, the 10-year survival of asymptomatic patients with PBC was 50% to 70%, and the median survival for symptomatic patients was 5 to 8 years from symptom onset. Approximately 49% of patients with PBC progressed to cirrhosis. With the widespread use of UDCA in PBC, progression to cirrhosis has decreased to approximately 13%.[4] Despite its efficacy in slowing the progression of disease, UDCA has no effect on the common and debilitating symptoms of fatigue or pruritus.

OBETICHOLIC ACID

In 2016, the FDA approved OCA as a second-line treatment of PBC as monotherapy in patients unable to tolerate UDCA or in combination with UDCA for those with an incomplete biochemical response. OCA is an analogue of chenodeoxycholic acid, a farnesoid X receptor agonist that works to reduce the toxic accumulation of bile acid.[10] The POISE trial, the only phase III clinical trial evaluating the efficacy of OCA in PBC, showed improvements in biochemical outcomes with the use of OCA in patients with suboptimal response or development of adverse events with UDCA. The primary end points studied were normalization of bilirubin and an ALP less than 1.67 times the upper limit of normal with at least a 15% decrease in serum ALP after 12 months of therapy. The three study arms included the placebo group, OCA 5 mg titrated up to 10 mg, and OCA 10 mg daily. Ten percent of the placebo group, 46% of the 5- to 10-mg OCA group, and 47% of the 10-mg OCA group met the primary end points ($P \leq .0001$).[11] Pruritus is a potentially severe adverse event associated with OCA, although it can usually be managed by dose adjustments or drug holiday.

SYMPTOMS
Fatigue

Chronic fatigue is the most common symptom of PBC and is associated with poor quality of life and decreased overall survival.[12,13] Severe fatigue causing significant impairment occurs in up to 85% of PBC patients. However, no correlation has been found between the severity of liver disease and fatigue. Fatigue is a nonspecific finding and etiologies other than PBC must be excluded.

Pruritus

Pruritus is a common symptom of cholestatic liver diseases including PBC. It is usually worse at night and may be triggered by certain fabrics, pregnancy, and heat.[4] In general, first-line treatment of pruritus in patients with PBC is cholestyramine, followed by rifampicin and naltrexone.[14] UDCA is nonefficacious for symptom control in these patients. In those with severe drug-resistant pruritus, LT is the only curative treatment.

Bone Diseases

Osteopenia in PBC is associated with low body index, suboptimal nutrition, and sarcopenia. Osteomalacia and osteoporosis may overlap in later stages of PBC. The incidence of osteoporosis in PBC ranges from 20% to 44% with increased prevalence with disease progression. Patients are at risk of bone fractures with incidence of 10% to 20%.[15]

Other Symptoms

Several autoimmune diseases can coexist with PBC including Sjögren syndrome and patients may present with sicca syndrome.

RISK ASSESSMENT

Once patients with PBC become symptomatic the median survival time is 5 to 10 years without LT. With decompensated disease, median survival decreases to 3 to 5 years.[16] Several risk scores have been developed to assess transplant-free survival in patients with PBC including the Mayo Risk Score, Barcelona, Paris I, Rotterdam, Toronto, Paris II, and more recently the GLOBE and UK-PBC scores.[17–24] These scoring systems incorporate different combinations of clinical and biochemical data for their calculations with the more recent scoring systems using objective data and focusing on treatment outcomes.

Mayo Risk Score

The Mayo Risk Score is a tool specific for patients with PBC used to estimate survival probability up to 7 years.[17] The model currently includes six variables: age, prothrombin time, bilirubin and albumin levels, presence or absence of edema, and dependence on diuretics. Other survival scores were more invasive requiring liver biopsies and have fallen out of practice. In 1989, Markus and colleagues[25] used the Mayo Risk Score to compare the probability of survival in patients with PBC who underwent LT with patients who were managed conservatively. They concluded that LT is an effective treatment option in patients with advanced PBC. At 2 years post-LT, patients with PBC at all levels of the Mayo Risk Score who underwent LT had a higher probability of survival compared with those who had not undergone LT. In 1989, Kim and colleagues[26] used the Mayo Risk Score to determine the optimal time for LT in patients with PBC and found that scores greater than 7.8 were associated with progressively increased post-LT mortality. Hospital and intensive care unit days and need for intraoperative blood transfusions were significantly greater in patients with higher risk scores. Hence, referral for LT in patients with PBC should be made when the Mayo Risk Score is around 7.8. The scoring system is also used to identify patients with PBC who are at risk of developing esophageal varices and who would benefit from a screening esophagoduodenoscopy.[27]

GLOBE Score

In 2015, Lammers and colleagues[23] developed and validated a new scoring system, the GLOBE score, to predict transplant-free survival of patients with PBC treated with UDCA for at least 1 year. Their study included more than 4000 patients from 15 liver centers in eight countries. They set out to improve the stratification system of patients with PBC into high- versus low-risk groups for LT or death. After univariate analysis they found several associations with their primary outcomes including older age, male sex, thrombocytopenia, elevated serum bilirubin, ALP, aspartate aminotransferase (AST), alanine aminotransferase (ALT), AST/ALT ratio and AST/platelet ratio index, and lower serum albumin levels after 1 year of UDCA. However, after multivariate analysis, only bilirubin, albumin, ALP, platelet count, and age were statistically significant. Hence, their scoring system is comprised of these five objective clinical and biochemical variables. Patients with GLOBE score less than or equal to 0.3 were labeled as UDCA responders and had a comparable life-expectancy with a matched general population. Those with GLOBE score greater than 0.3 were UDCA nonresponders and had decreased survival (hazard ratio, 5.51; 95% confidence interval, 4.52–6.72; $P<.0001$).[23] The GLOBE score is useful in identifying patients that should continue UDCA monotherapy versus those who may benefit from second-line treatment options.

UK-Primary Biliary Cholangitis

In 2016, Carbone and colleagues[24] presented the UK-PBC risk scores estimating the absolute risk of developing end-stage liver disease (ESLD) requiring LT at 5, 10, and 15 years from time of diagnosis. Their primary outcomes included death associated with liver disease, LT, and serum bilirubin greater than or equal to 100 μmol/L. More than 3000 patients with PBC treated at liver centers throughout Great Britain and the single major liver treatment center in Northern Ireland were included in their study. Like Lammers and colleagues,[23] they initially evaluated several variables that were associated with ESLD; however, after multivariate modeling baseline albumin and platelet count, and bilirubin, transaminases (ALT or AST), and ALP after 12 months of UDCA treatment were included in their risk score. They did not present thresholds for their risk scores arguing that scores should be individualized. They point out that certain risk scores confer different treatment implications for different patients. They do, however, note that clinicians may use the UK-PBC risk scores to evaluate which patients are at low risk of developing ESLD during a given timeframe and which patients would benefit from risk reduction with escalation of medical management using second-line therapy.[24]

TRANSPLANTATION

Liver transplant is currently the only cure for PBC. Between 1995 and 2006, a total of 111,975 patients were placed on the LT waitlist in the United States and 61,924 underwent LT of which 2736 (3.8%) had PBC as their primary listing diagnosis.[3] Until the 1980s, PBC was the most common indication for LT. Currently, in the era of viral hepatitides and increased awareness of nonalcoholic steatohepatitis, PBC has dropped to the sixth indication. In reviewing United Network for Organ Sharing data, Lee and colleagues[3] determined that although the number of liver transplants and the prevalence of PBC rose between 1995 and 2006, the number of liver transplants performed for PBC decreased by 20%. This discrepancy may be attributed to increased awareness, earlier diagnosis, the introduction and widespread use of UDCA to delay disease progression, or an increase in the number of patients transplanted for other indications.[28]

Cholestatic liver diseases, including PBC, are considered favorable indications for LT when grafts of both living donors (LD) or deceased donors (DD) are used, resulting in better post-LT outcomes when compared with viral and alcoholic hepatitides. Kashyap and colleagues[29] reviewed United Network for Organ Sharing data between 2002 and 2006, and found that the 1-, 3-, and 5-year patient survival among LD were 92.8%, 90.1%, and 86.4%, and among DD were 89.6%, 87%, and 85.1%. Furthermore, the 1-, 3-, and 5-year graft survival among LD were 85.6%, 80.9%, and 77.4%, and among DD were 85.2%, 82.5%, and 80.7%.

Indications for placement of a patient with PBC on the LT waitlist are similar to those for other causes of ESLD and include hepatocellular dysfunction with a Model for End-stage Liver Disease (MELD) score greater than or equal to 15, and cirrhosis complicated by ascites, hepatic encephalopathy, or variceal hemorrhage (**Box 1**).[30] Specific to patients with PBC, Mayo Risk Score of 7.8 and intractable pruritus even in the setting of preserved liver function may also be indications for LT evaluation.[26,31] Carbone and colleagues[32] set out to investigate the role of LT in PBC patients with fatigue. They concluded that although there was a significant decrease in degree of fatigue experienced by patients after LT, at 2 years post-transplant a significant proportion of patients continued to have impaired quality of life. Currently, fatigue is not recognized as an indication for LT.

Patients remain at risk for complications associated with PBC after LT, such as persistent fatigue, keratoconjunctivitis sicca and xerostomia, and osteoporosis. Exacerbation of osteoporosis occurs in all patients with PBC within the first year of LT, with highest incidence occurring during the initial post-LT period (20%–38%). Risk factors associated with bone fractures post-LT are pretransplant osteopenia, pretransplant bone fractures, female sex, and low serum albumin. The trabecular bone of the spine and ribs are affected most commonly.[33]

Liver Transplantation Waitlist and Primary Biliary Cholangitis

Currently, there are more than 14,000 patients on the waitlist for LT. Because of the inherent imbalance between supply and demand, the risk of dying while awaiting LT is 10% to 25%. Although patients undergoing LT for PBC have excellent results in terms of patient and graft survival, a recent study by Singal and colleagues[34] describes high waitlist mortality in patients listed for PBC when compared with most other etiologies. When compared with patients with primary sclerosing cholangitis, patients with PBC had higher overall and 3-month waitlist mortality independent of the MELD score at

---

Box 1
Indications for LT in patients with PBC

Mayo Risk Score of 7.8

MELD of $\geq$15

Cirrhosis with ascites, hepatic encephalopathy, and/or variceal hemorrhage

Intractable pruritus leading to decreased quality of life

time of listing (21.6% vs 12.7% and 5.0% vs 2.9%; $P<.001$). Patients with PBC were also more likely to be removed from the waitlist for worsening clinical conditions than patients with primary sclerosing cholangitis.[34] A Japanese group reported similar findings when comparing waitlist mortality in patients with PBC with patients with chronic hepatitis C virus infection. They found that patients listed for PBC had an 8-month shorter survival time on the transplant waitlist compared with patients listed for hepatitis C virus infection. However, after adjusting for MELD scores, the difference in survival was no longer significant and the two groups were comparable.[35]

RECURRENT PRIMARY BILIARY CHOLANGITIS

Recurrent PBC (rPBC) was first reported by Neuberger and coworkers in 1982.[36] Despite initial controversy, rPBC is now a recognized complication in patients who have undergone LT for PBC. Incidence of rPBC after LT is 21% to 37% at 10 years and approximately 40% at 15 years. Median range of recurrence is 3 to 5.5 years.[37] Recurrence of PBC does not seem to affect patient or graft survival in single-center studies.[38–40] Manousou and colleagues[41] report significant morbidity associated with recurrence of disease with median time to liver decompensation of 6.7 years. Rowe and colleagues[42] noted a median time to graft loss caused by recurrent disease of 7.8 years. Yet, no significant difference in survival has been found between patients with recurrence and those without recurrence. The incidence of rPBC may be underestimated by centers that do not perform protocol liver biopsies because recurrence may be present in the absence of abnormal liver biochemistries. PBC has been noted to recur after a second and third LT; yet, graft failure caused by disease recurrence remains low with subsequent LT.[43]

Diagnosis of Recurrent Primary Biliary Cholangitis

Histologic features
Unlike primary PBC, a diagnosis of recurrent disease cannot be made on biochemical features alone. Rather, the diagnostic hallmark of recurrent disease is histologic evidence of granulomatous cholangitis or florid duct lesions. Specifically, the following are characteristic portal tract lesions: mononuclear inflammatory infiltrate, formation of lymphoid aggregates, epithelioid granulomas, and bile duct damage (**Box 2**).[40]

Box 2
Criteria for rPBC diagnosis

PBC as indication for LT

Persistence of AMA

Other etiologies for graft failure excluded

Liver histology
  Bile duct damage
  Epithelioid granulomas
  Formation of lymphoid aggregates
  Mononuclear inflammatory infiltrate

Probable for rPBC: two of four portal tract lesions present.
Definitive for rPBC: three of four portal tract lesions present.

Adapted from Neuberger J. Recurrent primary biliary cirrhosis. Liver Transpl 2003;9(6):540; with permission.

Laboratory features

Up to one-third to one-half of patients with normal biochemistries may have abnormal allograft histology, whereas up to 5% of patients with abnormal biochemistries may have normal allograft histology.[40,44] AMA is a poor marker for recurrence because there is little correlation between the AMA serum titer and rPBC. Although there is a downward trend in concentration post-LT, overall levels remain elevated after LT in most patients. There does not seem to be a correlation between the titer of serum AMA and rPBC development.[45] In contrast, elevated IgM levels have been shown to be elevated in rPBC compared with patients without recurrence and can be used to identify who may require diagnostic liver biopsy.[46] Antiparietal cell antibodies have also been associated with rPBC. In one study, parietal cell antibodies were detectable in 41% of patients with PBC before LT, 47% post-LT, and in 100% of patients with rPBC.[47] Although a marker of primary PBC, elevation of ALP is nonspecific post-LT because elevated levels are found in other conditions, such as graft-versus-host disease, graft rejection, drug-associated cholestasis, biliary outlet obstruction, and viral coinfections.

Risk Factors for Recurrence

rPBC has been associated with donor and recipient age, type and number of HLA mismatches, and immunosuppressive regimen with calcineurin inhibitors; however, these associations remain controversial. The average age of patients undergoing LT for PBC is between 60 and 70.[48] Two studies have shown an association between younger age at LT and a greater risk for rPBC, whereas one other study showed an association between older recipient age and rPBC risk.[48,49] The Birmingham group concluded that there was no significant difference in donor age between patients with and without rPBC. The mean donor age in their study was less than 40 years old. However, two other studies concluded that increased donor age (50 years and 65 years) was an independent risk factor for rPBC.[48–50]

Human leukocyte antigen

The genetic contribution of PBC is supported by its familial clustering, high disease concordance among monozygote twins, and the increased prevalence of other autoimmune diseases in patients with PBC. The role of the HLA located in the polymorphic major histocompatibility complex with PBC susceptibility has been extensively studied.[38,41,48,50–53] The association between recurrence of PBC and the degree of mismatches between recipient and donor has also been evaluated with mixed results. Sanchez and colleagues[52] found that certain donor and recipient HLA alleles were associated with increased rates of rPBC, specifically donor alleles A1, B57, B58, DR44, DR57, and DR58, and the recipient allele B48.

In investigating graft mortality in LD LT, Harimoto and colleagues[51] found that grafts from male donors and four or more HLA mismatches were associated with graft loss caused by chronic rejection, immune-mediated reaction syndrome, obliterative portal venopathy, and veno-occlusive disease but not from rPBC. In contrast, another Japanese based study by Morioka and colleagues[50] evaluating LD LT in PBC found that a lower number of HLA-A, HLA-B, and HLA-DR mismatches was associated with an increased risk of rPBC. However, they found that a higher number of HLA-A, HLA-B, and HLA-DR mismatches was associated with increased mortality within 6 months of LT. Persistent ascites was also an independent risk factor for mortality. When comparing survival of patients whose donors were blood relatives (blood-relative donor) with patients whose donors were not blood relatives (non-blood-relative donor), they concluded that the blood-relative donor group had increased survival rates when compared with the non-blood-relative donor group at 1, 3, and 5 years post-LT. rPBC was observed only in blood-relative donor cases. In a separate study evaluating long-term follow-up in 100 patients transplanted for PBC a lack of HLA-B mismatch was associated with an increased risk for rPBC.[38] Several other studies have not found a significant association between HLA mismatches and LD LT or DD LT.[41,48,52,54]

Treatment

Immunosuppression

Immunosuppression after LT should prevent allograft rejection and optimize allograft function, while using the lowest effective dose of medication. Side effects associated with immunosuppression are numerous and cause significant morbidity, including infection, renal insufficiency, and malignancy. There are currently six classes of immunosuppression available to patients post-LT including corticosteroids, nucleotide synthesis inhibitors, calcineurin inhibitors, mammalian target of rapamycin inhibitors, interleukin-2 receptor blockers, and T-cell depleting agents. The calcineurin inhibitors have been studied most extensively in patients with PBC post-LT.

The role of immunosuppressive agents and rPBC remains controversial. Although some studies have failed to find an association between calcineurin inhibitors and rPBC, others have concluded that tacrolimus-based immunosuppression is associated with an increased risk of rPBC in DD LT and LD LT when compared with cyclosporine-based therapy.[38,41,49,55–58] Neuberger and colleagues[58] found that tacrolimus is associated with significant reduction in time to recurrence. The median time to rPBC was 10.2 years in the cyclosporine group, and 5.1 years in the tacrolimus group. In contrast, a systematic review by Gautam and colleagues[59] evaluated 16 studies addressing recurrence of PBC and did not find a significant difference between the two calcineurin inhibitors and recurrent disease. Similarly, Manousou did not find an association between tacrolimus or cyclosporine with rPBC; yet they did note a significant decrease in rate of disease recurrence with the addition of azathioprine to cyclosporine-based therapy.[41]

Ursodeoxycholic acid and recurrent primary biliary cholangitis

Currently there is no standardized protocol for treatment of rPBC. Because of its success as a temporizing treatment to prolong transplant-free survival in patients with primary PBC, UDCA has been evaluated for its efficacy post-LT.[60–62] Charatcharoenwitthaya and colleagues[62] followed patients with PBC undergoing LT at the Mayo Clinic to determine the efficacy of UDCA in rPBC and elucidate the significance of rPBC on overall patient survival. Normalization of ALP and ALT in patients with rPBC was approximately 52% in the UDCA-treated group, whereas normalization was only 22% in the untreated control group. Although treatment with UDCA post-LT may have improved liver function tests, they were unable to show an association with UDCA and patient or allograft survival. Bosch and colleagues[61] also evaluated the efficacy of starting UDCA post-LT and before onset of rPBC. In their study, liver biopsies were obtained at 1, 5, 10, 15, 20, and 25 years post-LT and when clinically indicated. Forty-four percent of patients who developed rPBC had normal levels of ALP at time of diagnosis. Furthermore, they found that even after multivariate analysis, recurrence of PBC was significantly lower in patients who were started on UDCA prophylactically compared with patients who did not receive prophylactic therapy (21% vs 62%; $P = .004$).

SUMMARY

With the discovery of AMA, the serologic hallmark of PBC, the prevalence of PBC has risen. Yet, the incidence of patients with PBC added to the LT waitlist does not correlate with this finding. This is likely caused by the widespread use of UDCA during early stages of disease. Furthermore, OCA has now been FDA approved for use in UDCA nonresponders. With more drugs being evaluated for PBC, transplant-free survival may continue to rise in this patient population. However, for those with ESLD and drug failure, LT is the only cure.

PBC is considered a favorable indication for LT.[63] rPBC is an adverse event associated with LT with incidence of up to 40% at 15 years.[37] Diagnosis of rPBC currently requires liver biopsy. There is no current protocol for treatment of rPBC. However, in one study, UDCA used prophylactically post-LT was associated with lower recurrence rates compared with patients who did not receive prophylactic therapy.[61]

REFERENCES

1. Gershwin ME, Mackay IR, Sturgess A, et al. Identification and specificity of a cDNA encoding the 70 kd mitochondrial antigen recognized in primary biliary cirrhosis. J Immunol 1987;138(10):3525–31.
2. Carbone M, Mells GF, Pells G, et al. Sex and age are determinants of the clinical phenotype of primary biliary cirrhosis and response to ursodeoxycholic acid. Gastroenterology 2013;144(3):560–569 e7 [quiz: e13–4].
3. Lee J, Belanger A, Doucette JT, et al. Transplantation trends in primary biliary cirrhosis. Clin Gastroenterol Hepatol 2007;5(11):1313–5.
4. Lindor KD, Gershwin ME, Poupon R, et al. Primary biliary cirrhosis. Hepatology 2009;50(1):291–308.
5. Mahl TC, Shockcor W, Boyer JL. Primary biliary cirrhosis: survival of a large cohort of symptomatic and asymptomatic patients followed for 24 years. J Hepatol 1994;20(6):707–13.
6. Angulo P, Batts KP, Therneau TM, et al. Long-term ursodeoxycholic acid delays histological progression in primary biliary cirrhosis. Hepatology 1999;29(3):644–7.
7. Lindor K. Ursodeoxycholic acid for the treatment of primary biliary cirrhosis. N Engl J Med 2007;357(15):1524–9.
8. Poupon RE, Lindor KD, Pares A, et al. Combined analysis of the effect of treatment with ursodeoxycholic acid on histologic progression in primary biliary cirrhosis. J Hepatol 2003;39(1):12–6.
9. Corpechot C, Carrat F, Bahr A, et al. The effect of ursodeoxycholic acid therapy on the natural course of primary biliary cirrhosis. Gastroenterology 2005;128(2):297–303.
10. Jhaveri MA, Kowdley KV. New developments in the treatment of primary biliary cholangitis: role of obeticholic acid. Ther Clin Risk Manag 2017;13:1053–60.
11. Nevens F, Andreone P, Mazzella G, et al. A placebo-controlled trial of obeticholic acid in primary biliary cholangitis. N Engl J Med 2016;375(7):631–43.
12. Al-Harthy N, Kumagi T, Coltescu C, et al. The specificity of fatigue in primary biliary cirrhosis: evaluation of a large clinic practice. Hepatology 2010;52(2):562–70.
13. Goldblatt J, Taylor PJ, Lipman T, et al. The true impact of fatigue in primary biliary cirrhosis: a population study. Gastroenterology 2002;122(5):1235–41.
14. Bhalerao A, Mannu GS. Management of pruritus in chronic liver disease. Dermatol Res Pract 2015;2015:295891.
15. Raszeja-Wyszomirska J, Miazgowski T. Osteoporosis in primary biliary cirrhosis of the liver. Prz Gastroenterol 2014;9(2):82–7.
16. Neuberger J. Primary biliary cirrhosis. Lancet 1997;350(9081):875–9.

17. Dickson ER, Grambsch PM, Fleming TR, et al. Prognosis in primary biliary cirrhosis: model for decision making. Hepatology 1989;10(1):1–7.

18. Pares A, Caballeria L, Rodes J. Excellent long-term survival in patients with primary biliary cirrhosis and biochemical response to ursodeoxycholic acid. Gastroenterology 2006;130(3):715–20.

19. Corpechot C, Abenavoli L, Rabahi N, et al. Biochemical response to ursodeoxycholic acid and long-term prognosis in primary biliary cirrhosis. Hepatology 2008; 48(3):871–7.

20. Kuiper EM, Hansen BE, de Vries RA, et al. Improved prognosis of patients with primary biliary cirrhosis that have a biochemical response to ursodeoxycholic acid. Gastroenterology 2009;136(4):1281–7.

21. Kumagi T, Guindi M, Fischer SE, et al. Baseline ductopenia and treatment response predict long-term histological progression in primary biliary cirrhosis. Am J Gastroenterol 2010;105(10):2186–94.

22. Corpechot C, Chazouilleres O, Poupon R. Early primary biliary cirrhosis: biochemical response to treatment and prediction of long-term outcome. J Hepatol 2011;55(6):1361–7.

23. Lammers WJ, Hirschfield GM, Corpechot C, et al. Development and validation of a scoring system to predict outcomes of patients with primary biliary cirrhosis receiving ursodeoxycholic acid therapy. Gastroenterology 2015; 149(7):1804–12.e4.

24. Carbone M, Sharp SJ, Flack S, et al. The UK-PBC risk scores: derivation and validation of a scoring system for long-term prediction of end-stage liver disease in primary biliary cholangitis. Hepatology 2016;63(3):930–50.

25. Markus BH, Dickson ER, Grambsch PM, et al. Efficacy of liver transplantation in patients with primary biliary cirrhosis. N Engl J Med 1989;320(26):1709–13.

26. Kim WR, Wiesner RH, Therneau TM, et al. Optimal timing of liver transplantation for primary biliary cirrhosis. Hepatology 1998;28(1):33–8.

27. Levy C, Zein CO, Gomez J, et al. Prevalence and predictors of esophageal varices in patients with primary biliary cirrhosis. Clin Gastroenterol Hepatol 2007;5(7): 803–8.

28. Carey EJ, Ali AH, Lindor KD. Primary biliary cirrhosis. Lancet 2015;386(10003): 1565–75.

29. Kashyap R, Safadjou S, Chen R, et al. Living donor and deceased donor liver transplantation for autoimmune and cholestatic liver diseases: an analysis of the UNOS database. J Gastrointest Surg 2010;14(9):1362–9.

30. Ahmed A, Keeffe EB. Current indications and contraindications for liver transplantation. Clin Liver Dis 2007;11(2):227–47.

31. Milkiewicz P, Wunsch E, Elias E. Liver transplantation in chronic cholestatic conditions. Front Biosci (Landmark Ed) 2012;17:959–69.

32. Carbone M, Bufton S, Monaco A, et al. The effect of liver transplantation on fatigue in patients with primary biliary cirrhosis: a prospective study. J Hepatol 2013;59(3):490–4.

33. Hay JE. Osteoporosis in liver diseases and after liver transplantation. J Hepatol 2003;38(6):856–65.

34. Singal AK, Fang X, Kaif M, et al. Primary biliary cirrhosis has high wait-list mortality among patients listed for liver transplantation. Transpl Int 2017;30(5):454–62.

35. Genda T, Ichida T, Sakisaka S, et al. Waiting list mortality of patients with primary biliary cirrhosis in the Japanese transplant allocation system. J Gastroenterol 2014;49(2):324–31.

36. Neuberger J, Portmann B, Macdougall BR, et al. Recurrence of primary biliary cirrhosis after liver transplantation. N Engl J Med 1982;306(1):1–4.
37. Khettry U, Anand N, Faul PN, et al. Liver transplantation for primary biliary cirrhosis: a long-term pathologic study. Liver Transpl 2003;9(1):87–96.
38. Jacob DA, Neumann UP, Bahra M, et al. Long-term follow-up after recurrence of primary biliary cirrhosis after liver transplantation in 100 patients. Clin Transplant 2006;20(2):211–20.
39. Neuberger J. Recurrent primary biliary cirrhosis. Liver Transpl 2001;7(7):596–9.
40. Neuberger J. Recurrent primary biliary cirrhosis. Liver Transpl 2003;9(6):539–46.
41. Manousou P, Arvaniti V, Tsochatzis E, et al. Primary biliary cirrhosis after liver transplantation: influence of immunosuppression and human leukocyte antigen locus disparity. Liver Transpl 2010;16(1):64–73.
42. Rowe IA, Webb K, Gunson BK, et al. The impact of disease recurrence on graft survival following liver transplantation: a single centre experience. Transpl Int 2008;21(5):459–65.
43. Jacob DA, Bahra M, Schmidt SC, et al. Mayo risk score for primary biliary cirrhosis: a useful tool for the prediction of course after liver transplantation? Ann Transplant 2008;13(3):35–42.
44. Sylvestre PB, Batts KP, Burgart LJ, et al. Recurrence of primary biliary cirrhosis after liver transplantation: histologic estimate of incidence and natural history. Liver Transpl 2003;9(10):1086–93.
45. Dubel L, Farges O, Bismuth H, et al. Kinetics of anti-M2 antibodies after liver transplantation for primary biliary cirrhosis. J Hepatol 1995;23(6):674–80.
46. Balan V, Batts KP, Porayko MK, et al. Histological evidence for recurrence of primary biliary cirrhosis after liver transplantation. Hepatology 1993;18(6):1392–8.
47. Ciesek S, Becker T, Manns MP, et al. Anti-parietal cell autoantibodies (PCA) in primary biliary cirrhosis: a putative marker for recurrence after orthotopic liver transplantation? Ann Hepatol 2010;9(2):181–5.
48. Silveira MG, Talwalkar JA, Lindor KD, et al. Recurrent primary biliary cirrhosis after liver transplantation. Am J Transplant 2010;10(4):720–6.
49. Liermann Garcia RF, Evangelista Garcia C, McMaster P, et al. Transplantation for primary biliary cirrhosis: retrospective analysis of 400 patients in a single center. Hepatology 2001;33(1):22–7.
50. Morioka D, Egawa H, Kasahara M, et al. Impact of human leukocyte antigen mismatching on outcomes of living donor liver transplantation for primary biliary cirrhosis. Liver Transpl 2007;13(1):80–90.
51. Harimoto N, Ikegami T, Nakagawara H, et al. Chronic immune-mediated reaction syndrome as the cause of late graft mortality in living-donor liver transplantation for primary biliary cirrhosis. Transplant Proc 2014;46(5):1438–43.
52. Sanchez EQ, Levy MF, Goldstein RM, et al. The changing clinical presentation of recurrent primary biliary cirrhosis after liver transplantation. Transplantation 2003;76(11):1583–8.
53. Invernizzi P, Ransom M, Raychaudhuri S, et al. Classical HLA-DRB1 and DPB1 alleles account for HLA associations with primary biliary cirrhosis. Genes Immun 2012;13(6):461–8.
54. Hashimoto E, Shimada M, Noguchi S, et al. Disease recurrence after living liver transplantation for primary biliary cirrhosis: a clinical and histological follow-up study. Liver Transpl 2001;7(7):588–95.
55. Jacob DA, Neumann UP, Bahra M, et al. Liver transplantation for primary biliary cirrhosis: influence of primary immunosuppression on survival. Transplant Proc 2005;37(4):1691–2.

56. Levitsky J, Hart J, Cohen SM, et al. The effect of immunosuppressive regimens on the recurrence of primary biliary cirrhosis after liver transplantation. Liver Transpl 2003;9(7):733–6.

57. Montano-Loza AJ, Wasilenko S, Bintner J, et al. Cyclosporine A protects against primary biliary cirrhosis recurrence after liver transplantation. Am J Transpl 2010; 10(4):852–8.

58. Neuberger J, Gunson B, Hubscher S, et al. Immunosuppression affects the rate of recurrent primary biliary cirrhosis after liver transplantation. Liver Transpl 2004; 10(4):488–91.

59. Gautam M, Cheruvattath R, Balan V. Recurrence of autoimmune liver disease after liver transplantation: a systematic review. Liver Transpl 2006;12(12):1813–24.

60. Guy JE, Qian P, Lowell JA, et al. Recurrent primary biliary cirrhosis: peritransplant factors and ursodeoxycholic acid treatment post-liver transplant. Liver Transpl 2005;11(10):1252–7.

61. Bosch A, Dumortier J, Maucort-Boulch D, et al. Preventive administration of UDCA after liver transplantation for primary biliary cirrhosis is associated with a lower risk of disease recurrence. J Hepatol 2015;63(6):1449–58.

62. Charatcharoenwitthaya P, Pimentel S, Talwalkar JA, et al. Long-term survival and impact of ursodeoxycholic acid treatment for recurrent primary biliary cirrhosis after liver transplantation. Liver Transpl 2007;13(9):1236–45.

63. Carbone M, Neuberger J. Liver transplantation in PBC and PSC: indications and disease recurrence. Clin Res Hepatol Gastroenterol 2011;35(6–7):446–54.

Moving?

Make sure your subscription moves with you!

To notify us of your new address, find your **Clinics Account Number** (located on your mailing label above your name), and contact customer service at:

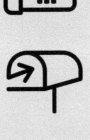

Email: journalscustomerservice-usa@elsevier.com

800-654-2452 (subscribers in the U.S. & Canada)
314-447-8871 (subscribers outside of the U.S. & Canada)

Fax number: 314-447-8029

Elsevier Health Sciences Division
Subscription Customer Service
3251 Riverport Lane
Maryland Heights, MO 63043

*To ensure uninterrupted delivery of your subscription, please notify us at least 4 weeks in advance of move.

Printed and bound by CPI Group (UK) Ltd, Croydon, CR0 4YY

03/10/2024

01040392-0020